Radiodiagnosis, Nuclear Medicine, Radiotherapy and Radiation Oncology

AF070315

Radiodiagnosis, Nuclear Medicine, Radiotherapy and Radiation Oncology

(With a Special Approach for Various Competitive Medical Examinations)

Author
Bipin Valchandji Daga MD (Radiodiag) DNB FRCR (London)
Assistant Professor
Department of Radiology and Imaging
Dr Vaishampayam Memorial Government Medical College
Solapur, Maharashtra, India

Co-Authors
Vaibhav Ramesh Shah MD (Radiodiag)
Assistant Professor
Department of Radiology and Imaging
Dr Vaishampayam Memorial Government Medical College
Solapur, Maharashtra, India

Sachin Valchandji Daga MS (Surg) DNB (Surg Gastro) Fellow in Liver Transplant
Consultant Surgical Gastroenterologist and
Hepatobiliary and Liver Transplant Surgeon
Asian Institute of Gastroenterology
Hyderabad, Andhra Pradesh, India

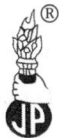

JAYPEE BROTHERS MEDICAL PUBLISHERS (P) LTD

New Delhi • London • Philadelphia • Panama

Jaypee Brothers Medical Publishers (P) Ltd.

Headquarters
Jaypee Brothers Medical Publishers (P) Ltd.
4838/24, Ansari Road, Daryaganj
New Delhi 110 002, India
Phone: +91-11-43574357
Fax: +91-11-43574314
Email: jaypee@jaypeebrothers.com

Overseas Offices

J.P. Medical Ltd.
83, Victoria Street, London
SW1H 0HW (UK)
Phone: +44-2031708910
Fax: +02-03-0086180
Email: info@jpmedpub.com

Jaypee-Highlights Medical Publishers Inc.
City of Knowledge, Bld. 237, Clayton
Panama City, Panama
Phone: +507-301-0496
Fax: +507-301-0499
Email: cservice@jphmedical.com

Jaypee Brothers Medical Publishers Ltd.
The Bourse
111, South Independence Mall East
Suite 835, Philadelphia, PA 19106, USA
Phone: + 267-519-9789
Email: joe.rusko@jaypeebrothers.com

Jaypee Brothers Medical Publishers (P) Ltd.
17/1-B, Babar Road, Block-B
Shaymali, Mohammadpur
Dhaka-1207, Bangladesh
Mobile: +08801912003485
Email: jaypeedhaka@gmail.com

Jaypee Brothers Medical Publishers (P) Ltd.
Shorakhute
Kathmandu, Nepal
Phone: +00977-9841528578
Email: jaypee.nepal@gmail.com

Website: www.jaypeebrothers.com
Website: www.jaypeedigital.com

© 2013, Jaypee Brothers Medical Publishers

All rights reserved. No part of this book may be reproduced in any form or by any means without the prior permission of the publisher.

Inquiries for bulk sales may be solicited at: jaypee@jaypeebrothers.com

This book has been published in good faith that the contents provided by the authors contained herein are original, and is intended for educational purposes only. While every effort is made to ensure accuracy of information, the publisher and the authors specifically disclaim any damage, liability, or loss incurred, directly or indirectly, from the use or application of any of the contents of this work. If not specifically stated, all figures and tables are courtesy of the authors. Where appropriate, the readers should consult with a specialist or contact the manufacturer of the drug or device.

Radiodiagnosis, Nuclear Medicine, Radiotherapy and Radiation Oncology

First Edition: **2013**

ISBN 978-93-5025-712-8

Printed at Rajkamal Electric Press, Plot No. 2, Phase-IV, Kundli, Haryana.

Dedicated to

My parents and teachers

Preface

Radiology is a specialized branch of medicine, essentially for a postgraduate study and consequently few medical students have adequate knowledge and/or experience of it. Most of the postgraduate medical entrance examinations now include MCQs on Radiodiagnosis, Nuclear Medicine, Radiotherapy and Radiation Oncology, hence, it has also become a must for all aspiring postgraduates to keep themselves abreast with these subjects.

Though there are many excellent books written for radiologists, radiotherapists, radiation oncologists and the nuclear medicine specialists, but they inevitably assume that the reader already has a working knowledge of the subject. Apart from this, medicine is becoming increasingly complex and future progress demands knowing and understanding several new and recent advances also.

With this in mind, this book is presented, written to assist the students to understand the practice of radiotherapy, radiation oncology, nuclear medicine, and radiodiagnosis, especially pertaining to postgraduate medical entrance examinations.

It has been simplified in the hope that it will be helpful to all those who would like to understand something of these specialties.

Bipin Valchandji Daga

Acknowledgments

I am thankful to:
- Dr Aditi B Daga
- Dr Srikantha S Rathi
- Dr Suresh M Bakle
- Dr Vivek A Choudhary

Contents

Section 1: RADIODIAGNOSIS

1. General Radiology and Radiology Physics   3
    Brief Historical Review: The Discovery of X-rays   3
    Various Modalities for Imaging   6
    Conventional Radiography   7
    Chemical Processing of an X-ray Film   14
    Digital or Computed or Filmless Radiography or Phosphor Plate Technology   14
    Picture Archiving and Communication System   15
    Contrast Radiography   17
    Barium Studies   17
    Nonbarium Studies   17
    Sialography   18
    Myelography   18
    Excretory Urography (Intravenous Urography, IVU, IVP)   18
    Urethrography   23
    Hysterosalpingography   24
    Xeroradiography   26
    Mammography   26
    Orthopantomography or Panoramic Radiography   27
    Ultrasonography/Ultrasound Study   28
    Color Doppler Imaging/Study   33
    Echocardiography   34
    Transesophageal Echocardiography   34
    Computed Tomography   35
    Special Application of Multislice CT   38
    Magnetic Resonance Imaging   42
    Radionuclide Imaging   47
    Emission Computed Tomography   47

Bone Densitometry 50
Extracorporeal Shock Wave Lithotripsy 51

2. Radiological Contrast Agents/Media — 60
Contrast Media for Barium Procedures 60
Contrast Media for Nonbarium Procedures 62
MR Contrast Media: Key Facts 66

3. Radiation Hazards and Protection — 68
Radiation Protection 79
Primary and Secondary Barriers for Radiation 82
Radiation Units 84

4. Pulmonary Radiology — 87
General Aspect 87
Common Abnormalities Noted on CXR 91
Role of CXR in Thoracic Trauma 98
Pediatric Chest 100
Congenital Lesions 100
Foreign Body Aspiration 106
Pulmonary Infections 106
Lung Collapse 112
Bronchiectasis, Industrial and Interstitial Lung Diseases 115
Neoplasms 122
Mediastinum 127

5. Cardiovascular Radiology — 131
Heart 131
Congenital Anomalies 138
Pulmonary Edema 142
Kerley Lines 143
Pulmonary Embolism 145
Pericardial Effusion 147
Pericardial Tumors 148
Aorta 149
Imaging in Peripheral Arterial Disease 160
Vascular Rings 161
Dysphagia Lusoria 162

6. Abdominal Imaging — 165

- Modalities Available for Abdominal Pathologies 165
- Important Preliminary Clinicoradiologically Terms 168
- Pneumoperitoneum 168
- Ascites 170
- Spleen 171
- Esophagus 172
- Stomach 179
- Small Intestinal 185
- Small Intestinal Neoplasms 192
- Appendix 193
- Colon and Rectum 194
- Blunt Trauma Abdomen 202
- Hepatobiliary System 204
- Focal Hepatic Lesions 206
- Gallbladder and Biliary Apparatus 209
- Imaging in Obstructive Jaundice 210
- USG 211
- CECT 212
- Radiology of Gallbladder and Biliary System Pathologies 215
- EHBA 219
- Pancreas 220
- Tumor Localization of GI NETs (Carcinoids and Pancreatic Endocrine Tumors) 224

7. Genitourinary Radiology — 226

- Imaging Keys 226
- Kidneys and Ureters 230
- Calculus Disease of Kidney 233
- Features of Hydronephrosis on IVU 235
- Papillary Necrosis on IVU 235
- Renovascular Hypertension 236
- Renal Infections 237
- Renal Tumors 239
- Wilms' Tumor versus Neuroblastoma 241
- Angiomyolipoma (Hamartoma) 242
- Renal Injuries 243
- Bladder and Urethra 243

Prostate and Testes 246
Testicular Tumor 247
Seminal Vesicle 248
Penile Imaging 248

8. Musculoskeletal Radiology 249

Imaging Protocols 249
Musculoskeletal Radiology: Differential Diagnosis 250
Congenital Skeletal Anomalies and Skeletal Dysplasias 255
Metabolic Bone Disorders 265
Bone Infections 272
Skeletal Trauma 275
Miscellaneous Musculoskeletal Radiology Diseases 277
Spondylolisthesis 277
Osteonecrosis/Osteochondritis 278
Differential Diagnosis of Hip Pain in Children 280
Disorders of Lymphoreticular and Hemopoietic System 282
Bone Tumors and Tumor-like Conditions 286
Joint Diseases 302
Soft Tissues 310

9. Endocrine Imaging 311

Thyroid 311
Adrenals 312

10. Head, Neck and Spine Imaging 317

General Aspect and Skull Radiograph 317
Radiological Investigations 322
Congenital Malformations of Brain 331
Neurocutaneous Syndromes (Phakomatoses) 335
Imaging in Dementia 340
Stroke and Vascular Disorders 340
Intracranial Infections 346
Diseases of Demyelination (Acquired) 350
Mesial Temporal Lobe Epilepsy Syndrome 352
Brain Tumors 353
Pituitary Imaging 363
Head Trauma 364

ENT Radiology 370
Ophthalmic Radiology 377
Neck Imaging 381
Spine Radiology 385

11. Obstetrics and Gynecological Radiology   396
Ultrasonography in Pregnancy 396
Transvaginal USG 397
Pathological Consideration in Obstetrics USG 400
Gynecology 407
Ovarian Neoplasms 408

12. Breast Imaging   411
Diagnostic Mammography versus Screening Mammography 411

Section 2: NUCLEAR MEDICINE

13. Radioactivity and Basics of Nuclear Medicine   421
What is Radioactivity? 421
What Is an Element? 423
Useful Terminologies 425
Basic Isotope Notation 427
Instrumentation 427
Radionuclides 428
Nuclear Stability and Radioactive Decay 431
Radionuclide Production 433
Radioactive Decay 433
Radioactive Isotopes 436
Diagnostic Uses 436

14. Nuclear Scans   437
Radionuclide Scans 437
Single Photon Emission Computed Tomography 438
Brain Scan 438
Salivary Gland Scan 440
Thyroid Scan 441

Parathyroid Scan 442
V/Q Scan 443
Myocardial Scan 443
Myocardial Perfusion Studies 444
Multiple Gated Acquisition Scan 445
Liver Scan 445
Biliary Scintigraphic Scan 446
Meckel's Diverticulum Imaging 447
Gastrointestinal Bleeding Studies 447
Renal Scan 448
Adrenal Scan 449
Testicular Scan 449
Bone Scan 449
Scintigraphic Scan for Neuroendocrine Tumors 453
Miscellaneous 453
Therapeutic Uses 454

Section 3: RADIOTHERAPY AND RADIATION ONCOLOGY

15. Radiation Oncology — 459
An Overview 459
What are Electromagnetic Rays? 459
What is Ionizing Radiation? 460
Cancer Biology 466
Principles of Radiation Therapy 467
Radiosensitizer and Radioprotector 471

16. Radiotherapy — 474
Schedule of Radiotherapy 474
Modes of Radiotherapy 476
Types of Radiotherapy Treatment 489
Recent Advances in Radiotherapy 498
Radiation Portals 504
Complications of Radiotherapy 504
Benign Diseases that can be Treated with Radiotherapy 507

Various Tumors and Viscera: Dose Limits 512
Guide to the Relative Radiosensitivity of Normal Tissue 513
Follow-up of Cancer Patients Receiving Radiotherapy 513

Section 4: NEWER ADVANCES AND INTERVENTIONAL RADIOLOGY

17. Newer Advances 517
Advances in CT Scan 517
Cardiac Computed Tomography 519
Cardiac Magnetic Resonance Imaging 520
Echo-Planar MRI: Ultrafast MR Sequence 523
Diffusion-weighted MRI (DWMRI) 524
Functional MRI 524
MR Spectroscopy (MRS) 524
Near Infrared Spectroscopy 526

18. Interventional Radiology 527
Digital Subtraction Arteriography 527
Catheter Angiography 528
Therapeutic Embolization 531
Particulate Embolic Agents 532
Bronchial Artery Embolization 532
Interventional GI Radiology 533
Interventional Neuroradiology 533
Ablation 534
Cavitron Ultrasonic Surgical Aspirator 536
Percutaneous Transcatheter Vascular Occlusion 537
Medical Tumor Ablation 539
Therapeutic Effects of Deep Heating 539
High-Intensity Focused Ultrasound 540

Index 543

Abbreviations

AP	:	Anteroposterior
IV	:	Intravenous
AVM	:	Arteriovenous Malformation
IVC	:	Inferior Vena Cava
BE	:	Barium Enema
IV-DSA	:	Intravenous Digital Subtraction Angiography
Ca	:	Cancer
CA	:	Carotid Artery
CXR	:	Chest X-ray
DM	:	Diabetes Mellitus
IVP	:	Intravenous Pyelogram
CABG	:	Coronary Artery Bypass Graft
KUB	:	Kidney Ureter Bladder
GB	:	Gallbladder
CBT	:	Computed Body Tomography
LBBB	:	Left Bundle-Branch Block
CCF	:	Carotid-Cavernous Fistula
MRI	:	Magnetic Resonance Imaging
CNS	:	Central Nervous System
OCG	:	Oral Cholecystogram
C-Spine	:	Cervical Spine
PA	:	Pulmonary Artery
CT	:	Computed Tomography
PE	:	Pulmonary Embolism
CTAP	:	Computed Tomography after Arterioportography
PSA	:	Prostate Specific Antigen
PTC	:	Percutaneous Transhepatic Cholangiogram
DSA	:	Digital Subtraction Angiography

BMD	:	Bone Marrow Density
DXA	:	Dual Energy X-ray Absorptiometry
RBC	:	Red Blood Cells
ECG	:	Electrocardiogram
RN	:	Radionuclide
ERCP	:	Endoscopic Retrograde Cholangiopancreatography
R/O	:	Rule out
RT	:	Radiotherapy
F/U	:	Follow-up
SBFT	:	Small Bowel Follow-Through
THA	:	Transient Hemispheric Attacks
GI	:	Gastrointestinal
UGI	:	Upper Gastrointestinal
GU	:	Genitourinary
USG	:	Ultrasound Sonography
HIDA	:	Hepatobiliary Iminodiacetic Acid
VCUG	:	Voiding Cystourethrogram
HCG	:	Human Chorionic Gonadotropin
v/q	:	Ventilation Perfusion Scan
IOUS	:	Intraoperative Ultrasound
VRSA	:	Vancomycin Resistant *Staphylococcus aureus*
WBC	:	White Blood Cells
ABPA	:	Allergic Bronchopulmonary Aspergillosis
NCRP	:	National Congress of Radiation Protection
ICRP	:	International Congress of Radiation Protection
TAI	:	Traumatic Aortic Injury
AAAS	:	American Association for the Advancement of Science
ADR	:	Adverse Drug Reaction
AR	:	Attributable Risk
ARR/ARD	:	Absolute Risk Reduction/Absolute Risk Difference
AYUSH	:	Department of *Ayurveda, Yoga* and Naturopathy, Unani, Siddha and Homeopathy
CDMS	:	Clinical Date Management System
CDSR	:	Cochrane Databases of the Systematic Review

Abbreviations

CIOMS	:	Council for International Organisation of Medical Science
CI	:	Confidence Interval
CONSORT	:	Consolidated Standards of the Reporting of Trials
COPE	:	Committee of Publication Ethics
CPCSEA	:	Committee for the Purpose of Control and Supervision of Experiments on Animals
CRO	:	Contract Research Organization
CSIR	:	Council for Scientific and Industrial Research
CTRI	:	Clinical Trial Registry of India
CV	:	Coefficient of Variation
DARE	:	Database of Abstracts of Reviews of Effects
DBT	:	Department of Biotechnology
DST	:	Department of Science and Technology
EBM	:	Evidence-Based Medicine
EC	:	Ethics Committee
EIND	:	Exploratory Investigational New Drug
EmBase	:	Excerpta Medica Database
FINER	:	Feasibility, Interesting, Novel, Ethical, and Relevant
FOGSI	:	Federation of Obstetric and Gynecological Societies of India
GIF	:	Good Impact Factor
IAEC	:	Institutional Animal Ethics Committee
ICC	:	Intraclass Correlation Coefficient
ICH	:	International Conference on Harmonization
ICMJE	:	International Committee/Council of Medical Journal Editors
ICMR	:	Indian Council of Medical Research
ICTRP	:	International Clinical Trial Registry Platform (Set-up WHO)
IDMC	:	Independent Data Monitoring Committee
IEC	:	Institutional Ethics Committee
IF	:	Impact Factor
IMRaD	:	Introduction, Methods, Results and Discussion
IND	:	Investigational New Drug
INSA	:	Indian Nation Science Academy
IPAB	:	International Pharmaceutical Abstracts
IRB	:	Institutional Review Board

JOGI	:	Journal of Obstetrics and Gynecology of India
KVPY	:	Kishore Vaigyanik Protsahan Yojana
LAR	:	Legally Accepted Representative
LR	:	Likelihood Ratio
MCI	:	Medical Council of India
MOOSE	:	Meta-analysis of Observational Studies in Epidemiology
MOU	:	Memorandum of Understanding
MRC	:	Medical Research Council (UK)
N/n	:	Number
NGO	:	Non-Government Organization
NIH	:	National Institute of Health
NIMS	:	National Institute of Medical Statistics
NLM	:	National Library of Medicine (USA)
NNH	:	Number Needed to Harm
NNT	:	Number Needed to Treat
NPV	:	Negative Predictive Value
OR	:	Odds Ratio
P/p/P/p	:	Probability
PASS	:	Power Analysis and Sample Size
PI	:	Principal Investigator
PPV	:	Positive Predictive Value
PSTF	:	Preventive Services Task Force (USA)
QUORUM	:	Quality of Reporting of Meta-analysis
RIA	:	Radioimmunoassay
R & D	:	Research and Development
RR	:	Relative Risk
SAE	:	Serious Adverse Reaction
SAS	:	Statistical Analysis System
SD	:	Standard Deviation
SEM	:	Standard Error of the Mean
SI	:	International System of unit (Systeme Internationale units)
SMART	:	Specific, Measurable, achievable, Relevant, and Time-bound
SMO	:	Site Management Organization
SNOSE	:	Sequential Numbered, Opaque, Sealed Envelopes

SOP	:	Standard Operating Procedure
SPSS	:	Statistical Packages for Social Sciences
TAKAR	:	Title, Abstract, Keywords, Acknowledgement, and References
UTRN	:	Unique Trial Registration Number (Provided by CTRI)
UTRN	:	Universal Trial Registration Number (Provided by ICRTP)
WAME	:	World Association of Medical Editors
WMA	:	World Medical Assembly
WOS	:	Women Scientists Scheme

Section 1

Radiodiagnosis

Chapter 1

General Radiology and Radiology Physics

BRIEF HISTORICAL REVIEW: THE DISCOVERY OF X-RAYS

Wilhelm Conrad Roentgen, a German physicist, discovered X-rays on **November 8, 1895**. The year 1995 became the **Centenary year** for X-rays. Roentgen was investigating the behavior of electrons in high-energy cathode ray tubes with air evacuated from the tube and the tube enclosed in black cardboard. A short platinum electrode was fitted into each end and on passing a high-voltage discharge through tube, he noticed a faint light glowing on a work bench about 3 ft away. He discovered that the source of the light was the fluorescence of a small piece of paper coated with barium platinocyanide. He concluded that some unknown type of ray was produced when the tube was energized. **We can imagine his excitement as he investigated the mysterious new ray**. He held his hand between the tube and the screen and, to his surprise, the outline of his skeleton appeared on the screen. By 28th December 1895, he investigated properties of the rays and was awarded the **first Nobel Prize for Physics in 1901**.

Tool/Procedure	*Discovered by*
1. X-rays	WC Roentgen
2. Color Doppler	Christian Doppler
3. CT scan	Godfrey Hounsefield
4. Nobel Prize for MRI (2003)	Peter Mansfield and Paul Lauterbur
5. Theory of NMR elucidated by	Felix Block and Edward Purcell
6. Arterial Cannulation and Angiography	Seldinger
7. PTCA	Grundzig
8. Cardiac catheterization	Werner Forssmann

Gamma (γ) rays have highest penetrating ability and least ionization potential

Types of Radiations and their Uses

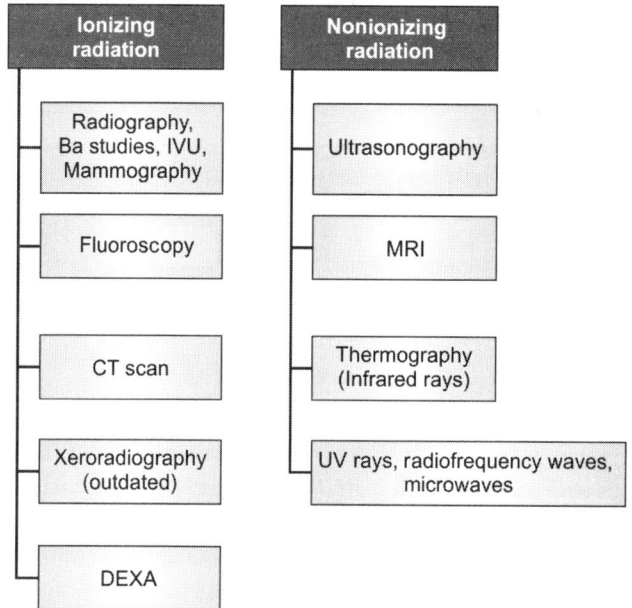

Atomic number	Number of protons in nucleus (Z)
Neutron number	Number of neutrons in nucleus (N)
Atomic weight or Mass number	Number of mass particles in nucleus (A) (A = N + Z)
Neutron excess	Excess of neutrons over protons (N − Z)

Types of ionizing radiation are:

Alpha radiation	• Particulate radiation • Consists of nucleus of helium atoms • Positively charged with "+2" • Least penetrating ability stopped by thin sheet of paper or skin • High LET radiation • They have highest ionizing potential • Predominant alpha emitter: Uranium, Plutonium.

Beta radiation		• Particulate radiation • Consists of electrons • Negatively charged with "–1" • More penetrating than alpha particles • Can pass through 1–2 cm of water or tissue or a few mm of aluminum • Predominant β-emitter: Phosphorus-32, Strontium-89, Yttrium-92.
Gamma radiation		• Are electromagnetic radiation (nonparticulate) • Highly penetrating • Can pass through the human body • Cannot be absorbed completely • Least ionization potential • Are emitted from nucleus in excited state (radioactive isotopes) • Predominant γ-emitter: Co-60, Radium-126.
X-rays		• Are electromagnetic radiation (nonparticulate) • Emitted when fast moving charged particles (like electrons) are stopped (like by anode) • Have penetrating power less than gamma rays but more than alpha and beta rays • Photoelectric effect is important for production of X-ray of diagnostic range • Compton effect is important for X-ray in CT and radiotherapy • Can pass through human body • Cannot be absorbed completely.
Neutrons		• Are uncharged particulate radiation • Present in nuclear reactors and at high altitudes • Have higher penetrating power • Water and paraffin wax are effective in absorbing it • Predominant neutrons emitter: Californium.

X-rays are produced mechanically, by making electrons strike a target, which causes the electrons to give up their kinetic energy as X-rays, while gamma rays are produced by nuclear disintegration of radioactive isotopes.

Points of difference	X-rays	γ-rays
Origin	Extranuclear – X-ray tube – Linear accelerator	Intranuclear Radioactive isotopes like Co-60, ^{99m}Tc
Penetrating power	Intermediate	Highest

Ionization potential	Intermediate	Least
Diagnostic use	– Radiography – Mammography – Contrast radiography (IVU, Ba studies, etc.) – Xeroradiography (Outdated) – Fluoroscopy – CT scan – DEXA	Nuclear scan/ Scintigraphy/ Gamma-imaging
Therapeutic use	Teletherapy (Ortho < Super < Megavoltage X-ray therapy)	Tele- as well as brachytherapy

VARIOUS MODALITIES FOR IMAGING

- Conventional radiography
- Computed/digital radiography
- Contrast radiography
- Thermography (Outdated)
- Xeroradiography (Outdated)
- Mammography
- Ultrasonography (USG)
- Computed tomography (CT)
- Magnetic resonance imaging (MRI)
- Radionuclide imaging/scintigraphy/nuclear scan
- Emission tomography (SPECT and PET).

Diagnostic imaging modality and resolution

Modality	Resolution	Typical imaging time	Radiation dose
Plane X-ray	<mm	<1 sec	Low
Mammography	<mm	<1 sec	High
Compound tomography (CT)	mm	Few seconds	High
SPECT and PET	0.5 – 1 cm	10 – 30 minutes	High
Digital radiography	mm	<1 sec	Low
MRI and MRS	mm	10 – 40 minutes	Nil

CONVENTIONAL RADIOGRAPHY

X-ray Production

X-rays are produced mechanically, by making electrons strike a target, which causes the electrons to give up their kinetic energy as X-rays (X-rays are produced extranuclearly).

While gamma rays are produced by nuclear disintegration of radioactive isotopes (Gamma rays are produced intranuclearly).

Properties of X-rays

- Affect photographic plate
- Bombard scattered/secondary radiations
- Chemical and biological changes produced
- Dual nature (emitted as well as absorbed)
- Electrically neutral
- Electromagnetic rays
- Fluorescence producing rays
- Gases ionized (indirectly)
- Highly penetrating
- Heterogeneous (polyenergetic)
- Heat energy produced (in small amount) on passing through matter
- High frequency
- Invisible rays
- Short wavelength (extremely short)
- Straight line traveling rays
- Speed same as that of light (3×10^8 m/s).

X-ray Tube

X-rays are produced whenever a stream of fast-moving electrons undergo rapid deceleration and these conditions prevail during operation of special thermionic vacuum tube called **hot filament or Coolidge X-ray tube**.

A typical X-ray tube is a thermionic diode consisting of a tungsten filament cathode, a tungsten target anode, an evacuated glass tube enclosure (**Pyrex glass**) and 2 circuits to heat the filament and to drive the space charge electrons to anode.

The underlying principles include
- A hot metal filament (cathode) gives off electrons by the process of thermionic emission.
- If no kilovoltage is applied, the emitted electrons remain near filament as an electron cloud or space charge.
- If kilovoltage is applied between the filament and target so as to place a negative charge on filament (cathode) and a positive charge on target (anode), space charge electrons are driven over to anode at high speed by the large potential difference. The electron stream crossing the gap between cathode and anode constitute the tube current, measured in milliamperes (mA).
- If supplied kilovoltage and resulting electron spin are high enough, the electron strikes and enters the target, their kinetic energy being converted to heat (99.4%) and X-ray (0.6%) and thus X-rays are produced.
- The wavelength of the characteristic radiations produced by the target of X-ray tube is not changed by the potential difference (kVp) applied.
- Intensity is proportional to $(kVp)^2$.
- The quantity of X-rays produced depends on atomic number of target material, kVp and mA, while the quality depends on kVp only.
- Heat dissipation in **stationary anode tube** occurs by absorption and conductivity, provided by massive copper anode.
- In rotating anode tube, absorption of heat by the anode assembly is undesirable because heat absorbed by the bearings of the anode assembly would cause them to expand, bind and get damaged. Because of this problem the stem, which connects the tungsten target to the remainder of anode assembly is made up of molybdenum, which has high melting point and is a poor conductor of heat.
- Thus in **rotating anode X-ray tube** the heat generated in rotating tungsten anode disc is dissipated by radiating through the vacuum to the wall of the tube, and then into the surrounding oil and tube housing.
- When an object is placed in the X-ray beam, it will cast a "shadow" on the film that will show some degree of enlargement.
- If X-rays were emitted from a point source, the magnification could be determined by ratio of target-film distance to the target-object distance, which is called **geometric magnification**.
- But in reality, X-rays are emitted from an area, the focal spot, hence the magnification that results with X-rays from focal spot, is called the **true magnification**.

Under usual radiographic situations, magnification of the image should be kept to a minimum. Two rules apply for this purpose:
1. Keep the object as close to the film as possible.
2. Keep the focus-film (X-ray machine to photographic plate) distance as large as possible.

X-ray filters are sheets of metal (aluminum filters are commonly used) placed in the path of X-ray beam near the X-ray tube housing to absorb low energy radiation before it reaches the patient. they are simple and inexpensive. their main function is to protect the patient from useless (low energy) radiation. they reduce skin exposures by as much as 80 percent. NCRP recommends an equivalent of 2.5 mm of aluminum permanent filtration for diagnostic X-ray beams of energy more than 70 kVp.

Heavy metal or k-edge filters are used to remove higher energy photons from the X-ray beam by taking advantage of the increased mass attenuation coefficient at the k-edge of certain elements. Compared to aluminum, k-edge filters enhance contrast, reduce patient dose, and increase tube loading.

An **X-ray beam restrictor** is a device that is attached to the opening in the X-ray tube housing to regulate the size and shape of an X-ray beam.

They are of three types:
1. Aperture diaphragm.
2. Cones and cylinders.
3. Collimators.

Closely collimated beams have two advantages over larger beams:
1. Less scattered radiation and thus improved film quality.
2. Smaller area of patient exposed and hence decreased patient exposure.

A major disadvantage of aperture diaphragm, cones and cylinders is the severe limitation they place on the number of available field sizes and hence have no role in modern radiology.

Collimator
Collimators are best general-purpose restrictors/ they offer following advantages:
- Light beam shows the center and exact configuration of the X-ray field.
- Accurate localization of the patient due to X-ray field illumination is permitted.
- It provides an infinite variety of rectangular X-ray fields.

Grid
Grid, a device invented by Dr Gustave Bucky in 1913, is the most effective way of removing scatter radiation from large radiographic fields.

Radiographic grid consists of lead foil strips separated by X-ray transparent spacers.

They are used to absorb scatter radiation (and not primary radiation) and to improve radiographic image contrast.

There are two types of grids—stationary and moving grids.

Chief advantage of moving grids is elimination of image of the lead strips from the film, but they require a little greater exposure factors.

Air gap technique is an alternative method of eliminating scatter radiation with large radiographic fields (obsolete).

The Five Basic Ways that an X-ray Photon can Interact with Atom/Matter

1. Photoelectric effect.
2. Coherent scattering.
3. Compton scattering.
4. Pair production.
5. Photodisintegration.

Element	Atomic number	K edge (keV)
Hydrogen	1	0.013
Carbon	6	0.28
Copper	29	9.0
Lead	82	88.0

Photoelectric Interaction

- The photoelectric effect is the predominant interaction with low energy radiation and with high atomic number absorbers.
- It generates no significant scatter radiation and produces high contrast in the image, but exposes the patient to great deal of radiation.
- The photoelectric effect is inversely proportional to cube of energy of incident photon and directly proportional to cube of atomic number of interaction material.
- It predominates in diagnostic radiology.
- The atom consists of a central nucleus and orbital electrons. The positively charged nucleus holds the negatively charged electrons in specific orbits, or shell. The innermost shell is called K-shell, and the more peripheral shells are named consecutively L, M, N, and so forth. These shells have limited electron capacity and specific binding energy.
- The K-shell can hold only two electrons.

When an incident photon, with little more energy than the binding energy of K-shell electron, encounters one of these electrons, it ejects it from orbit and the photon disappears, giving up all its energy to electron. This electron now flies into space and is absorbed. Thus the atom is now left with an electron void on the K shell, which is filled up soon by as an electron from adjacent shell drops into K shell, giving up energy in the form of X-ray photon. This is photoelectric effect.

Thus, it is the predominant interaction of low energy radiation with high atomic number absorbers, generating no significant scatter radiation, producing high contrast X-ray images, but exposing the patient to great deal of radiation.

X-rays are ionizing electromagnetic radiations, essentially produced when a stream of K shell electrons of an atom accelerated by a high voltage applied between the filament (cathode) and the target (anode), strikes the target and the electrons give up their energy producing **characteristic radiations,** i.e. the X-rays.

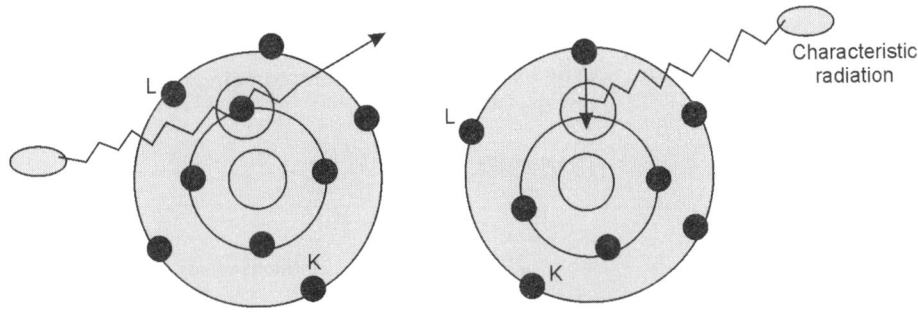

Linear attenuation co-efficient (LAC or μ) is equal to CT number for CT scanning and attenuation of X-rays depend on it.

Primary radiation: It goes from cathode to anode of X-ray tube. It comes direct from of X-ray tube. Except for the useful beam, the bulk of this radiation is absorbed in the tube housing.

Secondary radiation: It is radiation other than primary and is emitted by any matter irradiated with X-ray, which are often loose called scattered radiation.

Scattered radiation: Radiation, which during passage through a substance has been deviated in direction. It may also have been modified by an increase in wavelength (Compton effect). It is one form of secondary radiation.

Stray radiation: Secondary radiation and any radiation other than the useful beam coming from within X-ray tube housing (such as item radiation). This is the radiation against which special protection is needed. Useful beam is that part of primary radiation which passes through aperture, cone or other device for collimating X-ray beam.

Penetrating power of X-ray increases with decreased wavelength and increased frequency.

mAs controls film density of soft tissue resolution, while kVP controls image contrast and penetration of X-ray.

To increase contrast, reduce kV; to reduce contrast, increase kV (*a well-known rule*).

Compton Scattering

- When incident photon has enough energy to dislodge a loosely bound electron, the emerging photon, undergoes a change in direction—and it is called scattered photon.
- Thus, frequency and energy of the scattered photon is less than that of incident photon.
- These are responsible for scatter radiation, which constitute film fog, impairing image contrast.

In addition, therapeutic radiation acts by Compton effect [Compton effect predominates in CT scan and RT].

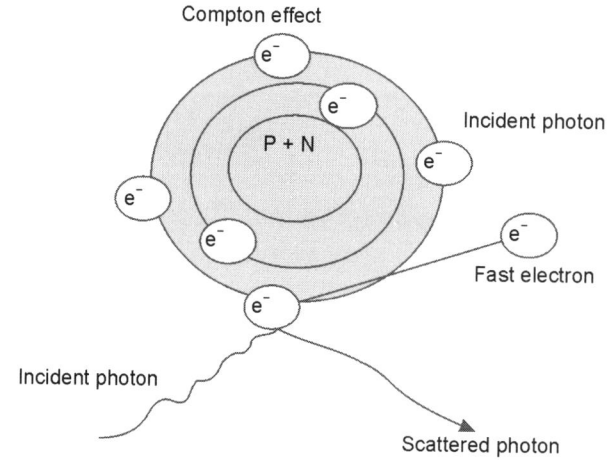

X-ray Film

There are following layers in an X-ray film:
- Supportive base made up of polyester plastic.
- Adhesive or Subbing layer for proper binding of the emulsion to the base.
- Emulsion containing silver halide (most commonly used is silver bromide). Crystals suspended in gelatin (**photosensitive layer**) – *the key component of a X-ray film.*

- Protective anti-abrasive supercoat of pure gelatin.
- Non-curl backing (only in single coated film) to prevent curling of the film.
- Antihalation layer of dye added to non-curl backing or to the base to prevent reflection and unsharpness.

The behavior of X-ray film (silver bromide emulsion) with respect to light spectrum (VIBGYOR) is known as its spectral response.

An X-ray film is far more sensitive to blue, violet and ultraviolet light than to the rest of the spectrum (monochromatic).

An *X-ray film is least sensitive to red light* and if sensitizers are added to X-ray film, the spectral response can be extended into green (up to 570 nm), known as orthochromatic emulsion, or even as far as the red (up to 700 nm) in polychromatic emulsion.

Films Used in Medical Imaging

1. **Double emulsion/coated (duplitized) films:** Have emulsion, applied to both sides of the plastic base in order to increase sensitivity, e.g.
   a. Direct-exposure (nonscreen type) films
      - Intra-oral **dental films**
      - Radiation monitoring films
   b. Screen type films (most commonly used type in **routine X-ray filming** and used with two intensifying screens).
2. **Single emulsion/coated films:** Have emulsion applied only to one side of its base. Their main advantage is high quality images. To identify the emulsion side of single-coated film a **small notch is provided** into one edge of each film. The emulsion side is facing if the film is held with the notch in the top right-hand corner, e.g.
   a. Screen type film (used with single intensifying screen)
   b. Photofluorographic film
   c. Cathode-ray tube (CRT) photography
   d. Subtraction film
   e. Laser imaging film
   f. Mammography film
   g. Computed tomography (CT) film
   h. Radionuclide imaging film
   i. Diagnostic ultrasound film
   j. Computed radiography (CR system) film.

CHEMICAL PROCESSING OF AN X-RAY FILM

X-rays film exposed to radiation → Develops $\xrightarrow{\text{Rinse}}$ Fixer → Washed
- Developer – major constituent – mixture of phenidone and hydroquinone
- Fixer – major constituent – sodium thiosulfate/ammonium thiosulfate.

Complex chemical processing of exposed film causes deposition of metallic silver on the film resulting in blackening of the film.

Intensifying Screens

Screens are composed of thin cardboard base coated with crystals of phosphorus (luminescent material).

These phosphorus have unique ability to emit light, when exposed to radiation. Hence screens are stuck to the inside of the cassette or film holder.

The aerial image is temporarily formed on the screen, resulting in various degree of brightness. These, in turn, ultimately produce corresponding difference in darkening of the radiograph.

Ninety-eight percent of the blackening of film exposed with screens may be photographic in origins, i.e. due to light. Rest 2 percent of the density is due to exposure to X-rays directly.

Hence, use of screens causes considerable reduction in the radiation exposure to the patient.

Phosphor composition/following chemicals can be used
- Calcium tungstate
- Barium lead sulfate
- Gadolinium ⎫
- Lanthavium ⎬ Oxybromide Oxysulfide
- Yttrium ⎭

DIGITAL OR COMPUTED OR FILMLESS RADIOGRAPHY OR PHOSPHOR PLATE TECHNOLOGY

It is one of the most modern imaging methods in which selective window settings of some image enhance visualization of lung fields, mediastinum or bones as desired.

Optic drum scanners/laser scanners can digitize conventional film radiographs.

Types

1. Phosphor plate CR (e.g. europium activated barium fluoride).
2. Selenium detection CR → Excellent quantum efficiency considerable dose reduction possible.
3. Large area, thin film transistor detector CR → Rapid image, excellent resolution.

Although it is most mature radiographic technology and uses conventional radiographic equipment but employs reusable photostimulable phosphor or selenium plate (europium-doped barium fluorohalide) instead of convocational film cassette.

Mechanism

The phosphor plate stores energy of incident X-ray as latent image
↓
On scanning the plate with LASER beams the stored energy is emitted as light, which is detected by a photomultiplier
↓
And converted to digital signal by digitizer
↓
This digital information is then manipulated, displayed and stored in whatever format desired on computer
The phosphor plate can be reused once latent image has been erased by exposure to whole light.

Major Advantages of CRS

- Linear photoluminescence dose response, which is much greater than that of conventional film
- Hide attitude
- Post processing of images possible
- Advantage of image archiving and transmission
- Excellent resolution.

PICTURE ARCHIVING AND COMMUNICATION SYSTEM

- A picture archiving and communication system (PACS) *aims to replace conventional analogue film and paper, clinical request forms and reports with a completely computerized electronic network* whereby digital images are viewed on monitors in conjunction with the clinical details of the patient and associated radiological report displayed in electronic format.

Types of PACS

a. Central PACS
b. Distributed PACS

- Thus, PACS must replace the function of traditional X-ray film, i.e. image acquisition, storage, transportation and display.
- True efficiency benefits can only be realized once a PACS is hospital-wide, as any more limited installation means running two systems in parallel, i.e. it entails continuing to produce conventional film and moving it around the hospital, as well as the cost of installing and maintaining a PACS.
- The hospital information technology (IT) network is likely to need upgrading to enable large amounts of image data to be transported and it is advisable to install multiple PACS 'drops' (work-station outlets) so that more PACS work-stations can easily be added at a later date.

Advantages of PACS

- Once correctly acquired into PACS, no image can ever be lost or misfiled and is always available when needed.
- It facilitates easy comparison of a patient's current and past examinations.
- All images remain accessible from the PACS archives day and night.
- Simultaneous multilocation viewing of same image is possible on any connected work-station.
- Image retrieval is infinitely quicker from PACS that is using conventional film.
- All images correctly and permanently reside under appropriate imaging study, remain in their correct orientation and are automatically chronologically ordered.
- Viewing of images on monitors allows many post processing soft copy manipulations, a range of different window width and level setting can be applied to CT images.
- Cost saving (major reduction in film budget, film packet cost and chemical processing).
- Substantial time saving incurred as never have to search for or retrieve films.
- It sets stage for introduction of teleradiology over a wide area of network.
- After hospital wide PACS, old films can be progressively removed from store.

Disadvantages of PACS

- Expensive technology
- Technological complexity
- Dedicated maintenance program required
- Hospital is no longer equipped to run a film-based service
- Changing from a hard copy to soft copy necessitates change of work pattern.

CONTRAST RADIOGRAPHY

Definition

Contrast radiography means radiography (taking X-rays films) with use of contrast (*for all practical purpose, broadly only two types of contrast agents are used, barium sulfate and waters soluble iodinated contrast agent*). Contrast is injected in some of other space or lumen of the body and films are taken.

BARIUM STUDIES

Barium studies form one of the still most commonly used radiological procedures.

Barium sulfate is inert and best for examination of GI tract, except in few settings like TO fistula and bemls perforation.

However, compared to barium sulfate, the major advantage of aqueous contrast agents is their rapid absorption from the interstitial spaces and peritoneal cavity.

This property makes them *uniquely useful for examining patients with suspected TO fistula and perforation of a hollow viscus*. No permanent deleterious effects from the presence of these aqueous contrast materials in the mediastinum, pleural cavity, or abdomen have been shown.

NONBARIUM STUDIES

Apart from Barium procedures (done for gastrointestinal imaging), other several procedures include:
- Sialography
- Intravenous urography (IVU)
- Urethrography
- Myelography
- Hysterosalpingography
- Fistulography
- Arteriography (Conventional and DSA)
- Venography.

> **Extremely *vital facts* to be remembered regarding radiological contrast agents:**
> - *Older contrast radiographic procedures like* Oral cholecystography (Iopanoic acid – telepaque, sodium iopodate-biloptin), bronchography (Dionosil), lymphangiography (methylene blue, lipiodol ultrafluid), and splenoportography *are outdated.*

- Today almost all contrast studies, i.e. radiological procedures including *contrast enhanced CT scan* are done with use of much safer **water soluble iodinated contrast media**, while older contrast media like Conray 280, myodil, lipiodol, hypaque, etc. are outdated.
- Both, ionic (e.g. Sodium and Meglumine salts of diatrizoate) and nonionic (e.g. Iohexol, Iopamidol, Ioversol, Metrizamide) water soluble iodinated contrast media are available but *low-osmolar nonionic water soluble iodinated contrast media* (LOCM) should be preferred whenever contrast media is to be injected in intravascular (as in IVU, CECT) or subarachnoid space (as in myelography).

SIALOGRAPHY

It is used to diagnose stones (sialolithiasis), chronic or recurrent inflammation, and tumors in parotid and submandibular glands. It is contraindicated in acute sialadenitis (parotitis) for fear of exacerbating the condition.

MYELOGRAPHY

It is the radiographic investigation of the spinal canal for the diagnosis of space occupying and obstructive lesions and requires the contrast agent to be injected into the subarachnoid space (which lies between pia mater and the arachnoid mater) usually following a lumbar puncture.

Either a **negative contrast** agent like air or oxygen is used or more usually a **positive** nonionic water soluble low osmolar, organic iodine compound (Iohexol).

Oily preparations like iophendylate (Myodil, Pantopaque) is abandoned as it is known to be toxic and causes **chronic adhesive arachnoiditis**. Amipaque (metrizamide) has replaced myodil (iophendylate) due to its advantages like freely miscible with CSF, flows along subarachnoid spaces around the nerve roots and is absorbed from subarachnoid space within 48 hours. It is isotonic with CSF in concentration usually used for lumbar myelography made up to a volume of 10 cc. It also has low viscosity and thus a narrow bone needle can be used reactions like headache, and nausea seldom last for more than 24 hours.

Iohexol (Omnipaque) is nonionic iodinated contrast agent commonly used today. Iohexol has more evenly distributed OH groups; hence, has less subarachnoid toxicity. Although arachnoiditis remains the most dangerous, but very rare complication if myelography.

Now, myelography has almost completely supplanted by MRI.

EXCRETORY UROGRAPHY (INTRAVENOUS UROGRAPHY, IVU, IVP)

Since 1929, when the first intravenous contrast agent was developed by Swick, excretory urography has been the primary modality for imaging the urinary tract.

The renal margins and parenchyma (*nephrogram*), as well as the entire collecting system (pye*logram*), including the ureters and bladder, can be visualized diagnostically.

After intravenous injection, whether by bolus or by infusion, these preparations leave the vascular system in two ways. First, rapid permeation of the capillary wall and equilibration with the extracellular fluid occurs. At the same time, contrast in the bloodstream undergoes glomerular filtration and subsequent excretion in the urine. As plasma contrast concentration falls as a result of ongoing renal excretion, there is a continual redistribution of the extracellular contrast into the vascular system.

The quality of the urogram depends on good pelvicalyceal concentration of contrast media as well as sufficient distention of the collecting system.

Indications

Infections, acute genitourinary pain, hematuria (microscopic or gross), renal transplantation, neurogenic bladder, congenital anomalies, and investigation of complications following a surgical procedure.

There are several indications for immediate urography. These include massive gross hematuria of unknown cause, and suspected ureteral calculus.

In the past, indications for urography have included the evaluation of hypertension. The hypertensive urogram involves obtaining coned-down films of the kidneys in a rapid sequence following bolus injection of contrast. The minimum series includes films at 1, 2, and 3 minutes post injection. The radiographic criteria for renovascular hypertension include delayed visualization of contrast in the collecting system on the affected side, decreased renal size, and delayed wash-out of contrast on the later films in the urogram. A secondary finding is that of notching of the proximal ureter on the involved side due to development of collateral flow via the periureteral plexus reconstituting the renal artery.

Recently, digital subtraction angiography has been claimed to provide good visualization of the renal arteries and may eventually become a satisfactory screening examination for renovascular hypertension.

The present day urogram is reliable test for functional assessment of the kidneys. But IVU has been replaced by DTPA/MAG$_3$ scan as best test for residual function of kidneys.

Useful information can be gained with regard to the presence or absence of obstruction in many patients with renal failure, assuming tomography is used for better visualization of the poorly opacified collecting systems. A better modality for evaluating such patients, however, is renal ultrasound, which is an excellent screening examination for suspected urinary tract obstruction. Its usefulness is based on its ability to detect hydronephrosis. However, it must be realized that there exist a significant number of conditions that can mimic or produce dilatation of the collecting system in the absence of obstruction. Renal sonography suggestive of hydronephrosis should be followed by additional diagnostic studies to confirm or exclude obstruction, which may mainly include CT scan, especially with respect to ureteric stones.

Contraindications

- Combined renal and liver failure
- Multiple myeloma
- Pregnancy
- Previous reactions to contrast media
- History of allergy
- Infancy
- Thyroid disease
- Renal failure
- Diabetes mellitus.

Patient Preparation

- Bowel preparation
- Informed consent
- Nil by mouth.

Both the plain film and the urogram should be exposed at 66 kV(p)-70 kV(p), although patients built is vital consideration.

Contrast Administration

Doses in the range of 17 g to 20 g of iodine for the average size adult will result in diagnostic studies if careful monitoring is performed.

In children, weight of the patient is a more prominent factor, and recommended doses are based on this parameter.

Iohexol (low-osmolar water soluble nonionic iodinated contrast media) are best for IVU.

Film Sequencing

- Plain film of abdomen
- 1-minute film (nephrogram)—seen due to contrast in collecting tubules
- 5-minute full view (pyelogram)—seen due to contrast in pelvicalyceal system
- Full view post voiding.

Tailoring

The usual sequences of films taken after injecting contrast are 5 (nephrogram), 15, 30/45 minutes and a postmicturition film.
Nephrogram is due to the contrast in nephrons.

Delayed films are essential when an obstructive nephrogram is seen on the routine early views. A recommended sequence for these delayed views is 30 minutes, 1 hour, 2 hours, 4 hours, 8 hours, and 24 hours. When obtaining delayed views, the patient should be instructed to void prior to exposure of the film so that a calculus at the level of the ureterovesical junction will not be obscured by the full bladder. Unless the degree of obstruction is extremely severe, at some point during this sequence of delayed films contrast can usually be seen columning in the ureter to the point of obstruction. If the degree of obstruction is such that there is no columning by 24 hours, further films are not indicated. In such patients further imaging modalities will be necessary to determine the anatomy of the obstructed system. These may include antegrade or retrograde pyelography.

Modifications in IVU Include

Rapid sequence IVU: Done in patients with suspected renovascular hypertension. Films taken at 1, 2 and 4 minutes after injection of contrast medium in addition to the routine filming sequence.

Infusion urography: Done in patients with compromised renal function 40–50 gram of iodine (as against 16 gram in usual procedure) is injected into 200–500 cc of glucose and given as infusion.

Diuretic urography: It is done in patients with PUJ obstruction. Patient is not dehydrated prior to procedure, IV furosemide injected immediately following contrast which causes copious contrast secretion, thus dilating the renal pelvis to greater extent and demonstrating the pathology nicely.

Abnormal Nephrogram

- **Rim nephrogram** (Rim of cortex receiving collateral blood flow)
    - Acute complete occlusion of main renal artery
    - Renal vein thrombosis
    - Acute tubular necrosis
    - Severe chronic urinary obstruction
- **Shell/rim nephrogram**
  Sever hydronephrosis

- **"Swiss cheese" nephrogram**
  Polycystic kidney disease (ADPKD)
- **"Sunburst" nephrogram** (Striated nephrogram with persistent radiating radioopaque streaks on delayed images)
  Infantile polycystic kidney disease
- **Striated nephrogram** (Streaky linear bands of alternating hyper and hypodensity parallel to axis of tubules and collecting ducts)
  - Acute ureteral obstruction
  - Acute pyelonephritis
  - Renal contusion
  - Renal vein thrombosis
  - Intratubular obstruction
  - Systemic hypotension
  - Autosomal recessive PCKD
  - Medullary sponge kidney
  - Medullary cystic disease
- **Dense persistent nephrogram**
  - Systemic hypotension
  - Intratubular obstruction/tubular damage
  - Renal artery stenosis
  - Renal vein thrombosis
  - Urinary tract obstruction
  - Focal parenchymal disease
- **Increasingly dense nephrogram**
  - Systemic arterial hypotension
  - Severe renal artery stenosis
  - Acute tubular necrosis
  - Acute renal vein thrombosis
  - Acute glomerular disease
  - Intratubular obstruction
  - Acute ureteral obstruction
- **Black nephrogram/negative pyelogram:** Hydronephrosis
- **Soap bubble nephrogram:** Hydronephrosis.

URETHROGRAPHY

Retrograde Urethrography/Ascending Urethrography

Direct retrograde examination is appropriate, particularly if the anterior urethra is of paramount interest. Although an uncommon procedure in the female, examination of the male urethra by this technique is frequently done to evaluate urethral trauma or obstruction secondary to inflammatory disease or neoplasm.

Opacification of the male urethra in retrograde fashion allows visualization of the anterior urethra but is usually accompanied by *relatively poor filling of the posterior urethra* because of the resistance encountered at the external sphincter. The anterior urethra will be well-defined and distended and the level of the external sphincter clearly identified. The posterior (membranous and prostatic) urethra, on the other hand, will usually not be well distended and anatomical landmarks will be more difficult to identify.

The appropriate contrast material should be water soluble, minimally irritating, and handled in a sterile manner. Methylglucamine diatrizoate or iothalamate is readily available in any radiology department and serves the purpose well.

> **Retrograde urethrography** depicts the membranous and anterior urethra better and is preferred approach your assessing inflammatory lesions and diverticuli of anterior urethra, while VCUG (MCU) is best for posterior urethra.

Voiding Cystourethrography/Micturating Cystourethrography/Descending Urethrography

The primary indications for cystourethrography are to evaluate the presence of vesicoureteral reflux and to investigate abnormalities of the bladder neck and the posterior urethra. Functional assessment of bladder contractility and micturition is also possible using this technique. When radiographic complete assessment of the urethra is of primary concern, cystourethrography should be used in conjunction with a retrograde urethral study. Current infection of the lower urinary tract is a contraindication to the procedure.

Indications

To demonstrate the various abnormalities in the neck of bladder and urethra:
- Recurrent UTI especially in children
- For complete assessment of cases of bladder diverticuli
- For demonstration of VUR
- For demonstration of bladder contractions and the control of micturition.

- The MCU is indicated in all boys under 1 year of age with UTI.
- Any child who requires imaging of kidneys and or urinary tract for whatever reason, with the exception of trauma cases, should undergo a USG examination as the first investigation.
- The MCU is however the definitive method of assessing prostatic urethra and bladder.
- It is necessary also in all boys to assess by MCU when there is any suspicion of urethral pathology.
- Congenital abnormalities affect both anterior and posterior urethra, the most common being hypospadias, which has little radiological importance.
- Posterior urethral valves is one of the most common GUT congenital abnormalities in males causing obstructive uropathy.
- USG usually strongly suggests the diagnosis and may detect complication like urinoma. This may, however, be followed by an MCU especially for confirmation and follow-up.

Voiding cystourethrogram or micturating cystourethrogram demonstrates the prostatic urethra to best advantage as it is better distended than the membranous and anterior urethra.

HYSTEROSALPINGOGRAPHY

Definition

Visualization of the uterine cavity and Fallopian tubes by using negative contrast media (normal saline in hydrosalpingosonography) or positive contrast media [Echovist in sonosalpingography and the iodinated nonionic low-osmolar contrast agent in hysterosalpingography (HSG)].

Ideal Time to Perform HSG

Between 7th and 10th day of menstrual cycle (postmenstrual, but preovulatory period) for following reasons:
- No risk of early pregnancy
- Isthmus is most easily distensible
- Tubal filling occurs readily.

Indications for HSG

- Infertility
- Recurrent miscarriage
- Congenital abnormalities
- Post-uterine and/or tubal surgery

- Abnormal uterine bleeding
- Evaluation after major pelvic trauma and/or surgery
- Prior to artificial insemination and *in vitro* fertilization, for tubal patency (other tubal patency tests are laparoscopic chromopertubation, CO_2 insufflation and hydrosonosalpingography test).

Contraindications for HSG

- Pregnancy
- Bleeding
- Immediate pre- and postmenstrual phases
- Recent untreated pelvic infection
- Tubal or uterine surgery within last 6 weeks
- Contrast medium sensitivity
- Recent D and C procedure
- Severe renal or cardiac disease
- Migrated IUCD.

Complications of HSG

- Pain
- Bleeding/hemorrhage
- Intravasation (venous)
- Vasovagal episode
- Pelvic infection
- Pregnancy irradiation
- Allergic reaction
- Transient nausea, vomiting and headache.

Genital Tuberculosis and HSG

Initially, fallopes are involved.
 In 50 percent of such cases, uterus is secondarily infected.

Tuberculous Salpingitis

Plain film: Calcification in region of tubes and ovaries.

HSG
- Bilateral tubal occlusion (isthmic or ampullary part)
- Tubal contours—smooth gross thickening of longitudinal mucosal folds
- Irregular or ragged outline
- Multiple strictures giving **'beaded' appearance** of fallopes
- Cavities or sinus tracts
- Rigid straight 'pipe-stem' appearance
- Tubointestinal and tubovesical fistulae

Uterine tuberculosis: Polypoidal lesions, hyperplastic endometrium, ragged saw-toothed uterine contour, shriveled and deformed uterus, and fibrosis. Venous or lymphatic intravasation.

XERORADIOGRAPHY

- In xeroradiography instead of an X-ray film, a thin layer of semiconductor is used to produce a latent image which is transferred onto paper.
- Characteristically the images have marked edge enhancement and good resolution.
- Thus in breast, blood vessels, ducts, and skin the small calcification and tumor edges stand out clearly.
- Hence, was commonly used in breast cancer detection.
- Further, it also gives a more uniform exposure.
- It also produces good images with low kV tungsten tube.
- The radiation dose is, however, 60 to 100 percent greater than with low dose film techniques.
- It is not in use nowadays and has been replaced totally by mammography.

MAMMOGRAPHY

It's a special radiographic technique for imaging of breasts, basically used for screening purpose.

It has replaced xeroradiography because apart the effect of greater depth dose due to the use of higher X-ray tube kilovoltage, the average glandular dose in xeromammography is about three to six times greater than in screen-film mammography.

The required image should have high contrast, high spatial resolution, and low noise.

It differs from routine radiographic technique in that *instead of tungsten filament;* molybdenum is used as *target material. Rhodium and rhenium* can also be used. This is because, molybdenum produces low energy X-ray beam after bombardment with electrons, which are must in mammography as it is used as a screening tool for breast lesions and its repeated use is likely and one of the predisposing factors for carcinoma breast is radiation itself.

It requires high soft tissue resolution (aim is to image breast tissues), low radiation *dose* (aim is to avoid radiation hazard to breast), special compression views (mediolateral view and craniocaudal are the most important one) and equal radiation exposure to all parts of breasts.

Hence, mammography X-ray tubes are *low kV-high mA output* tube, operated in the 22- to 35-kVp range, commonly have a rotating anode to achieve currents of the order of 100 mA, and usually have a **molybdenum target,** a thin **beryllium window** (less than 1 mm), as opposed to the more absorbing Pyrex glass used on routine X-ray tubes, and a molybdenum filter of about 0.03 mm thickness. Focal spots of 0.3 mm are required.

Overall detection rate of carcinoma breast by mammography is 58 to 69 percent and 8 percent only, if the lesion <1 cm in size. Hence, mammography is a screening modality and not the best diagnostic measure.

- The "triple assessment" for carcinoma breast includes–
  - Clinical examination
  - Mammography
  - FNAC/Biopsy
- In young females, mammography is not a good screening tool as young breasts are more dense, i.e. glandular tissue is more fatty in young females, hence in young females with family history/*BRCA-1; BRCA-2* gene caries MRI used.

Average or mean glandular dose on film screen mammography should be 2 mGy/0.2 rad or less.

1 mGy = 100 mrad = 0.1 rad

Indications for Mammography

- Before breast surgery, as it may avert an unnecessary biopsy demonstrating that the palpable mass has a characteristically benign appearance.
- Follow-up of breast cancer patients.
- Work-up a patient with metastases from an unknown primary.
- *Mammographic Screening is best screening method for carcinoma breast.*

ORTHOPANTOMOGRAPHY OR PANORAMIC RADIOGRAPHY

Pantomography is a special radiographic technique that produces a panoramic radiograph of a curved surface.

Orthopantomography (OPG) is currently the extraoral technique of choice in dental radiology as it depicts both the **upper and lower jaws** in their entirety together with the **floor of maxillary sinuses** and **temporomandibular joints** on a single film. The rounded configuration of the mandible and teeth makes them especially suitable for OPG. Pantomograms of jaw thus show the Tm joints on either side of film with the teeth laid out between them.

It is a modified form of tomography where jaws are positioned in a predetermined image layer, which is thinner in the anterior region. The patient is in chair and remains stationary throughout the examination. The X-ray film holder and the tube both rotate during the exposure. The film holder has a protective lead front, considerably lower than the film. The film is exposed through a narrow slit in its holder. The film moves across this slit and the X-ray tube rotates and the radiographic image is laid out as the film passes by the tube in much the same way that paint is applied to a wall with a roller.

The resulting image is flattened out image of a curved surface, but it is sensitive to errors of positioning, in particular of incisor teeth, leading to increased distortion and blurring.

ULTRASONOGRAPHY/ULTRASOUND STUDY

Jean-Daniel Colladon a Swiss physicist/engineer discovered sonography with an underwater bell in 1826. He accurately determined the speed of sound through water.

In 1881, **Pierre Curie** found a connection between electrical voltage and pressure on crystalline material. This was the breakthrough that was needed to create the modern ultrasound transducer.

Ian Donald, invented and improved on many devices used in pregnancy and fetal development. During World War II, he became interested in radar and sonar. He became known in the 1950s when a woman with a diagnosis of inoperable stomach cancer came to his attention. He studied the case with his new equipment and found that she had an ovarian cyst, which was safely removed. He became the father of obstetric ultrasound. He also invented the B-mode scanner. He was able to detect a twin pregnancy.

Dr. John Wild and John Reid modified standard medical imaging equipment and produced a hand held B-mode instrument that could swing side to side and get cross views from various angles to detect breast tumors. This type of unit was the forerunner of the modern machines used today as they produced the first breast ultrasound. They also invented an A-mode scanner for the detection of ovarian cancer.

- Ultrasound is a sound with a frequency greater than **20, 000 cycles/sec** (Hertz, Hz).
- Thus, sounds with a frequency above 20 kiloHertz (20 kHz) are called ultrasonic (beyond the range of human hearing).
- The sounds used for sonar are well into the ultrasonic range, with frequencies of 2 to 20 megaHertz (MHz).
- Medical sonography employs frequencies between 1 MHz and 20 MHz.
- It does not involve use of ionizing radiation (the greatest advantage).

- The piezoelectric crystals in the ultrasound probe are nothing but innumerable dipoles arranged in geometric pattern and electric field causes sudden change in their physical dimensions (shape) by realigning them, thereby starting a series of vibrations that produce sound waves.
- Thus, by the virtue of **piezoelectric effect** in the ultrasound probe one form of energy (electric energy) is converted in to another form (sound energy) the body/organs parts are imaged.
- It works on pulse echo principle and B-mode is used for transmission during all routine including abdominal ultrasonography.
- **Real-time B-scans** allow body structures which are moving to be investigated. The simplest type of scanner is just a speeded up version of the 2-D B-scan, allowing a rapid series of still pictures to be built up into a video of the movement.
- The probe or the transducer is any device that converts one form of energy to another. In case of ultrasound, the transducer converts electric energy to mechanical energy and vice versa.
- The ultrasound transducer uses the **principle or property of piezoelectricity** which occur naturally in some materials whereby an applied electric field produces a change in linear dimensions.
- **Quartz, natural ceramic** is a naturally occurring piezoelectric material having the unique ability to respond to the action of an electric field by changing shape and to the change in polarity of voltage applied by generating small potentials and thus producing an ultrasound image.
- Currently **Lead zirconate titanate (PZT), synthetic ceramic** is the most widely used material in the ultrasound sound transducers/probes replacing the firstly discovered Barium titanate. Although some naturally occurring materials possess piezoelectric properties (e.g. quartz) but most crystals used in medical ultrasound are man made with artificial ones, known as Ferroelectrics.
- These ceramic crystals are made up of innumerable tiny dipoles but, to possess piezoelectric characteristics, the dipoles must be arranged in specific geometric configuration which requires to be heated to a high temperature to be strong electric field. The curie temperatures for several crystals to possess the piezoelectric crystals property is as follows: Quartz 573°C, Barium titanate 100°C, PZT-328°C, PZT-365°C.

In most diagnostic applications, frequencies in the range 2 to 20 MHz are commonly used.

The various frequencies used for various body parts are as follows:
1. **1.5 to 2.5 MHz**—Abdomen in obese patients and transcranial studies.
2. **3 to 7 MHz**—Abdomen, heart and obstetric USG (2nd and 3rd trimester).
3. **7 to 15 MHz**—Superficial tissues like thyroid, breast and scrotum, orbital, transrectal, transvaginal and transesophageal or endoscopic ultrasonography.
4. **> 20 MHz**—Eye (anterior chamber especially) skin and intravascular USG (IVUS).

The frequencies of ultrasound required for medical imaging are in the range **2 to 20 MHz**. These frequencies can be obtained by using **piezoelectric** materials. When an electric field is placed across a slice of one of these materials, the material contracts or expands. If the electric field is reversed, the effect on the material is also reversed. If the electric field keeps reversing, the crystal alternately contracts and expands. So a rapidly alternating electric field causes the crystal to vibrate.

The piezoelectric effect occurs in a number of natural crystals including **quartz**, but the most commonly used substance is a synthetic ceramic, **lead zirconate titanate**. The crystal is cut into a slice with a thickness equal to half a wavelength of the desired ultrasound frequency, as this thickness ensures most of the energy is emitted at the fundamental frequency.

> **Dictum:** *Higher the frequency of an ultrasound probe, better are superficial structures seen.*

- Percentage of the beam reflected at the tissue interface depends on the tissue's acoustic impedance and the angle of incidence of the beam.
- Two factors determine the acoustic impedance of the tissue, density of the tissue and the velocity of ultrasound. But as the velocity of ultrasound in tissues is almost constant (1540 m/s), reflection of the ultrasound beam (change in impedance) is mainly dependant on density.
- More the dense a tissue is, more will be the acoustic impedance, reflection of the ultrasound beam will be more, producing more acoustic shadow.
- The acoustic impedance of bone is maximum in our body (7.8 Rayls); hence it produces dense/maximum acoustic shadow.
- Calculus also produces acoustic shadow.
- Medium acoustic impedance (in standard unit):
    1. Air   0.000429
    2. Water   1.50
    3. Blood   1.59
    4. Fat   1.38
    5. Muscle   1.70
    6. Bone   6.50

Clear liquids allow ultrasound to pass directly through without much alteration, so that echoes that come from tissue behind liquid are usually enhanced (brighter). This is known as **"acoustic enhancement"**.

Dense materials such as bones or calculi cast shadows on the structures behind them, as the ultrasound waves do not go through them. This is known as **"acoustic shadowing"** (Postacoustic shadow). Postacoustic shadow is of immense importance in detecting gallbladder and renal calculi. To quote a classical example, **WES triad** (Wall Echo Shadow) is diagnostic sign of gallstones on ultrasonography, where wall of gallbladder, echo of calculus, and postacoustic shadow of the calculus seen together is diagnostic of cholelithiasis.

Air (Gas) can present a variety of sonographic patterns; beams can be scattered, reflected, refracted and absorbed and may hence also produce acoustic shadowing. But, it produces *dirty* postacoustic shadow, hence, air can be said to the *enemy of ultrasound* and whenever air/gas comes ultrasound fails to image the underlying organ. To quote common examples regarding this we can recall that for detecting of pancreatic lesions and ureteric calculi, CT is far superior to ultrasonography because bowel gas shadow degrades imaging by ultrasound [CECT for pancreatic lesions and NCCT for ureteric stones].

Fat is echogenic but does not produce acoustic shadows.

Dictum: Air *is enemy of ultrasonography, hence, it is not good for imaging of lungs, pancreas, ureters, etc.*

The percentage of the beam reflected at the tissue interface depends on the tissue's acoustic impedance and the angle of incidence of the beam.

Thus lungs, bone, air, fat are echogenic (white) while blood, water, bile are anechoic (Black).

How things look on USG		
Hyperechoic	Hypoechoic	Anechoic
Air	Bile	Cyst
Bone	Chronic hemorrhage	–
Acute hemorrhage	Abscess	–
Fat	Tumors (Most)	–
Stones	–	–
Liver hemangioma	–	–

Ultrasound is often the only investigation necessary in confirming calculi in GB.

Its sensitivity is so high that careful correlation between the clinical presentation and ultrasound findings has to be made to ensure that unnecessary treatment, especially cholecystectomy is not carried out in asymptomatic patients. A sensitivity of around 90 percent is claimed in diagnosis of acute appendicitis and its complications by ultrasound.

Ultrasonography is investigation of choice for
- Hydrocephalus in infants
- Gallstones
- Acute cholecystitis (although theoretically HIDA scan is best)
- Screening for rotator cuff injuries (Best initial investigation, although MRI is best)
- Renal colic in pregnancy
- Minimal ascites
- Obstetrics indications
- Adenomyomatosis of gallbladder (Comet-tail sign)
- CHPS
- Intussusception
- Screening tool of choice for blunt trauma abdomen (in FAST protocol)
- Hydronephrosis
- Initial test of choice for obstructive jaundice
- Initial test of choice for acute abdominal pain
- Verical calculus
- DDH
- Popliteal cyst
- Retinal detachment and vitreous hemorrhage
- Choroidal melanoma.

Theoretic Safety Risks from Ultrasound

Ultrasound continues to be the major technique for imaging in pregnancy, especially the second and third trimester. Theoretic safety risks from ultrasound energy include thermal damage (due to a rise in temperature) and cavitation (production and collapse of gas-filled bubbles) with subsequent tissue injury.

However, no confirmed deleterious biologic effects on patients or instrument operators caused by exposure at intensities typical of present diagnostic US instruments have been reported. It has no radiation (ionizing) hazard.

Transrectal Ultrasonography

Prostatic Lesions
- Transrectal ultrasonography (TRUS) is an **excellent** adjuvant to physical examination, it does not serve as a screening investigation. However, the combination of digital rectal examination (DRE) and serum PSA level is more sensitive then TRUS.

- But once suspected, prostatic carcinoma is most effectively confirmed by TRUS-guided needle biopsy.
- The staging accuracy of TRUS does not match the accuracies attainable by MRI, especially **endorectal coil MR** (ERMR).
- TRUS-guided biopsy is the best utility of TRUS for prostatic lesions.
- CT is not recommended for routine tumor staging as it is insensitive and nonspecific. **CT** is useful in advanced cancer for evaluation of adenopathy and metastases.
- **Major role of MRI** is in local staging of disease.

Ca Rectum
- In rectal carcinoma the depth of penetration can be best achieved with TRUS, while the involvement of perirectal nodes can be better assessed by MRI in addition to depth of penetration.

Seminal Vesicle Lesions

COLOR DOPPLER IMAGING/STUDY

When ultrasound is reflected from a moving surface, the frequency of the sound is altered slightly in a manner that depends on the speed of movement of the surface. This is due to the **Doppler effect.**

The Doppler effect is now commonly used in ultrasound imaging to examine the movement of liquids, such as blood flow in arteries and veins, allowing the location of blockages to be determine precisely. Another common medical application is in fetal heart monitoring and cardiac ECHO.

In Color Doppler Imaging areas of blood flow are represented as color within image.

When the ultrasound waves strike upon the moving RBCs, they are not reflected; they are scattered in all directions and hence the blood vessels are seen as echo-free structures.

It has become common practice to represent flow towards transducer as red and flow away as blue.

Velocity information in special form and color flow helps in diagnosis.

Many indices of waveform analysis have been devised including resistance index (RI) and pulsatilty index (PI), the commonly used ones.

The ***main advantages of Color Doppler imaging*** include:
- Confirmation that a structure is a vessel or that a known vessel is patent. It shows vessels that are too small to be seen by 2D image.
- Direction of flow can be easily confirmed, as important in the portal vein.

- It also permits the assessment of number and distribution of vessels within a tissue volume which is important to second blood flow signals from vessels like renal accurate and uterine arteries and in assessment of vascularity in and around focal lesion.
- Doppler frequency shift data also needed to measure blood flow velocity directly.

It is investigation of choice for
- Diagnosis of deep venous thrombosis
- For assessment of fetal wellbeing during 2nd and 3rd trimester pregnancy
- Best screening modality for common carotids and extracranial part of internal carotid artery
- Vein of Galen malformation (Present in neonates)
- Peipheral vascular diseases (e.g. Burger's disease)
- Portal hypertension ("sinusoidal" wave form of portal vein and "triphasic" waveform of hepaticvein is lost and flow in portal vein becomes centrifugal
- One of the screening test of choice for renal artery stenosis
- Midgut volvulus (whirlpool sign).

ECHOCARDIOGRAPHY

Echocardiography is a safe, painless, portable and relatively inexpensive method of acquiring high quality tomographic images of the heart in a variety of patients. It is "first-test" of choice in the noninvasive examination of cardiac anatomy and function.

Posterior structures (pulmonary veins, the atria and their appendages and atrioventricular valves) are especially well imaged by transesophageal echocardiography (TEE) and hence the thrombi, which are common in atria and their appendages (especially the left atrial thrombus) can be easily detected.

TRANSESOPHAGEAL ECHOCARDIOGRAPHY

Even in the hands of experienced echocardiographers, some portion of the adult population, *due to obesity, chronic obstructive lung disease, or abnormalities of thoracic musculoskeletal anatomy*, may not be amenable to transthoracic (i.e. precordial, apical, suprasternal, or subcostal) echocardiographic imaging. In these patients, the development of transesophageal methods has permitted superior visualization of certain portions of cardiac anatomy. In particular, *assessment of structures near the esophagus (left atrium, right atrium, interatrial septum, atrioventricular valves, pulmonary veins, and aorta)* may be visualized from transesophageal windows.

Common Indications

- Detailed assessment of LA for thrombus
- Diagnosis of dissection of thoracic arch (preferred in hemodynamically unstable patients)
- Assessment of LV function perioperatively
- Assessment of cardiac surgical repairs perioperatively
- Detailed assessment of native or prosthetic mitral valve
- Assessment interatrial septum
- Assessment of heart valves in known or suspected endocarditis
- Assessment of aortic valve
- Assessment of some forms of CHD
- Assessment of some right sided cardiac lesions
- General echo indications in 'hard to image' patients
- It is also a cardiovascular monitoring technique
- It is the *most sensitive and practical technique* for detection of myocardial ischemia in the perioperative period.

COMPUTED TOMOGRAPHY

(**Synonym:** CAT scan-computed axial tomography)

Godfrey N. Hounsfield (1973), while working with central research laboratories of EMI *(Electromusical instruments)* England, first described an elaborate technique in which X-ray transmission readings were taken through the head at a multitude of angles. He got a Nobel Prize of Medicine in 1979 for describing this first effective scanning system, which was called EMI scanner, the **Generation I Computed tomography (CT) machine.**

The *fundamental concept* in CT is that the internal structure of an object can be reconstructed from multiple projections of the object.

For obtaining image by CT scan things required are an *X-ray source, detectors and associated electronics*, all mounted on a gantry, or a frame that mechanically moves to produce the scan.

Hounsfield originally developed *first generation scanners*. In this machine the X-ray beam is collimated to dimensions of roughly 2 × 13 mm. Here 13 mm is the slice thickness, X-ray tube and detectors system moves continuously across the patient, making 16 multiple measurements during translation. At the end of each translation, X-ray tube and detector system are rotated 1 degree and the translation is repeated. Major disadvantage is long scanning time. It requires 5 minutes to gather 28,800 ray sums.

Such instruments have been designed along 3 lines, since their introduction by Godfrey Hounsfield.

1. **Generation II CT machine:** Scanners in which the X-ray tube and detectors are made to move in translate rotate type of mechanical motion.
2. **Generation III CT machine:** Scanners that employ a rotating motion in which the detectors and X-ray beam rotate around the object.
3. **Generation IV CT machine:** Scanners in which detectors are stationary and the X-ray source is moved around the object.

The first modification was simply to convert the X-ray beam to a fan shape with diverting angle of between 3 and 10 degrees. Also *more detectors are used*, so number of angular rotations could be decreased and an adequate number of views obtained in much shorter intervals such *second generation scanners* were able to obtain a scan in periods as short as 18 seconds.

Next development involved widening the X-ray divergent angle so that it could entirely compass the object without performing any translatory motion. Thus rotate only scanner was developed referred to as the *third generation scanner*. It can produce scan in 1 to 10 seconds. This advent of *spiral or helical CT* in 1989 was a dramatic development, which helped CT to mature into a true volume imaging modality. It combines continuous gantry rotation with continuous table feed. It thus eliminates interscan delay. Spiral CT can be *single or multiple slice* machine.

The pursuit of faster scanning and higher resolution in volume scanning led to **concept of multislice CT**. The technological innovation of the new millennium is the world of spiral CT. A **multislice CT system** in contrast uses multiple detector rows and can therefore acquire multiple slices per rotation ranging from 4, 8, 16, 32 to 64 slices per sec. Speed of gantry rotation is increased, resulting in overall increase in scan speed. This reduction in scan time allows larger volumes to be scanned in the same time and same volume in much reduced time or in the same time at a narrower collimation leading to higher axial resolution.

Removing detectors from rotating gantry and mounting them in stationary positions around the patient allowed a further decrease in scanning time. These machines are named *fourth generation scanners*. In this scanner the X-ray tube is on continuously during a scan and each detector receives X-ray beam for a significant portion of the scan cycle.

Basic principle of CT is linear attenuation of X-rays

CT tissues
↓
Anatomy, physiology, biochemistry, pathology
↓
μ (Radiation absorption)/LAC
↓
Signal intensity
↓
CT image depends mainly on X-ray absorption

CT Number/HU Value

Basic principle of CT is linear attenuation of X-ray.

Incident X-rays are linearly attenuated by their interaction with orbital electrons of tissues. Measurement of attenuation of emerging/detected beam → gives density of intervening tissues and this density forms basis of signal intensity variation obtained in X-ray tomograms.

For unenhanced CT, there is an essentially linear relationship between voxel signal intensity (image brightness) and the **X-ray linear attenuation coefficient**, which is scaled relative to air and water and converted to an integer.

This is expressed in Hounsfield units (HU), which range from −1000 to +4000.

Actually the linear attenuation coefficient of each pixel converted to a new number is called a "CT number" which allows computer to present the information gathered as picture/image with large gray scale.

It is to honor Hounsfield; CT numbers are also called **Hounsfield units (HU)**.
- Air has a value of −1000 HU
- Fat of −120 to −200 HU
- Water of 0 HU
- Soft tissues of 20–60 HU
- Blood of 50–60 HU
- Bone of + 1000 HU

$$HU\ value = \text{Magnification constant} \frac{(\text{Pixel linear attenuation coefficient} - \text{Water linear attenuation coefficient})}{\text{Water linear attenuation coefficient}}$$

CECT makes use following phases of iodinated contrast medium, vascular enhancement, tissue opacification, and opacification of urinary tract/bowel lumen/cisternal spaces.

Computed tomography (CT) consists of directing X-rays at an object from multiple orientations and measuring the decrease in intensity along a series of linear paths. This decrease is characterized by **Beer's Law**, which describes intensity reduction as a function of X-ray energy, path length, and material linear attenuation coefficient. A specialized algorithm is then used to reconstruct the distribution of X-ray attenuation in the volume being imaged.

Generation of CT	CT machine
First generation CT (Outdated)	EMI scanner
Second generation CT (Going out of use)	Conventional CT
Third generation CT (Most common type in India at present, but rapidly being superceded by MDCT)	Spiral helical CT (It can be single or multislice CT)
Fourth generation CT (No beam-hardening artefacts)	MDCT (Multidetector CT)
Electron beam CT/Ultrafast CT/Real-time CT/mSec CT	EBCT

SPECIAL APPLICATION OF MULTISLICE CT

- CTA
- Triple phase CT of liver and pancreas
- Cardiac CT
- Coronary calcium scoring ("Noninvasive coronary angiography")
- CT perfusion
- CT enteroclysis
- Virtual colonography
- CT urography.

HU value scale					
Hypodense			Isodense	Hyperdense	
−1000	−50–100	0–10	20–40	50–60	1000
Air	Fat	Water	Soft tissue	Blood	Bone

Unenhanced/Noncontrast (NCCT)/Precontrast/Plain CT scan is investigation of choice for
- Acute SAH (As the age of blood advances, its density decreases as it gets degraded into its degradation products, i.e. oxyhemoglobin → deoxyhemoglobin → methemoglobin → hemosiderin, hence for chronic bleeds CT is not good).
- Head injury
- Intracranial calcification
- Fractures of pelvis/vertebral fractures/fractures of facial bones
- Minimal pneumoperitoneum
- Ureteric calculi (most sensitive investigation for acute renal colic)
- Detecting calcification (e.g. as in retinoblastomas, ovarian dermoids, hydatid cysts, corpus callosal lipomas, neuroblastoma, etc.)
- CT PNS for sinonasal polyps and recurrent chronic sinusitis and pre-FESS noncontrast CT for "Road-map".

Contrast-enhanced/ CECT is investigation of choice for
- Calcified tumors:
    - Oligodendroglioma
    - Craniopharyngioma
    - Central neurocytoma
    - Retinoblastoma.
- Lung carcinoma (Except pancoast tumor)
- Mediastinal tumors (Except posterior mediastinal tumors, which are neurogenic)
- Pancreatic lesions (Except neuroendocrine tumors of pancreas)
- Staging of renal cell carcinoma (Except for RCC with renal/IVC thrombosis)
- Abdominal adenopathy
- Small bowel tumors
- Blunt trauma abdomen
- Advanced Ca prostate (staging)
- Penetrating (stab injury) abdominal trauma with stable patient
- Sensitive and specific screening tool for renal artery stenosis
- Juvenile angiofibroma
- Ca maxilla
- Focal hepatic lesions–triple phase CECT (except for FNH)
- Small bowel tumors (CT better than enterolysis)
- Diverticulitis and abscess

- Complicated appendicitis
- Screening tool of choice for acute mesenteric ischemia.

High Resolution Computed Tomography

Basic Principles

Three factors which significantly improve the spatial resolution of CT such that it can be described as high resolution computed tomography (HRCT) and be used for studying the greater details of lung parenchyma/petrous temporal bone are:
1. High spatial reconstruction or edge enhancing or sharp or "bone algorithm" (for image reconstruction, as it reduces image smoothing and makes structure visibly sharper).
2. Narrow beam collimation (reduces volume averaging within the section and so increases spatial resolution causing marked effect on appearance of lungs, notably the vessels and bronchi).
3. Small field of view.

This makes HRCT an ideal modality for correct identification of subtle diffuse abnormalities of lung parenchyma even in very early stage and thus evaluating interstitial lung disease in the best manner. It is also helpful in imaging of temporal bone.

* Slice thickness of 1 mm is ideal for HRCT.

Clinical Applications

- Lung diseases:
  - Bronchiectasis
  - Interstitial and diffuse lung diseases
  - Emphysema.
- Temporal bone imaging:
  - Ossicular chain disruption
  - Cholesteatoma
  - Mastoiditis and petrositis
  - Fracture of facial canal.
- HRCT is of proven value in the diagnosis of diffuse lung disease (like interstitial lung diseases), particularly in the early stages when the chest radiograph is normal and for follow-up.
- HRCT clearly depicts distribution and higher definition of appearances of pulmonary parenchymal disease.

- Nowadays HRCT is used for detection of bronchiectasis, and surgery is undertaken without preoperative bronchography. Severity and extent of bronchiectasis is demonstrated.
- HRCT can identify regions most suitable for biopsy at a time when the chest radiograph is normal.
- Mediastinal or chest wall involvement by lung pathway may also be demonstrated.

Safety Aspect of Computed Tomography

Examination	Effective total dose (mSv)
Chest X-ray	0.06
Skull X-ray	0.2
Pelvis X-ray	0.65
Lumbar spine X-ray	1.3
Upper GI series	2.45
Abdomen X-ray	0.55
Barium enema	4–9
IVP/IVU	1.6
Extremities	0.01
Enteroclysis	1.5
CT chest	8
CT abdomen	10
CT head	3.5
Bone scan	4.2
MCU	1

Mechanism for dose reduction at CT

- X-ray beam filtration
- X-ray beam collimation
- X-ray tube current modulation and adaptation for patient body habitus (automatic exposure control)
- Peak kilovoltage optimization
- Improved detection system efficiency
- Noise reduction algorithms

Advantages

- Less time of acquisition
- High spatial and temporal resolution
- Best to detect calcification
- Best to detect cortical bony lesions and fine osseous details
- Extremely sensitive to detect free air in abdomen/pleural space/cranial.

Disadvantages

- Modality that gives highest radiation dose (Ionizing radiation hazard)
- No multiplanar capability, only axial images possible (except for MDCT)
- Contrast related toxicity
- Due to *'beam hardening'* artifact not good for posterior fossa tumors
- Poor soft tissue resolution compared to MRI.

MAGNETIC RESONANCE IMAGING

(**Synonym:** NMR–nuclear magnetic resonance)

- It is a noninvasive method of mapping the internal structure of body by producing images by the virtue of gyromagnetic property of protons, with the greatest advantage of **not using ionizing radiation** for imaging.
- It employs radiofrequency (rf) or radiowaves waves/radiation in the presence of carefully controlled magnetic fields in order to produce high quality cross sectional images of body in any plane.
- It portrays the distribution of hydrogen nuclei and parameters relating to their motion in water and lipids.
- Prucell, *pioneer of MRI*, took the advantage of the fact that 60 percent our body is made up of water, i.e. protons. Nuclei of certain atoms (protons or neutrons) when placed in a magnetic field, absorb and emit energy of a specific frequency.
- Almost all images produced to date have been by the virtue of **gyromagnetic property of protons and the nuclear magnetism of hydrogen nucleus (or proton)**, which is a particularly favorable nucleus from magnetic resonance imaging (MRI) standpoint, and is present in virtually all biological material. Because nuclei are spinning, they respond to magnetic couple like gyroscope to their axes, are tilted so that they come to rotate at exactly same frequency about the magnetic field; direction of movement is **known as 'precession'**.

Larmor equation is $f = \gamma B$:

Where f = resonant frequency
 γ = gyromagnetic ratio
 B = applied field.

Magnetic **field strengths used for clinical imaging** currently range from **0.2 Tesla (T) to 8 T**.

- **Michael Faraday** (1791-1867) created a complete cage of metal or metallic meshwork. If a region in space is completely surrounded by a Faraday Cage (MRI rooms), ambient electromagnetic waves are effectively screened from enclosed region. Copper or Aluminum foils can transform any room into Faraday Cage. A continuous sheet or wire-mesh of copper or aluminum is used to shield the MRI rooms so as to protect the imager from external electromagnetic radiations, which is known as **Faraday Cage**. All NMR examinations including MRI imaging and MRI spectroscopy have to be performed in a Faraday Cage to prevent radiofrequency waves from ambient sources from interfering with reception of radio waves emitted from the sample (patient) during examination.
- The induction coils (transmitter/receiver coils) used in MRI are **Maxwell coils**.

Principle of MR Imaging

Pulse of oscillating radiofrequency (rf pulse) field is applied on a **group of protons** (a body part) placed in a strong **magnetic field** ⇒ this produces a resonant effect on protons, called magnetic resonance (providing that the frequency of oscillation of protons is equal to their precession frequency) ⇒ this resonant effect on protons causes change in magnetization due to absorption of rf energy from **transmitter coil** causing motion of elementary magnets to be disturbed so that direction of total nuclear magnetization is altered ⇒ and as the altered net magnetization returns to equilibrium in exponential manner it induces a small voltage in **receiver coil** which is placed next to the patient → this small **electrical voltage signal induced** in receiver coil following an rf pulse is known as free induction decay or FID, the magnitude and length of which is determined by nuclear relaxation times which reflect molecular motion ⇒ and then the FID, i.e. electrical signal produced in receiver coil is **digitized and analyzed** in a **computer** using a complex mathematical technique called Fourier analysis, to produce **amazing images**.

When Protons flip towards RF pulse it results in:
- T1 Spin lattice relaxation
- T2 Spin spin relaxation.

The first of these relaxation times, T1 or the longitudinal relaxation time, represents the time taken by the system of nuclei to return to thermal equilibrium after the rf pulse (For T1, TE and TR are short).

The second T2 or transverse relaxation time represents the characteristic decay time of FID and is due to irresponsible dephasing of initially coherent precession of nuclei, which follows the rf pulse (For T2, TE and TR are long).

Unlike CT images in which contrast is determined by differences in one parameter (the linear X-ray attenuation coefficient mu), **multiple parameters influence MRI Signal including nuclear or proton density, T1 and T2**.

In human tissue T1 is usually 10 times longer than T2.

A local change in magnetic field homogeneity, e.g. due to local iron or deoxyhemoglobin content, causes a reduction in T2 which is called T2*.

The induction coil in MRI unit is made up of **niobium-titanium**.

The principle pulse sequences are:
- Partial saturation (PS) or gradient or field echo
- Spin echo
- Inversion recovery.

Technical advances in the form of high field strength MRI machines [(3T) and ultrafast MRI pulse sequences (Echo planar imaging)] have included improvements in spatial resolution, contrast and speed imaging and major advances have related to development of MRI for following special uses:
- **Diffusion weighted MRI (DWRI):** Excellent for acute and hyperacute.
- **MR Volumetry:** Excellent for mesial temporal sclerosis (Temporal lobe epilepsy)
- **Functional MRI (Bold-blood oxygen level dependent MRI):** For cognitive function of brain and physiological studies
- **MR tractography** (Diffusion tensor imaging): For WM tracts
- **MRCP:** Excellent screening tool for biliary anomalies, sclerosing cholangitis, etc.
- **MR angiography:** Excellent for imaging almost all vessels
- **Flair sequence:** Excellent for chronic SAH.

The summary of How MRI works
- Random movement in the hydrogen atoms in the absence of magnetic field
- Alignment of hydrogen atoms in the presence of a strong magnetic field
- Realignment of the hydrogen atoms in the presence of radiofrequency wave/pulse
- When the radiofrequency is switched off, the atoms return to their original position and release energy in the form of electrical voltage signal

- This electrical signal (produced in receiver coil) is digitized and analyzed in a computer, to produce MR images.

- Water (CSF) looks white (Hyperintense) on T2 (***Hint to remember** → World War-2)
- Thus, CSF looks hyperintense on T2 weighted image and hypointense on T1 weighted image.

Substance	T1 weighted	T2 weighted
Water/Vitreous/CSF	black	Light gray or white
Fat	White	Light gray
Muscle	Gray	Gray
Air	Black	Black
Fatty bone marrow	White light	Gray
Brain: White matter	Light gray	Gray
Brain: Gray matter	Gray	Very light gray

Advantages

- No use of ionizing radiations (radiowaves are used in MRI).
- Greater inherent soft tissue contrast (e.g. tumors of brain including cerebral metastases are usually better demonstrated on MRI than on CT due to greater inherent soft tissue contrast).
- Provide direct multiplanar imaging, which helps to define the relationship of the tumor to adjacent structures, and thus helps in planning of surgery (e.g. facilitates the distinction between intra-axial and extra-axial tumors).
- MRI is vastly superior to CT in evaluating posterior fossa tumors as CT is frequently hampered by **'beam-hardening' artifact** from the base of skull.
- Vascular imaging possible without use of intravenous contrast.

Disadvantages

- Longer time of acquisition
- Claustrophobia
- Metal is absolutely contraindicated
- Costly
- Not the best for detecting calcification or air.

Applications of MRI are many, but amongst the commonly imaged parts are brain, spine and musculoskeletal tissues.

> **Dictum:** Whenever it comes to nervous tissue imaging (e.g. brain, spinal cord, nerves, sympathetic and parasympathetic chains), MRI is best.

MRI is investigation of choice for
- Empty sella syndrome
- Hyperacute and acute infarct (DWMRI)
- Chronic SAH (MRI with FLAIR sequence)
- To detect cerebral metastases (CEMRI and DWMRI)
- Demyelinating and dysmyelinating diseases of brain (e.g. Multiple sclerosis, SSPE, motor neuron disease, central pontine myelinolysis, etc.)
- Congenital brain anomalies (e.g. Arnold Chiari malformation, etc.)
- To differentiate between arachnoid cyst and epidermoid cyst (DWMRI)
- All brain tumors, especially the posterior fossa tumors
- All spinal cord pathologies (e.g. Prolapsed intervertebral disc, metastases, spinal cord tumors, traumatic paraplegia, transverse myelitis, etc.)
- Imaging of breast with silicon implants
- Juvenile angiofibroma (Invasive one)
- Ca nasopharynx (CT better for delineating skull base/bony erosion)
- All bone tumors (except osteoid osteoma, for which CT is better)
- Avascular necrosis
- Bone marrow edema
- Cartilage, meniscal, or ligament injuries
- Rotator cuff injury
- Preoperative evaluation of carcinoma endometrium and cervix (CEMRI)
- Early detection of Ca prostate
- Assessment of depth of penetration and perirectal nodes in rectal cancer
- Dissection of aorta/ aortic aneurysm
- RCC with tumor thrombus in renal vein or IVC (CEMRI)
- Vascular rings and anomalies.

Contraindications to MRI

- Cochlear implants
- Intraocular metallic foreign body
- Aneurysmal clips
- Cardiac pacemakers (absolute contraindication)
- Prosthetic heart valves
- Bone implants
- Claustrophobia (Phobia of closed spaces).

Dictum: *Metal is enemy of MRI, however, TITANIUM is a metal compatible with MRI.*

RADIONUCLIDE IMAGING

This encompasses γ-scans (isotope scans/scintigraphy), SPECT and FDG-PET scan. Isotope scanning is discussed in section B.

EMISSION COMPUTED TOMOGRAPHY

Conventional planer imaging provides only a 2-dimentional projection of a 3-dimentional presentation of activity. Emission computed tomography (ECT) provides an *in vivo* 3-dimensional distribution of radiopharmaceutical within the body. It also provides improved image contrast and quantification.

It includes
- Single photon emission computed tomography (SPECT)
- Positron emission tomography (PET).

Single Photon Emission Computed Tomography

It involves detection of gamma (γ) rays emitted singly from radionuclide like ^{99m}Tc and thallium 201. It is 3-dimensional examination. Most of its use is in brain and heart. Perfusion studies and functional imaging of brain is possible with it.

Positron Emission Tomography/18-FDG-PET Scan

Positron is a positively charged electron.

Basic principle: Coincidence detection of paired high energy (511 keV) annihilation gamma photons from **positron emitting radionuclides** like carbon-11, nitrogen-13, oxygen-15 and fluorine-18.

Agent used: Fluorine-18 (F-18) is most commonly preferred. To make the agent to go specifically to the site of interest, F-18 is coupled with deoxyglucose which gets more concentrated in malignant cells as they have much more metabolic demand compared to normal cells.

Mechanism: PET compounds are radiolabeled with positron emitting radionuclides and injected into patient. The compound concentrates at the target and after some time positron is emitted. Positron after being emitted by the given agent combines with an electron in the tissue resulting in formation of high energy **annihilation photons**, which are emitted in diagonally/exactly opposite directions; in turn detected by coincidence circuit through simultaneously arriving detectors on opposite sides of patient. An electronic collimation occurs through coincidence circuit (thus, **no need of lead collimators**) hence has better resolution and sensitivity than SPECT. Thus, technically the patient is injected with the 18F-FDG iv and after about 45 minutes imaged with PET camera.

Imaging time → 1-10 minutes.

Positron emission tomography (PET) camera: Routine gamma camera is not used for PET imaging. PET detectors are made up of special material, called **BGO (Bismuth germinate) crystals**, which sensitively and specifically detects the high energy (511 keV) gamma photons produced after electron and emitted positron combine with each other.

Advantages

- The kind of radiopharmaceutical that can be used most physiological molecules in body are made of carbon, nitrogen and oxygen, enabling them to be labeled with "11C, 13N and 15O and 18F" which are position emitters.
- It is a *'unique tool'* to study and quantify physiological and pathological function of human tissues and organs.
- Imaging modality that permits noninvasive *in vivo* examination of metabolism (biochemical imaging), blood flow, electrical activity and neurochemistry.
- Only radiological modality with which *metabolic imaging* is possible.
- Most accurate noninvasive method of detecting and evaluating most cancers.

PET Scan (Summary)
- PET is a functional scan.
- Routinely, *18-FDG is agent of choice for* PET scanning (^{18}**FDG-PET scan**).
- F^{18} has half-life of 112 minutes.
- Rubidium^{82} is especially preferred for myocardial PET.
- Scanning time for PET scan is 45 minutes.
- **Cyclotron** machine is required for F^{18} production.
- The detectors in PET camera are usually made-up of Bismuth germinate–BGO crystals (unlike that of gamma camera, in which detectors are made up of sodium iodide – NaI).
- PET CT fusion scan has revolutionized oncoimaging, especially for follow-up of cancers.

Clinical Applications

- **Oncology** (Glucose and oxygen utilization of tumors measured)
  - Breast cancer
  - Colon cancer recurrence
  - Lung cancer and pancreatic cancer
  - To differentiate benign from malignant solitary pulmonary nodule (SPN)
  - Differentiation of incidentalomas from metastasis in adrenals
  - Best to detect lymph node metastasis anywhere in the body (especially from head and neck cancer)
  - Best to detect metastases anywhere is body except cerebral metastases, for which MRI is best.
- **Cardiology:** Quantification of myocardial blood flow and best to differentiate between a salvageable and nonsalvageable myocardium.
- **Neurology:** (Metabolic and functional assessment, cerebral blood flow quantification).
  - Stroke
  - Encephalopathies
  - Brain tumor
    i. Residual/recurrent tumor versus neurosis
    ii. Response to chemoradiation
    iii. Prediction of patient's average survival in it
    iv. Lymphoma staging

Pearls
- Cardiac PET perfusion imaging is performed with 13N-ammonia or 82Rb (Rubidium-82) and metabolic or viability imaging is performed with 18F-FDG.
- Abnormal 18F-FDG activity may represent malignancy but is not pathognomonic and may represent inflammation, infection, or granulomatous disease.
- Diffuse FDG activity may be seen in the thyroid, but focal activity should raise the suspicion of thyroid cancer.
- Cancers that avidly accumulate FDG are larynx, esophagus, non-small-cell lung, colorectal cancer, melanoma and lymphoma.
- Conversely, some malignancies do not accumulate 18F-FDG well, such as prostate, carcinoid, and mucinous cancers.
- The limit of spatial resolution for PET scans is about 5 to 8 mm.
- In a SPN (Solitary Pulmonary Nodule), Standard Uptake Value (SUV) > 2.5 favors malignancy.

BONE DENSITOMETRY

- It is currently the most accurate bone density measurement technique or a method for predicting patients at risk of osteoporotic fracture (Gold Standard).
- **Bone density measurement techniques are:**
    - **Radiogrammetry:** Cortical thickness measured from a PA hand radiograph and subjected to a variety of mathematical formulae for estimating skeletal status and cortical bone volume. Its drawback is that it doesn't provide an absolute measurement of bone density.
    - **Photodensitometry:** In single absorptiometry (SPA), a single energy source of 125-I used to produce a highly collimated beam of low energy photons and the absorbed radiation is detected by Na T scintillation counters. An area measurement of bone mineral density as well as bone mineral content can be obtained by SPA.
    - **Quantitative computed tomography (QCT):** A measurement of pure trabecular bone mineral density (BMD) in lumbar spine is obtained using a conventional computed tomography (CT) scan. Its advantages over other BMD measuring techniques include: a pure measurement of trabecular bone (sensitive) and measurement of bone that does not include any extraneous calcification that may artefactually increase BMD. A disadvantage is higher radiation dose than DXA.
    - **Dual photon absorptiometry (DPA):** With DPA it became possible to measure BMD and body composition regionally as well as in the whole body. A radionuclide source (153 Gd) is used to produce two discrete energies by using which the different attenuation values of bone and soft

tissue could be calculated. It was a simple, accurate precise technique and required only a low dose of radiation. But it had a number of drawbacks, like problem with longitudinal measurements, long scanning time and poor image quality.

- **Dual energy X-ray absorptiometry (DXA)**
- DXA has superseded DPA and is now the most commonly used technique for measuring BMD throughout the world.
- It provides a very useful noninvasive clinical tool to evaluate and monitor bone mineral density and body composition in both adults and children.
- The result is accurate and precise, with added advantage of very low radiation dose to the patients.
- The first generation DXA scanners used a pencil beam of X-rays coupled to a single detector and although a low radiation dose is produced it has an increased scan time as compared to latest generation of DXA scanners.
- The development of **Fan beam DXA scanners (2nd generation DXA)** has provided faster scan times and improved image resolution and quality and ability to measure vertebral deformity.
- With dedicated software, measurements of forearm, small animals, periprosthetic bone and vertebral height can be obtained or spinal morphometric X-ray absorptiometry (**MXA**) for vertebral deformities can be performed.
- The principle of DXA is very similar to DPA, but it uses a beam or X-ray emitted from an X-ray tube rather than an isotope source to provide dual energies.
- With energy switching system there is simultaneous calibration of emergent X-ray beam by a rotating wheel containing internal reference standards for bone, soft tissue and air.
- The K-edge filter systems require photon counting discriminating detectors but, with energy switching technique, current integratory detectors are used. In K-edge filters (cerium or samarium) the output of contrast potential X-ray tube is filtered to produce energies of 40 and 70 keV, while in rapid switching technique, switching between 70 and 140 kVp is done to produce energies of 45 and 100 keV.

EXTRACORPOREAL SHOCK WAVE LITHOTRIPSY

- The development of extracorporeal shock wave lithotripsy (ESWL) by Eisenberger and Chaussy in Munich in 1980 revolutionized the treatment of upper tract renal calculi.
- The first generation lithotripter was an electrohydraulic machine in which a shock wave induced by the underwater discharge of 20 kV across a spark gap.
- Second generation ultrasonic/electromagnetic lithotripter machines have proved to be the simplest and most successful.

- **Complications:**
  - Some degree of ureteric obstruction, as multiple stone fragments build up in distal ureter.
  - Failure of treatment
  - Rapid recurrence of calculus, may be due to residual fragments acting as nidus
  - Renal contusion, perinephric hemorrhage, fracture transverse process (due to misdirected shock waves) are rare
  - Increased incidence of long-term hypertension.

Endoscopic Retrograde Cholangiopancreaticography

It has become primary method of direct cholangiography and has developed considerable therapeutic potential also.

A side viewing endoscope is required and the pancreatic tree should be visualized before the biliary tree. The number of side branches of the pancreatic duct opacifying at ERCP decreases with age.

Advantages

PTC include less patient discomfort and fever complications, and a success rate, which is independent of the biliary tract. It also offers ability to examine the upper gastrointestinal tract, the papilla of vater, and the pancreatic duct.

Disadvantage

The procedure is more prone to technical failure than percutaneous transhepatic cholangiography. PEP (Post ERCP Pancreatitis) is one of the most common complications.

Pancreatic pseudocysts and esophageal varices are *contraindications* for ERCP.

Recent Advances

- Digital mammography, sonomammography, mammography scintigraphy.
- Tissue harmonic imaging (USG of focal lesions in liver)
- IVUS (Intravascular ultrasonography) – needs > 20 MHz probe
- EBCT (Electron Beam CT/Generation V CT/ultrafast CT/mSec CT)
- Virtual endoscopy (Multislice CT with navigator software fecal tagging and colonic distension with in air makes it possible)
- MR and CT enteroclysis for small bowel imaging

Chapter 1 ❖ General Radiology and Radiology Physics

- Fetal MRI (especial for complex cranial anomalies)
- Intraoperative MRI
- PET–CT fusion (Revolution in oncoimaging especially due to function and anatomical fusion scanning.

Key indications for various radiological investigations

Radiological tool	Prime indications
IVP/IVU	– Renal tuberculosis
	– Renal anomalies
Esophagography	– TO fistula (Water-soluble contrast study)
	– Motility disorders (initial evaluation)
	– Dysphagia
HSG	– Infertility^Q
(Postmenstrual-	– Congenital uterine anomalies
preovulatory period)	– Tubal block
Urethrography	– PU valves (RGU)
	– VUR (RGU)
	– Trauma
	– Stricture
Ultrasound	– Hydrocephalus in infants^Q
	– Thyroid nodule
	– Initial evaluation of rotator cuff injury/subacromial bursitis/bicipital tendinitis^Q
	– Synovial cysts
	– Pleural/Pericardial effusion^Q
	– First investigation done for acute abdomen and obstructive jaundice^Q
	– Congenital hypertrophic pyloric stenosis and intussusception
	– Gallstones^Q
	– Adenomyomatosis of Gallbladder ("Comet tail" sign)
	– Initial evaluation of focal liver lesions
	– Initial evaluation of blunt trauma abdomen (FAST protocol)^Q
	– Minimal ascites^Q
	– Cystic hygroma
	– Prostatic pathologies (TRUS)
	– Seminal vesicle pathologies (TRUS)
	– Staging of early rectal/pancreatic head malignancies (EUS)
	– Neuroectodermal pancreatic tumors—insulinoma and gastrinoma (EUS)
	– Scrotal pathologies
	– Developmental dysplasia of Hip^Q

CT Scan

HRCT (Bone algorithm)
Lungs:
- ILD
- Bronchiectasis
- Emphysema

Temporal bone:
- Petrositis
- Mastoiditis
- Ossicular chain disruption
- Cogenital anomalies [e.g. Mondani's malformation]
- EAC osteoma
- Cholesteatoma
- Fracture facial canal

Noncontrast CT (NCCT)
- *Initial test of choice for acute stroke*
- *Fractures:*
    - Skull (Head injury)
    - Facial bones
    - Vertebral
    - Pelvis
    - Talus
    - Scaphoid
- *Acute hemorrhage*
    - Intratumoral
    - Intracerebral
    - Intraventricular
    - EDH/SDH
    - Acute SAH
- *Minimum air:*
    - Pneumoperitoneum
    - Pneumocephalus
    - Pneumomediastinum
- Calcification anywhere in body
- Ureteric calculi

CTA (CT angiography)
- Screening of intracranial internal carotid (ICA) lesions
- Screening of circle of Willi's lesions
- Chronic abdominal angina
- Pulmonary embolism

- Noninvasive coronary angiography
- Coronary anomalies
- Pulmonary sequestration
- Rapid screening tool for aortic lesions
- Sensitive and specific screening tool for renal artery stenosis

CT brain
- Oligodendroglioma
- Screening for cortical venous thrombosis (Empty delta sign in lateral sinus thrombosis)
- Evaluation of an acute change in mental status
- Evaluation of an focal neurologic findings
- Conductive hearing loss
- Craniopharyngioma
- Craniosynostosis
- Krabbe's disease (Globoid cell dystrophy)

CECT neck
- Staging of Ca larynx
- Staging of Ca thyroid
- Cold abscess
- Nodal characterization

CT PNS
- Chronic recurrent sinusitis (NCCT)
- Noninvasive fungal sinusitis (NCCT)
- Sinonasal polyps (NCCT)
- Pre-FESS CT (NCCT)
- Neoplasms of maxilla (CECT)
- Juvenile angiofibroma (CECT)
- Screening for Glomus jugulare (Phlep sign)
- CSF rhinorrhea (CT cisternography)

CT orbit
- Metallic foreign body (NCCT)
- Optic drusen
- Retinoblastoma (CECT)

CECT chest
- Screening detection and staging of lung cancer
- Lung hamartoma
- Pleural lesions
- Diaphragmatic hernia

- Anterior and middle mediastinal lesions
- Congenital labor emphysema
- Congenital adenomatoid lung malformation
- Morgagni's hernia
- Mediastinal lymph node characterization
- Tubercular pericarditis
- Calcified cardiac tumors

CECT abdomen
- Blunt trauma abdomen (FAST USG for screening only)
- Abdominal lump
- Abdominal wall hematoma
- Advanced rectal/esophagus/stomach/bladder cancer
- Detection and staging of Ca gallbladder and small bowel tumors
- Focal hepatic lesions
- Adrenal imaging (Nonfunctional lesions)
- Renal carcinoma detection and staging
- Oncocytoma (Central stellate scar)
- Renal and perirenal infections
- Complicated ADPKD
- Mesenteric cyst
- Enteric duplication cyst
- Abdominal lymph node and peritoneal TB
- Diverticulitis and diverticular abcess
- Subdiaphragmatic abscess
- Bowel obstruction evaluation
- Complicated appendicitis
- Appendicitis epiploicae

CECT pelvis
- Adnexal mass
- Ovarian dermoid
- Ca urinary bladder
- Advanced prostatic cancer staging
- Sacrococcygeal teratoma

MRI

MRI advantages
- Superior soft tissue contrast resolution—excellent pathological discrimination
- No ionizing radiation
- Direct multiplanar imaging (transverse, coronal, sagittal, any oblique)
- Noninvasive—vascular studies can be performed without contrast

MRI disadvantages
- Expensive
- Long scan times
- Audible noise (65–115 dB)
- Isolation of patient (cloustrophobia monitoring of ill patients)
- Exclusion of patients with pacemakers and certain implants

Cranial MRI
- Chronic hemorrhage (GRE < FLAIR)
- Sensitive most for acute and hyperacute ischemic stroke (DWMRI)
- Demyelinating disorders (e.g. MS, ALS, SSPE, SACD, SMON, CPM, ADEM, PML, PVL, PRES, etc.)
- Infectious processes (encephalitis, meningitis)
- Abscesses
- Brain neoplasms (supra as well as infratentorial)
- Neurofibromatosis
- DAI
- Vascular disorders (AVM's, aneurysms, vasculitis, Moya-moya disease)
- Metastasis
- Internal auditory canal pathology
- Pituitary pathology
- Hydrocephalus especially in adults
- Cranial nerve pathology (e.g. vestibular Schwannoma)
- Congenital anomalies (for anatomical review)
- Epilepsy (seizures in general)
- Parameningeal tumors
- Low CSF volume headache

Spine MRI
- Cauda equina syndrome
- Tethered cord
- Arachnoiditis
- Marrow-replacing processes
- Degeneration disk disease
- Discitis
- Congenital anomalies
- Radiculopathy
- Spinal cord tumors
- Trauma/contusion
- Syringomyelia
- Metastasis
- Vascular disorders

- Cord edema
- MS plaques
- Traumatic paraplegia
- Retroperitoneal tumor with spine extension
- Pott's spine
- Myelomalacia

Musculoskeletal MRI
- Meniscal pathology
- Ligament/tendon injury
- PVNS
- Muscle/nerve impingement
- Rotator cuff tear
- Avascular necrosis
- Labral tears (shoulder, hip)
- Chondromalacia
- Inflammation (acute osteomyelitis)
- Primary bone tumors
- Spinal metastases
- Soft tissue tumors
- Perthe's disease
- Cartilage injury

Breast MRI
- Screening in young females (as glandular tissue is more than fat in young breasts)[Q]
- Breast with silicone implants (Augmented breast)
- Sensitive most investigation to detect DCIS

Chest MRI
- Imaging of Pancoast's tumor (superior sulcus tumor)[Q]
- Imaging of posterior mediastinal masses
- Demonstration of vascular sling[Q]
- Investigation of choice in aortic dissection[Q]
- Best diagnosis for dissecting aorta (aortic dissection)[Q]

Cardiac MRI
- Vascular rings (e.g. Double aortic arch; Aberrant right subclavian; Pulmonary sling)
- Post-up complex cyanotic congenital heart diseases[Q]
- ARVD
- Coarctation of aorta
- Cardiomyopathies (*in general*)

- Malignant cardiac tumors
- Pericardial malignancies

Abdominal MRI
- Investigation of choice for a pregnant lady with upper abdominal mass[Q]
- The most sensitive and specific investigation for renal artery stenosis
- Preoperative staging of endometrial and cervical cancer[Q]
- Anorectal sepsis, anorectal malformation and anorectal tumors
- RCC with suspected RV or IVC invasion
- Fetal cranial abnormalities
- Liver pathologies

MRA (Gd-enhanced MRA > PC or ToF MRA)

- Best for circle of Willis lesions
- AVMS
- Aneurysms
- Aortic lesions
  - Aneurysms
  - Dissection
  - Takayasu's
- Vascular rings
- Carotid lesions
- Carotid body tumors
- Paragangliomas (South Peeper appearance)

- Renal artery stenosis
- Acute mesenteric ischemia (Laparotomy test)
- Cortical venous thrombosis (MR venography)
- Vertebral artery dissection/thrombosis
- Corticocavernous fistula (Pulsatile exophthalmos)
- Coronary artery aneurysms

Note: 'Q' as a superscript indicates 'vital indications'

Chapter 2

Radiological Contrast Agents/Media

CONTRAST MEDIA FOR BARIUM PROCEDURES

Barium Sulfate

Barium sulfate is unique among the contrast media by the virtue of being a suspension rather than a solution.

Its inert nature and insolubility in water have made it for 50 years contrast media of choice for gastrointestinal tract.

The contents of barium powder include
- Suspending agent
- Flavoring agent
- Dispersible agent
- Wetting agent
- Defoaming agent
- Humectants
- Acidifiers
- Preservative.

Ba Study	Done for	Barium preparation used	Indications
Ba swallow	Esophagus	• 80 percent W/v–Single contrast • 200–250 percent W/v–Double constrast (High density low viscosity)	• Initial study for dysphagia • Screening study for motility disorder • Hiatus hernia
Ba meal	Stomach and duodenum	• Low density (80–100% W/v)–Single contrast • High density low viscosity (250% W/v)–Double contrast	• Second line study for CHPS • Second line study for ulcers • Linitus plastic and chronic gastric volvulus • Annular pancreas • SMA syndrome
BMFT	Small bowel	50–60 percent W/v medium density Ba containing suspending agent	• Malabsorption • Intestinal TB • Strictures • Worm infestation
Enteroclysis (small bowel enema)	Better than BMFT for small bowel	• Single contrast: 20 percent W/v $BaSO_4$ Susp. • Double contrast: 200–250 percent W/v ē methyl cellulose	Best study for non-neoplastic lesions of small bowel
Ba enema	Large bowel	• Single contrast: 15–20 • Double contrast: 55–75 percent W/v	• Initial study of choice for Hirschsprung • Best for diagnosing diverticulosis, sigmoid volvulus and polyps • Second line for intussusception

Water Soluble Radiological Media

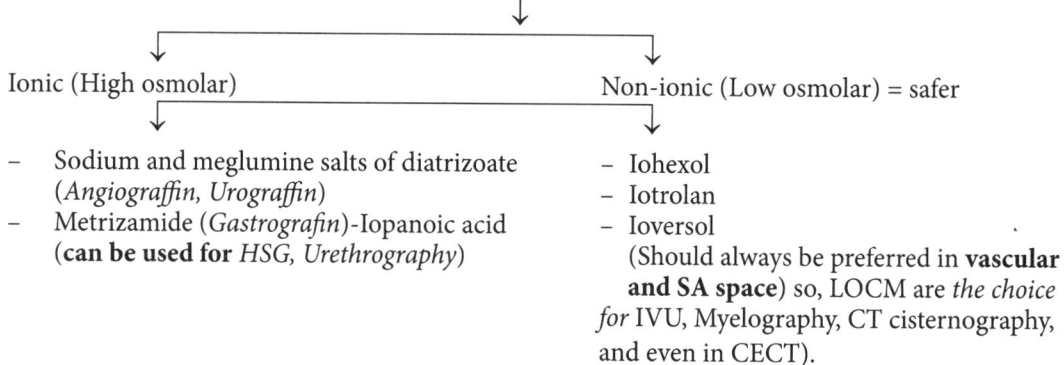

- Ionic (High osmolar)
  - Sodium and meglumine salts of diatrizoate (*Angiograffin, Urograffin*)
  - Metrizamide (*Gastrografin*)-Iopanoic acid (**can be used for** *HSG, Urethrography*)

- Non-ionic (Low osmolar) = safer
  - Iohexol
  - Iotrolan
  - Ioversol
  (Should always be preferred in **vascular and SA space**) so, LOCM are *the choice for* IVU, Myelography, CT cisternography, and even in CECT).

CONTRAST MEDIA FOR NONBARIUM PROCEDURES

Radiological procedure	Contrast (Dye) used
Intravenous urography/pyelography (IVU/IVP)	Outdated contrast media like Conray 420, i.e. sodium iothalamate and metrizoate (outdated).*
	Currently used ionic (Sodium or Meglumine salts of Diatrizoate) or nonionic contrast media (Iohexol, iopamidol, iomeprol, ioversol, iodixanol)
	Nonionic are best preferred
Esophagography (Ba Swallow)	Barium, Gastrografin (outdated), water-soluble iodinated contrast agent in suspected case of TO *fistula*.
Hysterosalpingography	Conray 280, i.e. Meglumine iothalamate (outdated), currently used is Meglumine salt of Diatrizoate (Angiografin 65%)
For intestinal obstruction or perforation	Gastrografin, water-soluble iodinated contrast agent (preferred)
Sialography	Lipiodol (Neohydiol) is outdated. Use water-soluble ionic/nonionic contrast agent used
Urethrography	Conray 280, i.e. Meglumine iothalamate (outdated), currently used is water soluble contrast agent like Meglumine salt of Diatrizoate (Angiografin 65%)
Cisternography	Iohexol (Omnipaque)
Myelography	Myodil (outdated), currently used is iohexol (Omnipaque) – outdated study

Contd...

Contd...

Lymphangiography	Methylene blue, Lipiodol
Splenoportography	75 percent sodium metrizoate–outdated study
Bronchography	Dianosil (Propylidone)–outdated studies
Intravenous cholangiography	Biligrafin (Meglumine ioglycamate)–outdated studies
• DSA/CECT	Water soluble nonionic low osmolar contrast media (LOCM), e. g. iohexol
• MRI	Gadolinium, Gadodamide, Gd-BOPTA, Gd-EOB DTPA, MIONS, SPIO, USPIO
• Ultrasound	Microbubbles (Echovist, Levovist, Albunex, perfluoropropane microbubbles)

*Currently Conray is completely obsolete from use, and now either ionic or nonionic iodine contrast media are used (nonionic preferred over ionic).

Basic Uses of Iodinated Water Soluble Contrast Media

- Angiography (Conventional angiography, DSA, CT angiography)
- Parenchymal staining/enhancement (CECT)
- Renal excretion (IVU)
- Luminal filling (Cystography, VCUG).

Adverse Effects of Iodinated Contrast Media

Issues pertaining to safety of contrast media include:

1. Hemodynamic effects
   - Hemodilution
   - Increased circulating volume
   - Vasodilation
   - Decreased systemic vascular resistance
   - Increased peripheral blood flow
   - Negative inotropic effect.
2. Contrast reactions
   - Nonidiosyncratic (e.g. hyperosmolality, chemotoxicity)
   - Idiosyncratic reactions (e.g. anaphylactoid reactions).

> The initial treatment of an anaphylactic contrast medium reaction in an adult should begin with a 0.2 to 1 mL subcutaneous injection of 1:1000 epinephrine.
> The risk for all adverse reactions was 3 percent for LOCM and 12 percent for HOCM.

3. Clotting tendency
4. Organ toxicity (e.g. Contrast induced nephropathy-CIN).

Strategies for Preventing Contrast Induced Nephropathy

Currently recommended strategies	• Employ noniodinated contrast studies • If iodinated, use low-osmolar or iso-osmolar contrast media • Provide adequate time between contrast procedures • Minimize contrast volume • Parenteral hydration • Avoid nonsteroidal anti-inflammatory drugs
Strategies that may work	• Iso-osmolar contrast media • N-acetylcysteine • Hemofiltration • Sodium bicarbonate • Calcium channel blockers • Theophylline • Ascorbic acid • Prostaglandins
Strategies that do not work	• Mannitol • Furosemide • Dopamine • Atrial natriuretic factor • Fenoldopam • Hemodialysis

Range of anaphylactoid reactions			
Reaction	Incidence	Clinical features	Management
Minor reaction	5–15 percent	Flushing, nausea, vomiting, headache, arm pain, mild urticaria	Self-limiting Occasionally oral anti-histaminic (for urticaria), a tranquilizer or an analgesic
Intermediate Reaction	0.5–2 percent	More severe degrees of above symptoms, hypotension or bronchospasm	Reassurance Chlorpheniramine (for urticaria), diazepam (for anxiety), salbutamol; inhalation for bronchospasm, hydrocortisone (100-500 mg IV/IM), adrenaline (0.3-1 mL of 1/1000 solution IM/Sc)
Severe life-threatening reaction	0.2% (HOCM) 0.04% (LOCM)	Laryngeal edema, Severe bronchospasm, Convulsions, Unconsciousness, Pulmonary edema, Cardiac dysrhythmias/arrest, Cardiovascular and pulmonary collapse	Secure airway, Oxygen/artificial respiration, IV fluid infusion, Adrenaline (gives most rapid and reliable relief from bronchospasm, angioneurotic edema, and other anaphylactoid symptoms, **main therapeutic agent**, should be the essential treatment to be administered as soon as possible), A powerful diuretic like frusemide (for pulmonary edema), Corticosteroids, Chlorpheniramine, Diazepam and barbiturates for convulsions, Vasopressors (nor-adrenaline, dopamine, metaraminol) for hypotension, Sodabicarb to correct acidosis, Atropine (0.6–1.2 mg IV/IM) for vasovagal reactions, bradycardia and cardiac failure

Contrast Agent Used for MRI/MR Contrast Agents

- Gadolinium
- Gd EOB-DTPA
- Gd BOPTA/dimeglumine
- Mn DPDP
- Iron oxide particles
  - MIONS
  - SPIO (superparamagnetic iron oxide)
  - USPIO
- Perflubron
- Intravenous gadolinium—DTPA and other gadolinium chelates are widely used in MRI.
- Another class of agents, magnetic iron oxide nanoparticles (MIONS) have been seen to lodge within reticuloendothelial system and reduce the signal intensity from normal parenchyma in liver and spleen but not from tumors and as a result lesion conspicuity can be greatly increased.
- GD-DTPA on the other hand, after IV injection, circulates within the vascular system but does not cross the normal blood-brain barrier. They cross the abnormal BBB.

MR CONTRAST MEDIA: KEY FACTS

- The heavy-metal element gadolinium forms the basis of all currently approved iv MR contrast agents.
- Gadolinium is a ***paramagnetic substance***, which means that it reduces the T1 and T2 relaxation times of nearly water protons, resulting in a high signal on T1W images and a low signal on T2W images.
- Gadolinium is chelated to DTPA (diethylenetriaminepentaacetic acid) which allows safe renal excretion.
- Approximately, 0.2 mL/kg body weight is administered intravenously.
- Gadolinium-DTPA does not normally cross the intact BBB immediately but will enhance lesions lacking a BBB and areas of the brain that normally are devoid of the BBB (pituitary, choroid plexus).
- However, gadolinium contrast has been noted to slowly cross an intact BBB if given over time and especially in the setting of reduced renal clearance.
- Generally well-tolerated; severe allergic reactions are rare but have been reported.
- The adverse reaction rate in patients with a prior history of atopy or asthma is 3.7 percent, however, the reaction rate increases to 6.3 percent in those patients with a prior history of unspecified allergic reaction to iodinated contrast agents.

- Gadolinium contrast material can be administered safely to children as well as adults, although these agents are generally avoided in those under 6 months of age.
- Renal failure does not occur.
- ***Nephrogenic fibrosing dermopathy*** is a rare but unique side-effect of gadolinium.
- Gd-enhanced MRA is better than 3D-TOF or phase contrast MRA.
- It is advisable to prefer Gd-MRA, especially for complex vascular lesions, indeterminate focal lesions and infective lesions.
- **Common clinical applications of contrast enhancement MRI are:**
  - Diagnosis of small acoustic neuromas
  - Tumor recurrence identification
  - Meningiomas
  - Relationship of tumor to tentorium
  - Differentiating tumors of high and slow grades
  - Distinguishing tumor from edema (greatest advantage)
  - Demonstration of metastatic spread
  - Distinguish between 'active' and 'inactive' lesions such as in multiple sclerosis
  - With MRI there is no need for an intrathecal contrast agent because the contrast between spinal cord and CSF is excellent on MRI and IV Gd-chelates are used to distinguish between intramedullary and extramedullary tumors and separating tumor from edema as in brain.
- Oral GD-DTPA has been used as a labeling agent to identify loops of bowel and so assist with diagnosis of lesions in abdomen.
- Perflubron (PFOB) is approved by FDA for oral use, but due to its high cost is not widely used.

Chapter 3

Radiation Hazards and Protection

VITAL TOPICS
- Radiation protection biologic effect of radiation—somatic and genetic effects, intermediate and late effects.
- Evaluation of radiation hazards and methods of protection.
- Maximum permissible dose.
- Radiation protection rules in India—ICRP recommendation—dose equivalent limits.
- Personnel monitoring—films badge pocket dosimeter—TLD.

INTRODUCTION
- G_2-M interphase is when the cell is most radiosensitive.
- The cell is vulnerable to radiation in the stage of mitosis (M), less so during synthesis (S) and relatively insensitive during resting periods.
- Radiosensitivity of a cell also depends on its histological type and oxygenation of the tissues.
- Tumor is seen somewhat more sensitive to radiation than normal tissues due to difference in ability to repair sublethal DNA.
- In target tissue, radiation damages DNA and **generates free radicals** from cell water that causes damage to cell membranes, proteins and organelles.
- Since, DNA is the most sensitive vital subcellular target of ionizing radiation, rapidly dividing cells are more radiosensitive than quiescent cells (Law of Radiobiology).

Cell Cycle and Radiation

- G_2-M interphase is most radiosensitive *(G_2-M interphase >G_2 >M)*.
- The cell is vulnerable to radiation in the stage of mitosis (M), less so during synthesis (S) and relatively insensitive during resting periods.
- 'S' phase is the most radioresistant phase of cell cycle.
- But, 'S' phase is the most chemosensitive phase of cell cycle.
- Radiosensitivity of a cell also depends on its histological type and oxygenation of the tissues.

Radiobiology

- Four important processes that occur after radiation exposure can be summarized as the "four R's" of radiobiology.
  - The ***first*** is *repair*. Repair is temperature dependent and is thought to represent the enzymatic mechanisms for healing intracellular injury.
  - The ***second*** R is *reoxygenation*, a process whereby oxygen (and other nutrients) are actually better distributed to viable cells following radiation injury and cell killing.
  - The ***third*** R is *repopulation*, the ability of the cell population to continue to divide and to replace dying and dead cells.
  - The ***fourth*** R is *redistribution*, which reflects the variability of a cell's radiosensitivity over the cell cycle.
- Radiosensitivity can vary through the cell cycle by as much as a factor of 3.
- The G1 phase has the most variable length of all the phases of the cell cycle.
- For most cell lines, cells that have a short G_1 period are most sensitive at the G_2/mitosis interface, less sensitive in G_1, and most resistant toward the end of the synthesis (S) period.

Sources of Radiation Exposure

Natural	Man-made
Cosmic rays, radioisotopes	Medical and dental: X-rays
Environmental: (Terrestrial and Atmospheric)	Occupational exposure
Internal: K-40, C-14	Nuclear: Radioactive fallout
Miscellaneous	Television sets
	Radioactive dial
	Watches
	Isotope tagged products
	Luminous markers

- Of the total radiation exposure to the population, about 85 percent occurs naturally.
- It is estimated that man derives about 50 mrad per year from terrestrial radiation. It has been calculated that a commercial jet pilot receives about 300 mrad per year from cosmic radiation. From atmospheric radiation it is about 2 mrad per year.
- All in all, it is estimated that the **total natural radiation** to which the average person is subjected comes to approximately 0.1 rad per year.
- When optimum radiographic techniques are employed, the skin dose to the patient from **a single X-ray film varies roughly from 0.02 to 3.0 rad. (Approximately it is 0.6 rads).**
- The amount radiation received from outer space and background radiation has been estimated to be 0.1 rad per year, which apparently does not, at present, constitute a hazard.

Biologic Effects of Radiation

- Stochastic (*Somatic*: Short-term and long-term)
- Nonstochastic (Genetic)

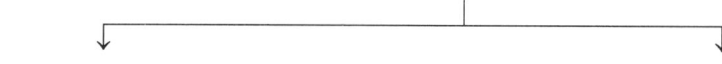

Effects of radiation

Stochastic effects	Nonstochastic effects
Threshold dose not known	Threshold dose known
Dose-independent effects	Dose-dependent effects
Possibility of occurrence rises with rise in dose	Severity increases with rise in dose
Nondeterministic effects,	Deterministic effects,
e.g. Mutations and carcinogenesis	e.g. Cataract, dermatitis, lung fibrosis

Somatic/Acute/Deterministic/Nonstochastic Effects

Deterministic/nonstochastic effects are the effects not subjected to the laws of chance or probability. There is a threshold dose below, which the effect does not occur of. Dose significantly above the threshold will inevitably produce the effect, and its severity increases with radiation dose, e.g. somatic effects and radiation accidents.

Immediate effects (short-term):
- Skin erythema
- Radiation sickness
- Acute radiation syndrome/sickness.

Delayed effects (long-term):
- Radiation dermatitis and radiation recall phenomenon
- Basal and squamous cell carcinoma skin
- Constrictive pericarditis
- Myocardial ischemia and fibrosis
- Radiation pneumonitis
- Peritubular fibrosis in kidney
- Esophagitis, gastroenteritis and colitis
- Intestinal ischemia, ulceration and atrophy
- Cataract
- Retinal damage
- Radiation necrosis of brain
- Transverse myelitis
- Infertility.

Genetic/Chronic/Nondeterministic/Stochastic

Nondeterministic/stochastic are the effects that obey the laws of chance or probability. *The risk of an effect occurring is increased as exposure to radiation increases (linear relationship exists between radiation dose and chance of stochastic effects)*, but the effect is not inevitable. Also the severity of effects is not related to dose received. There is no threshold dose below, which the effect does not occur, **e.g. induction of cancer and genetic effects,** i.e. Chromosomal mutations and leukemias and tumors.

Dermatological Effects
- Skin reaction can be seen with two weeks of fractionated radiotherapy (RT).
- Erythema is the *earliest observed* feature followed by desquamation (dry/moist).
- Chronic reaction can be seen starting at 6 to 12 months after irradiation.
- Atrophic, easily damageable epidermis, hyperpigmentation, thin skin with hair loss also occurs.
- Rarely malignant change in the skin can occur.

Gastrointestinal Tract Effects
Radiation enteritis is one of the most feared complications of abdominal and pelvic radiation. In fact, the toxic potential of this therapeutic modality is often the limiting factor in treating various abdominopelvic malignancies.

Site	Acute	Chronic
Esophagus	Esophagitis	Strictures, fistula
Stomach	Gastritis, ulcers	Submucosal fibrosis, perforation
Liver	Hepatitis	Hepatitis, necrosis
Intestine	Enteritis, ulcerations	Fibrosis, fistula
Rectum	Proctitis	Fibrosis, ischemia, bleeding, fistula

Carcinogenesis

A number of cases of cancer of thyroid have been reported in children who had some years previously received X-ray treatment for disorders like thymus enlargement, infected tonsils, etc. These treatments were given in early infancy and now are practically discontinued. However, radiation exposure during childhood, especially infancy, for some reason or other, has been linked to further risk of development of *thyroid cancer*. Most common secondary malignancy due to exposure to radiation is, however, leukemia, followed by ca thyroid and skin malignancy.

Postradiation Transverse Myelitis

Reaction of spinal cord is similar to brain necrosis.
Progressive and irreversible leg weakness and loss of bladder function and sensation.
Usual time of onset of symptoms is 12 to 24 months, but can occur as early as 6 months after radiation.
No correlation between Lhermitte's sign and transverse myelitis.

Effect on Embryo

The '10-day rule' advice that any X-ray examination involving the abdomen of a woman of child-bearing age should be carried out within 10 days of the onset of menstruation.

The period when the fetus is **most sensitive** to hazardous effect of ionizing radiations is at **8 to15 weeks' gestation**, when the rate of DNA proliferation within brain is at the maximum.

The hazardous effect mainly includes spontaneous abortion within the first few weeks after conception, and major effect is also likely to be an increase in incidence of Down's syndrome or slight reduction in IQ.

Whole body exposure (Rads)	Effects
0–25	No detectable clinical effect
25–50	Possible blood cell changes
50–100	Blood cell changes, some injury, possible radiation sickness, no disability
100–200	Nausea, diarrhea, possible radiation sickness, shortening of life expectancy
250 to gonads	Temporary sterility
300 localized	Loss of hair, reddening of skin
400	Nausea and vomiting in 1–2 hour, permanent sterility, death in 50 percent of exposed population in 30 days
600	Death in 100 percent cases
1000	Death in 2 weeks
3000	Death in 2 days

Radiation Sensitivity of Some Human Tissues in Descending Order
- Embryo **(high sensitivity)**
- Fetus
- Lymphatic and hematopoietic organs (lymphocytes, RBCs, platelets)
- Bone marrow
- Intestinal tract
- Ovaries (ova)
- Testicles (sperm cells)
- Capillaries
- Mucous membrane and salivary glands
- Hair follicles
- Bone growth zone (Epiphysis)
- Breasts
- Eye lens
- Sweat and sebaceous glands
- Epidermis
- Thyroid
- Liver and kidneys
- Adult bones
- Cartilage
- Lungs and serous membranes
- Vagina

- CNS (Brain and spinal cord)
- Peripheral nerves
- Muscle **(Low sensitivity)**.

Radiation, induced necrosis and similar changes are best assessed by biopsy of the particular affected tissue of organ.

Total Body Irradiation—Acute Effects

Prodromal radiation syndrome, central nervous system, cardiovascular syndrome, gastrointestinal syndrome, hematopoietic syndrome, mean lethal dose, treatment of radiation accidents.

Clinical manifestations of acute total body irradiation depend on the total body dose.
- At total body doses between 2–8 Gy, death may occur 2 to 4 weeks after exposure from bone marrow failure. This is known as **hematopoietic syndrome**.
- At doses between 5 and 12 Gy, death may occur in a matter of days as a result of the **gastrointestinal syndrome**. A total body dose of >10 Gy is uniformly fatal unless supportive therapy is given.
- At doses above >100 Gy, death occurs usually 24 to 48 hours later from neurologic and cardiovascular failure. This is known as **cerebrovascular failure**.

Specific Nonstochastic Effects

Hematopoietic Syndrome

The hematopoietic syndrome encompasses the medical conditions that affect the blood. Hematopoietic syndrome conditions appear after a gamma dose of about 200 rads (2 Gy). This disease is characterized by depression or ablation of the bone marrow, and the physiological consequences of this damage. The onset of the disease is rather sudden, and is heralded by nausea and vomiting within several hours after the overexposure occurred. Malaise and fatigue are felt by the victim, but the degree of malaise does not seem to be correlated with the size of the dose. Loss of hair (epilation), which is almost always seen, appears between the second and third week post exposure. Death may occur within 1 to 2 months after exposure. The chief effects to be noted, of course, are in the bone marrow and in the blood. Marrow depression is seen at 200 rads; at about 400 to 600 rads (4 to 6 Gy) complete ablation of the marrow occurs. In this case, however, spontaneous regrowth of the marrow is possible if the victim survives the physiological effects of the denuding of his marrow. An exposure of about 700 rads (7 Gy) or greater leads to irreversible ablation of the bone marrow.

Gastrointestinal Syndrome

The gastrointestinal syndrome encompasses the medical conditions that affect the stomach and the intestines. This medical condition follows a total body gamma dose of about 1000 rads (10 Gy) or greater, and is a consequence of the desquamation of the intestinal epithelium. All the signs and symptoms of hematopoietic syndrome are seen—with the addition of severe nausea, vomiting, and diarrhea which begin very soon after exposure. Death within 1 to 2 weeks after exposure is the most likely outcome.

Central Nervous System

A total body gamma dose in excess of about 2000 rads (20 Gy) damages the central nervous system, as well as, all the other organ systems in the body. Unconsciousness follows within minutes after exposure and death in a matter of hours to several days. The rapidity of onset of unconsciousness is directly related to dose. In one instance in which a 200 msec burst of mixed neutrons and gamma rays delivered a mean total body dose of about 4400 rads (44 Gy), the victim was ataxic and disoriented within 30 seconds. In 10 minutes he was unconscious and in shock. Vigorous symptomatic treatment kept the patient alive for 34 hours after the accident.

Other Acute Effects

Several other immediate effects of acute overexposure should be noted. Because of its physical location, the skin is subject to more radiation exposure, especially in the case of low energy X-rays and beta rays, than most other tissues. An exposure of about 300 R (77 mC/kg) of low energy (in the diagnostic range) X-rays results in erythema. Higher doses may cause changes in pigmentation, loss of hair, blistering, cell death, and ulceration. Radiation dermatitis of the hands and face was a relatively common occupational disease among radiologists who practiced during the early years of the twentieth century.

The gonads are particularly radiosensitive. A single dose of only 30 rads (300 mGy) to the testes results in temporary sterility among men. For women, a 300 rad (3 Gy) dose to the ovaries produces temporary sterility. Higher doses increase the period of temporary sterility. In women, temporary sterility is evidenced by a cessation of menstruation for a period of 1 month or more, depending on the dose. Irregularities in the menstrual cycle, which suggest functional changes in the gonads, may result from local irradiation of the ovaries with doses smaller than that required for temporary sterilization.

The eyes too, are relatively radiosensitive. A local dose of several hundred rads can result in acute conjunctivitis.

Dosages are in Roentgen Equivalent Man (Rem)
- 0–25 No injury evident. First detectable blood change at 5 rem.
- 25–50 Definite blood change at 25 rem. No serious injury.
- 50–100 Some injury possible.
- 100–200 Injury and possible disability.
- 200–400 Injury and disability likely, death possible.
- 400–500 Median Lethal Dose (MLD) 50 percent exposures fatal.
- 500–1,000 Up to 100 percent exposures fatal.
- 1,000–over 100 percent fatal likely.

Example dosages and resulting symptoms when an individual receives an exposure to the whole body within a twenty-four hour period.

100 to 200 Rem

First day	No definite symptoms
First week	No definite symptoms
Second week	No definite symptoms
Third week	Loss of appetite, malaise, sore throat and diarrhea
Fourth week	Recovery is likely in a few months, unless complications develop because of poor health

400 to 500 Rem

First day	Nausea, vomiting and diarrhea, usually in the first few hours
First week	Symptoms may continue
Second week	Epilation, loss of appetite
Third week	Hemorrhage, nosebleeds, inflammation of mouth and throat, diarrhea, emaciation
Fourth week	Rapid emaciation, generally 50 percent mortality

Over the years, numerous recommendations regarding occupational exposure limits have been developed by the International Commission on Radiological Protection (ICRP) and other radiation protection groups. In general, the guidelines established for radiation exposure have had two principle objectives: (1) to prevent acute exposure; (2) to limit chronic exposure to "acceptable" levels.

Current guidelines are based on the conservative assumption that there is no safe level of exposure. In other words, even the smallest exposure has some probability of causing a stochastic effect, such as cancer. This assumption has led to the general philosophy of not only keeping exposures below recommended levels or regulation limits but also maintaining all exposure "**as low as reasonable achievable**" (**ALARA**).

The ALARA is a basic requirement of current radiation safety practices. It means that every reasonable effort must be made to keep the dose to workers and the public as far below the required limits as possible.

Late Effects—Nonspecific life-shortening

Carcinogenesis

Latent period—Dose response curve in animals - leukemia - breast cancer - thyroid cancer - bone cancer - skin cancer - lung cancer - other tumors - malignancies in prenatally exposed children.

Radiation Effects in the Developing Embryo and Fetus

- Intrauterine death
- Congenital abnormalities including neonatal death - growth retardation - elective booking of 10-day rule. Practical threshold for therapeutic abortion. Effects of radiation on the skin, bones and cartilage and kidneys.

Tolerance Doses

TD5/5–5 percent patients having complication in 5 years.
TD50/5–50 percent patients having complication in 5 years.

	Tolerance doses (TD5/5 – TD50/5) to whole organ irradiation			
	Single dose (cGy)		Fractionated dose (cGy)	
	TD5/5	TD50/5		
Bone marrow	200	1000	4000	5000
Eye (lens)	200	1000	600	1200
Lung	700	1000	200	3000
Kidney	1000	2000	2000	3000
Liver	1500	2000	3500	4000
Skin	1500	2000	3000	4000
Heart	1800	2000	4000	5000
Lymphoid	200	500	4000	5000
GI	500	1000	5000	6000
Spinal cord	1500	2000	5000	6000

Sr No	Organ	Minimal tolerance dose (TD5/5)	Maximal tolerance dose (whole organ) (TD5/50)
1.	Bone marrow (Whole)	250	450
2.	Bone marrow (Segmental)	3000	4000
3.	Testis	600	1000
4.	Liver	2500	4000
5.	Stomach	4500	5500
6.	Intestine	4500	5500
7.	Brain	5000	6000
8.	Spinal cord	4500	5500
9.	Heart	4500	5500
10.	Lung	3000	3500
11.	Kidney	1500	2000
12.	Fetus	200	400

- In routine fluoroscopy a dose of 4 rad is delivered to a part of body in about 1 minute.
- The International Commission on Radiological Protection (ICRP), the International Atomic Energy Agency (IAEA) and the WHO have been active in this field and it has been recommended that the genetic dose to the whole population from all sources additional to the natural background radiation, should not exceed 5 rem over a period of 30 years.
- It is estimated that man derives about 50 mrad per year from terrestrial radiation.
- It has been calculated that a commercial jet pilot receives about 300 mRad per year from cosmic radiation.
- From atmospheric radiation it is about 2 mrad per year.
- All in all, it is estimated that the total natural radiation to which the average person is subjected comes to approximately 0.1 rad per year.
- When optimum radiographic techniques are employed, the skin **dose to the patient from a single X-ray film** varies roughly from 0.02 to 3.0 rad.
- The amount of radiation received from outer space and background radiation has been estimated to be 0.1 rad per year, which apparently does not constitute a hazard at present.
- According to National Council on Radiation Protection (NCRP) an individual's lifetime effective dose equivalent in rem should not exceed the value of his or her age in years.

RADIATION PROTECTION

- Radiation protection is the youngest branch of hygiene called *radiation-hygiene*.
- The basic principle of radiation principle is ALARA (As Low As Reasonably Achievable radiation dose).
- The **permissible dose** from man-made sources **should not exceed 5 rad/year**.
- Of the man made sources, the X-ray constitutes the greatest hazard.
- According to National Council on Radiation Protection (NCRP) the dose limit for the occasionally exposed individual is 0.5 rem/year, or 1/10th of MPD for the occasionally exposed.
- The NCRP recommends a total dose equivalent limit of 0.5 rem (50 mSv) for embryo fetus during pregnancy.
- The NCRP recommends a total dose equivalent limit (excluding medical exposure) of 0.5 rem (50 mSv) for the embryo, fetus. Once a pregnancy becomes known, exposure of the embryo-fetus should be no greater than 0.05 rem (0.5 mSv) in any month (excluding medical exposure).

NCRP Recommendation of Radiation Dose Limits

Class of exposed individual	Rems	mSv
Occupational exposures (annual)		
Stochastic effects	5	50
Nonstochastic effects		
Lens of eye	15	150
All other areas (e.g. red marrow, breast, lung, gonads, skin, and extremities)	50	500
Lifetime cumulative exposure	1 (x age in year)	10 (x age in year)
Public exposure (annual)		
Effective dose equivalent limit	0.5	5
Dose equivalent limits for lens of eye, skin, and extremities	5	50
Trainees under 18 years of age		
Effective dose equivalent limit	0.1	1
Dose equivalent limit for lens of eye, skin, and extremities	5	50
Embryo-fetus exposures		
Total dose equivalent limit	0.5	5
Dose equivalent limit in a month	0.05	0.5

- Excluding background and medical exposures, but including both internal and external exposures
- **Rem = rads × quality factor (R)**

- Because the quality factor for X-rays is 1, hence rad = rem
- In fact at diagnostic energy level the rad, rem and Roentgen usually will be considered.

The NCRP recommends a total dose equivalent limit per year of 50 mSv for occupationally exposed individuals.

The NCRP recommends a total dose equivalent limit (excluding medical exposure) of 0.5 rem (50 mSv) for the embryo-fetus. Once a pregnancy becomes known, exposure of the embryo-fetus should be no greater than 0.05 rem (0.5 mSv) in any month (excluding medical exposure).

Latest ICRP recommendations for maximum permissible dose for various groups are:
Occupational exposure (Radiation workers) → 20 mSv/year.
Public (in general) → 1 mSv/year.
Pregnancy → 2 mSv for declared term.

ICRP Recommendations for the Dose Limits

Application	Occupational	Public
Effective dose	20 MilliSv (2 rem/year)	1 milliSv/year (100 mrem)
Annual equivalent dose in		
Eye lens	150 mSv (15 rem)	15 mSv (1.5 rem)
Skin	500 mSv (50 rem)	50 mSv (5.0 rem)
Hands and Feet	500 mSv (50 rem)	50 mSv (5.0 rem)

ICRU: International Commission on Radiation Units recommend guidelines for radiotherapy.

ICRP: International Commission for Radiation Protection recommend guidelines for radiation protection.

- The permissible dose from man-made sources **should not exceed 5 rad a year.**
- Of the man-made sources, the X-rays constitute the greatest hazard.
- In routine fluoroscopy a dose of 4 rad is delivered to a part of body in about 1 minute. This implies unnecessary X-ray examinations should be avoided, especially in case of children and/or pregnant women.
- Lead aprons (0.5 mm of lead) will reduce the intensity of scattered radiation by 90 percent and should be worn by all the workers associated with X-ray procedures regularly.
- The **International Commission on Radiological Protection** (ICRP), the International Atomic Energy Agency (IAEA) and the WHO have been active in this field and it has been recommended

that the **genetic dose** to the whole population from all sources additional to the natural background radiation, should not exceed **5 rem** over a period of 30 years.
- Radiation exposure during childhood, especially infancy for some reason or the other has been linked to further risk of development of thyroid cancer.
- Palliation of metastatic disease is a substantial component of radiation oncology, and a vital aspect of cancer patient care in general, **severe pain** and debilitation resulting from untreated metastases have a significant impact on the patient's quality of life, but on health care and economics as well standard treatment is **30 Gy in 10 fractions**. However, there are recent trials, which have found 8 Gy in single sitting to be as effective, however, current standard in 30 Gy on 10 sittings only.
- **ALARA**—As Low As Reasonably Achievable Radiation dose, is a newer concept for decreasing radiation hazards.

Regulatory Limits for Occupational Exposure

Many of these recommendations ICRP and other groups have been incorporated into the regulatory requirements of countries around the world. In the United States, annual radiation exposure limits are found in Title 10, part 20 of the Code of Federal Regulations, and in equivalent state regulations. For industrial radiographers who generally are not concerned with an intake of radioactive material, the Code sets the annual limit of exposure at the following:
- The more limiting of:
    - A total effective dose equivalent of 5 rems (0.05 Sv)
    - The sum of the deep-dose equivalent to any individual organ or tissue other than the lens of the eye being equal to 50 rems (0.5 Sv).
- The annual limits to the lens of the eye, to the skin, and to the extremities, which are:
    - A lens dose equivalent of 15 rems (0.15 Sv)
    - A shallow-dose equivalent of 50 rems (0.50 Sv) to the skin or to any extremity.

The **shallow-dose equivalent** is the external dose to the skin of the whole-body or extremities from an external source of ionizing radiation. This value is the dose equivalent at a tissue depth of 0.007 cm averaged over and area of 10 cm^2.

The **lens dose equivalent** is the dose equivalent to the lens of the eye from an external source of ionizing radiation. This value is the dose equivalent at a tissue depth of 0.3 cm.

The **deep-dose equivalent** is the whole-body dose from an external source of ionizing radiation. This value is the dose equivalent at a tissue depth of 1 cm.

The **total effective dose equivalent** is the dose equivalent to the whole-body.

Declared Pregnant Workers and Minors

Because of the increased health risks to the rapidly developing embryo and fetus, pregnant women can receive no more than 0.5 rem during the entire gestation period. This is 10 percent of the dose limit that normally applies to radiation workers. Persons under the age of 18 years are also limited to 0.5 rem/year.

Nonradiation Workers and the Public

The dose limit to nonradiation workers and members of the public are 2 percent of the annual occupational dose limit. Therefore a nonradiation worker can receive a whole body dose of no more that 0.1 rem/year from industrial ionizing radiation. This exposure would be in addition to the 0.3 rem/year from natural background radiation and the 0.05 rem/year from man-made sources such as medical X-rays.

How We Protect Ourselves from Radiation? [Radiation Protection]

The best rule of radiation protection is *time*, *shield*, and *distance* (TSD). These basic principles are always adhered to protect oneself from radiation. The time to work with radiation should be kept as short as possible, hence if anyone has to work with radiation (preloaded brachytherapy), he should finish his work as quickly as possible. The second principle is shielding, meaning the person should be shielded from the radiation source by an appropriate shielding material (of appropriate thickness according to energy of radiation HVL) made up of lead or tungsten. The radiation source should be kept as far as possible by the use of long forceps so that the personnel would get minimal dose by a principle called *inverse square law*.

PRIMARY AND SECONDARY BARRIERS FOR RADIATION

Primary barrier is any barrier that intercepts the useful X-ray beam, e.g. Walls and floor of room. Secondary barrier is any that intercepts leakage and scatter radiation, e.g. Ceiling.

Materials for Radiation Protection

- Lead (aprons, gloves, and shields)
- Barium concrete
- Concrete
- Brick

Lead Aprons

- Lead aprons (0.5 mm of lead) reduce the intensity of scattered radiation by 90 percent and should be worn by all the workers associated with X-ray procedures regularly.
- Increasing the density, atomic number, or electrons per gram of the absorber decreases the transmitted photons.
- Lead has high atomic number and density.
- Atomic number of lead is 82 and its K edge is 88, hence it produces maximum photoelectric effect and absorbs maximum incident radiations.
- Other barriers are compared to lead in terms of their "lead equivalence".
- Higher the attenuation coefficient, the lower the number of transmitted photons.
- Gram for gram, tin is a better absorber of X-rays than lead between 29–88 keV.
- Hence tin attenuates more radiations per unit weight than lead and recently tin has come in use for making protective aprons. Thus, a lighter tin apron gives the same protection as a standard lead apron.
- Lead has high atomic number (82) and density and its K edge is 88, hence it produces maximum photoelectric effect and absorbs incident radiations to such an extent that it is routinely used as radiation barrier/shielding and other barriers are compared to lead in terms of their "lead equivalence".
- In advanced radiotherapy centers, most of the brachytherapy equipment have inbuilt protection devise called remote *after loading system*. Hence in centers with remote afterloading equipment, the chance of exposure to radiation is very remote. But despite of these safety measures the radiation personnel are monitored closely by personal monitors (film badges) every month, dosimeters, and thermoluminiscence dosimetery (TLD). Moreover if a person accidentally exposed to radiation, the blood lymphocytes of the victim are analyzed for the karyotypic evidence of chromosomal damage. The maximum permissible dose of radiation for man is 2 rems per year; but for the radiation workers a dose up to 5 rems can be permissible.

Radiation Dosimetry

Protection from primary radiation and leakage radiation and scattered radiation is very important issue and **Dosimetry** refers to the detection and measurement of ionizing radiation.

Dosimeter → a device to monitor/measure radiation exposure. Today TLD is the most often used dosimeter.

Emission of Light by X-rays is by 'Three' Methods:
1. Fluorescence—immediately following interaction
2. Phosphorescence—after a time interval
3. Thermoluminescence—only upon heating at 300 to 400°C

Thermoluminescence Dosimeter

- It is a personnel radiation-monitoring device
- The thermoluminescence material most commonly used is lithium fluoride
- Calcium sulfate was used previously
- Quantity of light emitted (brightness) is proportional to the radiation dose received
- It determines radiation exposure only and not exposure rate
- It detects dose of X-rays and gamma ray received
- It is energy nondependable
- It is reusable
- Thermoluminescence → Liberating stored energy in form of light.
  Thermoluminescence Dosimeter (TLD) material exposed to radiation → Heated at 300°C in special oven → Light emitted → Photoelectric cell → Electron current → Photomultiplier tube → Meter calibrated in rem.

Applications → For personnel monitoring:
- In Radiotherapy
- In Radiodiagnosis
- In CT dosimeter
- Geologists—age of rock.

RADIATION UNITS

Old Units
- Becquerel (Bq)   -   Unit of activity (1 Bq = 1 disintegration per second)
- Curie (Ci)   -   Was unit of activity formerly (1 Bq = 27 picocuries)
- Roentgen   -   Unit of exposure (1 mrad = 0.001 rad)
- Rem   -   Unit of absorption

New SI Units
- Coulomb per kg   -   Replaced Roentgen
- Gray   -   Replaced Rad (1 rad = 0.01 Gy)
- Sievert   -   Replaced Rem (1 Sv = 100 rems)

Dose equivalent (H) = Grays (D) × Quality factor (Q)

Chapter 3 ❖ Radiation Hazards and Protection

For	Old unit	New unit (SI)
Radioactivity	Curie	Becquerel
Radiation exposure	Roentgen	Coulomb/kg
Absorbed dose	Rad (Radiation absorbed dose)	Gy
Dose equivalent	REM (Radiation equivalent of man)	Sievert (SV)
Effective dose	—	MSV

- **R Roentgen**, the unit of exposure of radiation in air; meaning 1 Roentgen [R] = 1 electrostatic unit (esu) charge/0.001293 gm of air at STP; SI unit 1 R = 2.58×10^{-4} Coulomb/kg.
- **cGy** centiGray [1 cGy = 1 rad]
- **Gy** Gray SI unit of absorbed dose [1 Gy = 100 cGy or 100 rads]; 1 Gy = 1 joule/kg of air
- **rad** radiation absorbed dose [now called cGy]; 1 erg/gm
- **rem** rad equivalent man used most commonly for radiation protection [1 rem = 100 mrem]
- **Ci** Curie unit of radioactivity; 1 Curie (Ci) = 3.7×10^{10} disintegrations/sec
- This is a standard to measure rate or radioactive decay; based on disintegrations of 1 gram of radium or 3.7×10^{10} disintegrations per second
- **mCi** milliCurie; 1 mCi = 3.7×10^{7} disintegrations/sec
- **Bq** Becquerel SI unit of radioactivity; 1 Bq = 1 disintegration/sec
- **Sv** Sievert SI unit of absorbed dose equivalent used mainly for protection purpose [1 Sv = 100 rem]
- **Kerma** (Kinetic energy released per unit mass) is commonly used for estimation of dose rate in brachytherapy.

Absorbed Dose

- The amount of radiation energy absorbed into a given mass of tissue.
- Absorbed dose is the radiation quantity used to express the concentration of radiation energy actually absorbed in a specific tissue. This is the quantity that is most directly related to biological effects.
- Dose values can be in the traditional unit of the rad or the SI unit of the gray (Gy).
- The rad is equivalent to 100 ergs of energy absorbed in a gram of tissue and the gray is one joule of energy absorbed per kilogram of tissue.

$$1 \text{ gray (Gy)} = 100 \text{ rads}$$
$$10 \text{ mGy} = 1 \text{ rad}$$
$$1 \text{ mGy} = 100 \text{ mrad}$$

Dose Equivalent

- Measures the energy per unit mass times adjustments for the type of radiation involved (quality factor) and the biological response in the tissue (a weighting factor).
- Equivalent dose converts dose into an estimate of risk.
- They are quantities that can be measured and expressed in terms of the more fundamental physical quantities like energy. Dose equivalent, in the unit, Sievert (Sv), is a quantity that expresses the relative biological impact of the radiation by including a radiation weighting factor (W_R). The relationship is:

$$\text{Dose equivalent (Sv)} = \text{Dose (Gy)} \times W_R$$

The value of the radiation weighting factor (W_R) is a characteristic of each specific type of radiation.

Effective Dose

Effective dose is becoming a very useful radiation quantity for expressing relative risk to humans, both patients and other personnel. It is actually a simple and very logical concept. It takes into account the specific organs and areas of the body that are exposed. The point is that all parts of the body and organs are not equally sensitive to the possible adverse effects of radiation, such as cancer induction and mutations.

For the purpose of determining effective dose, the different areas and organs have been assigned tissue weighting factor (W_T) values. For a specific organ or body area the effective dose is:

$$\text{Effective Dose (Gy)} = \text{Absorbed Dose (Gy)} \times W_T$$

Chapter 4

Pulmonary Radiology

GENERAL ASPECT

Bronchopulmonary Segments
- Right upper lobe = Apical, anterior and posterior
- Right middle lobe = Medial, lateral
- Right lower lobe = Apical/superior, medial basal, posterior basal, lateral basal and anterior basal
- Left upper lobe = Apicoposterior, anterior, superior lingular and inferior lingular
- Left lower lobe = Apical/superior, posteromedial/posterior basal, lateral basal and anterior basal

Acquiring a Chest X-ray (CXR)
- Usually, a CXR is taken by using kV between 80 and 120 with a FFD of 6 feet (1.85 m) reduces magnification and produces sharper image.
- Using a low kVp (60–80 kV) produces a high contrast film with miliary shadowing and calcification being seen more clearly.
- With high voltages (120–170) the films are of lower contrast with increased visualization of hidden areas of lung, better penetration of mediastinum and better demonstration of normal, vessel markings and abnormal opacities [High kV radiography has been now supplanted by contrast-enhanced computed tomography (CECT)].
- 1 rad = 1 rem = 0.01 mSv
- The effective dose equivalent from resulting from chest radiographic examination is 0.02 to 0.06 (6 mrem or mrad)
- One CT thorax (8 mSv) is equivalent to 400 CXR

Special chest radiographic views	Use
Lordotic view	To detect lesions of = middle lobe (like collapse) and collection in fissure and subtle infiltrates in UZs.
Oblique views	To demonstrate = retrocardiac space, the posterior CP angles and the chest wall, with pleural plaques being clearly demonstrated.
Decubitus view	To demonstrate = small amount of pleural fluid, that is not seen on PA view.
Paired inspiratory and expiratory views	To demonstrate = air trapping, small pneumothorax, interstitial shadowing, diaphragm movements, and inhaled foreign body in childern.
Lateral view	Retrosternal space is best seen in lateral view. Mediastinal lesions. Fissural effusion and middle lobe collapse
Oblique view	The retrocardiac space is seen well on oblique view. Rib lesions.
Films exposed in expiration or at the end of expiration	To demonstrate air trapping, particularly in pediatric practice for any patient suspected of having inhaled a foreign body. To demonstrate a small pneumothorax and interstitial shadowing.

Special Chest Radiographic Views

- Good visualization of the apices of lung requires projection of clavicles upward, as in the *apical view* (**apicogram**) with the X-ray tube angled up 50 to 60°, or downward, as in the *lordotic view* with the patient in lordotic PA position in which a middle lobe collapse is seen clearly as a well-defined triangular opacity. A lordotic view is useful to detect lesions of middle lobe (like collapse) and collection in fissure and subtle infiltrates in Uzs.
- *Oblique views* are taken usually to demonstrate the retrocardiac space, the posterior costophrenic (CP) angles and the chest wall, with pleural plaques being clearly demonstrated.
- *Decubitus view* shows small amount of pleural fluid, which is not seen on PA view.
- *Paired inspiratory and expiratory views* are important in demonstrating air trapping, small pneumothorax, interstitial shadowing, diaphragm movements, and inhaled foreign body in children.
- Retrosternal space is best seen in lateral view while the retrocardiac space is seen well on oblique view.
- Films exposed *in expiration* are invaluable in the investigation of air trapping, particularly in pediatric practice for any patient suspected of having inhaled a foreign body. It may also enhance the demonstration of a small pneumothorax and interstitial shadowing.

- Paired views (inspiratory and expiratory films) are very important for children with a possible diagnosis of an inhaled foreign body.

Normal Chest Radiograph

- If the film is well-centered, the medial ends of the clavicles are equidistant from the vertebral spinous processes at the T4/5 level.
- With low kV film the vertebral bodies and the disk spaces should be just visible down to the T8/9 level through the cardiac shadow.
- Trachea is midline in its upper part, and then deviates slightly to the right around aortic knuckle.
- Central dense shadow seen on the PA chest film comprises the mediastinum, heart, spine and sternum.
- With good centering 2/3rds of the cardiac shadow lies to the left of midline and 1/3rd to the right. The normal cardiothoracic ratio is less than 50 percent in adults and 60 percent in children.
- In 97 percent of subjects the left hilum is higher than the right and in 3 percent they are at the same level. The normal hila should be of equal density and similar size with clearly defined concave lateral borders. Of all the structures in the hilum only the pulmonary arteries and upper lobar veins contribute significantly to hilar shadows on plain radiographs.
- Lung fields and costophrenic angle should be clear.
- The horizontal fissure is seen on PA view running from the hilum to the region of 6th rib in axillary line. Both oblique fissure commence posteriorly at the level of T4 or T5, passing through hilum and the left is steeper and finishes 5 cm behind the anterior CP angle, whereas the right ends just behind the angle.
- In most patients the right hemidiaphragm is higher than the left. This is due to the heart depressing the left sided and not to the liver pushing up the right dome. A difference greater than 3 cm in height of the two domes is considered significant.
- The bronchial vessels are normally not visualized on the plain chest film. The peripheral lung markings are mainly vascular, veins and arteries having no distinguishing characteristic.

Hila

These are composed of:
- Lymph nodes
- Pulmonary arteries and their main branches
- Upper lobar pulmonary veins
- The major bronchi.

The lower lobe pulmonary veins do not cross the hila in their course to left atrium and hence do not contribute to hilar shadow.

Mediastinal Outline

The superior vena cava (SVC) and innominate vessels form the right superior mediastinal shadow; a dilated aorta may contribute to this border. The SVC and the right atrium usually form the right inferior mediastinal, i.e. the right heart border.

On left side the superior mediastinal border is less sharp and formed by the subclavian artery above the aortic knuckle. The main pulmonary artery (pulmonary conus) and the left ventricle form the left inferior mediastinal, i.e. the left heart border. The area between the main pulmonary artery and the left ventricle is occupied by additional structures if they are slightly enlarged, namely left atrial appendage and the right ventricular outflow tract.

Trachea

Trachea is a straight tube which starts at C6 vertebral level as continuation of larynx, passes downward and backward in the midline and ends at carina, i.e. T4–T5 vertebral level which also corresponds to sternal angle of Louis, by dividing into right and left bronchi.

- Tracheal length is 6 to 9 cm.
- The upper limits of normal for its coronal and sagittal diameters in ducts on plain chest radiograph are 21 and 23 mm, respectively, for women, and 25 and 27 for men.
- Normal *subcarinal angle* is 60 to 75°.
- In children, the angles of division symmetrical, but in adults the right main stem bronchus has a steeper angle (40°) than the left (25°).
- The carinal angle is widened in left atrial enlargement due to elevation of left main stem bronchus.
- It starts at the level of C6 vertebra and ends at T4, having 6 to 9 cm length.
- It divides at carina into two main bronchi.
- Normal diameter of trachea on CT scan is:

	Male	*Female*
Coronal	23 mm	20 mm
Sagittal	21 mm	18 mm

On expiration, it reduces in width by about 10 percent and in length by about 20 percent and carina moves upwards by about 1 cm. During inspiration/recumbency the carinal angle (normal 60°) increases by about 10 to 15°. Clinical significance of these variations on respiration/change of position is that distal tip of intratracheal tube may appear in satisfactory position on inspiratory film but on expiration it may extend into right main stem bronchus and block the left bronchial orifice. Also this makes the splaying of carinal angle a nonideal detector of left atrial enlargement or carinal nodes.

$$\text{Tracheal index} = \frac{\text{Coronal diameter of trachea}}{\text{Sagittal diameter of trachea}}$$

- In females and children, it is = 1. In males, it is <1. When it goes below 0.6, it is called **Saber sheath trachea**.
- Tracheal bifurcation is known as carina. It is not visible on lateral view. It is seen well on left anterior oblique view.
- The tip of correctly positioned endotracheal tube (ETT) lies in the mid-trachea approximately 50 to 70 mm above the carina. The carina is usually at the level of 5th or 6th thoracic vertebral body. This distance is needed to ensure that it does not descend into the right main stem bronchus with flexion and extension of neck, and that it does not ascend into the larynx when the head and neck are extended.
- A tracheostomy may be needed for long-term ventilatory support and it should be parallel to the long axis of trachea, approximately one-half to 2/3rd the diameter of trachea, and positioned at least several cm from the carina.

COMMON ABNORMALITIES NOTED ON CXR

Poland's syndrome is characterized by unilateral absence or hypoplasia of the pectoralis major resulting in unilateral transradiancy and an abnormal anterior axillary fold, ipsilateral hand and arm anomalies (particularly syndactyly) with or without absence of pectoralis minor, rib anomalies, and hypoplasia or absence of the breast (amastia) and nipple (athelia).

Localized Rib Expansion
- Fibrous dysplasia
- Myeloma
- Gaucher's disease
- Eosinophilic granuloma
- Hemangioma

- Chondroma
- Brown tumor
- Aneurysmal bone cyst

Rib destruction is usually accompanied by extrapleural soft tissue mass and the causes include:
- Infection (osteomyelitis and actinomycosis)
- Soft tissue tumors in overlying part
- Tumors of adjacent part of lung and pleura
- Bone tumors like Ewing's sarcoma, chondrosarcoma, osteosarcoma
- Metastases
- Lymphoma
- Myeloma.

Differential Diagnosis of Unilateral Hypertranslucent of Lung

- Normal (increased density of contralateral lung, e.g. pleural effusion/thickening, consolidation)
- Rotation or scoliosis
- Mastectomy
- Congenital, absence of pectoralis major
- Polio
- Pneumothorax
- Congenital hyperinflation (McLeod's syndrome, congenital lobar emphysema)
- Compensatory emphysema (lobar collapse, lobectomy)
- Obstructive emphysema (foreign body, tumor)
- Bullous emphysema
- Absent or hypoplastic pulmonary artery
- Obstructed pulmonary artery (tumor, embolus).

Differential Diagnosis of Opaque Hemithorax

- Technical : Rotation, scoliosis
- Pleural   : Massive/large hydrothorax, pleural thickening, and mesothelioma
- Pulmonary : Collapse, consolidation (massive) fibrosis
- Congenital : Pulmonary agenesis

- Mediastinal : Gross cardiomegaly, tumors
- Surgical : Pneumonectomy, thoracoplasty
- Diaphragmatic hernia

Differential Diagnosis of Miliary Mottling

A miliary pattern describes the presence of small, discrete, rounded, pulmonary opacities measuring 2 mm in diameter.

Thus, miliary mottling has wide-spread small discrete opacities of similar size 2–4 mm in diameter. It can be fine or coarse miliary mottling.

Causes of miliary shadowing:
- Infection
  - TB
  - Coccidioidomycosis
  - Blastomycosis
  - Histoplasmosis
  - Chickenpox
- Dust inhalation
  - Tin
  - Barium
  - Beryllium
  - Silicosis
  - Coal worker's pneumoconiosis
- Hemosiderosis
- Hyaline membrane disease (HMD)
- Histiocytosis X
- Metastasis
- Alveolar microlithiasis
- Bronchiolitis obliterans
- Sarcoidosis
- Secondary hyperparathyroidism
- Amyloidosis
- Miliary carcinomatosis

Differential Diagnosis of Calcific Foci in Lungs

- Infective: Tuberculosis
  Histoplasmosis
  Coccidioidomycosis
  Chickenpox
  Actinomycosis
  Hydatid cyst
  Abscess (Chronic)
- Tumors: Metastasis (osteosarcoma, chondrosarcoma, cystadenocarcinoma)
  Benign (AV malformation, hamartoma, carcinoid)
- Miscellaneous (hematoma, infarction, mitral valve disease, broncholith, alveolar microlithiasis)
- Rare (hypercalcemia, silicosis, sarcoidosis, RA, amyloidosis, osteopathia racemosa).

Note

Bull's eye calcification (Dense central nidus or laminated calcification) → granuloma (Granulomatous lesion).

Popcorn calcification → hamartoma.

Eggshell nodal calcification → Silicosis, sarcoidosis, histoplasmosis, blastomycosis, scleroderma and amyloidosis.

Bronchogenic carcinoma (6–7%) → *Granular calcification* in larger tumors and *amorphous or cloud like calcification* especially in small peripheral tumors.

Pulmonary metastasis calcification is very unusual except in metastasis from osteosarcoma, chondrosarcoma.

Differential Diagnosis of Cavitating Pulmonary Lesions

- *Developmental:* Sequestration, bronchogenic cyst, congenital cystic adenomatoid malformation (CCAM)
- Traumatic lung cyst
- Pulmonary hematoma
- Infections (TB, *Staph, Klebsiella,* histoplasma, amoebic, hydatid, fungal)
- Pneumatocele
- Abscess
- Sarcoidosis
- Pulmonary infarct

- Bullae, blebs
- Malignant: Primary, secondary, lymphoma, metastasis
- Pneumoconiosis
- Connective tissue disorders: Wegener's granulomatosis, RA, Caplan syndrome.

Note: Cavitation may occur in metastases from any primary site, but is more common in squamous carcinomas and sarcomas. Cavitation in subpleural, metastasis is recognized cause of spontaneous pneumothorax.

Calcification is most commonly seen in metastasis from osteosarcoma, and rarely in chondrosarcoma and mucinous adenocarcinoma.

Differential Diagnosis of Honeycombing of Lungs

Destroyed, fibrotic and cystic lungs representing complete loss of acinar and bronchiolar architecture as the end stage of fibrosing lung disease with lung cysts measuring about 3 mm to 1 cm in size.

It implies end stage disease.

Causes of Honeycombing in Lungs
- Sarcoidosis
- Interstitial lung disease
- Extrinsic allergic alveolitis (Cryptogenic)
- Idiopathic (UIP)
- Storage disorders
- Histiocytosis (eosinophilic granuloma)
- Amyloidosis
- Pneumoconiosis
- Drugs → Bleomycin, Busulfan, Nitrofurantoin
- Collagen vascular diseases → SLE, Scleroderma, RA, Sjögren's syndrome
- Cystic fibrosis
- Oxygen toxicity
- Tuberculosis.

Patterns of Interstitial Lung Diseases (ILD)

Reticular Pattern
- Fibrosing alveolitis
- Asbestosis

- Sarcoidosis
- Chronic allergic alveolitis
- Langerhan's cell histiocytosis
- Lymphangioleiomyomatosis.

Nodular Pattern
- *Silicosis*
- Coal worker's pneumoconiosis
- Sarcoidosis
- TB
- Subacute extrinsic allergic alveolitis.

Reticulonodular Pattern
- Langerhan's cell histiocytosis
- Sarcoidosis
- Spread of tumor via lymphatics.

Septal Pattern
- Interstitial pulmonary edema
- Spread of tumor via lymphatics.

"Ground-glass" Pattern
- Pneumocystis carinii pneumonia (PCP)
- Nonspecific interstitial pneumonia
- Idiopathic pulmonary hemorrhage (Diffuse pulmonary hemorrhage)
- Alveolar proteinosis
- Eosinophilic pneumonia
- Collagen vascular diseases, e.g. Scleroderma, Wegener's granulomatosis
- Subacute extrinsic allergic alveolitis.

Interstitial Lung Diseases Affecting Upper Zone
- Allergic bronchopulmonary aspergillosis (ABPA)
- Extrinsic allergic alveolitis
- Coal workers pneumoconiosis
- Langerhan's disease
- Ankylosing spondylitis
- Sarcoidosis
- Silicosis.

ILDs Primarily Affecting LZs
- Fibrosing alveolitis
- Asbestosis
- Interstitial pulmonary edema
- Lymphangitis carcinomatosa.

Differential Diagnosis of 'Ground-glass' Haze on X-ray Chest in a Neonate
- Left-to-right shunt produces hyperemic lung fields.
- As **hyaline membrane disease (HMD)** progresses, influx of plasma renders the lungs more radio-opaque, reticulogranular shadowing becomes more confluent and ground glass haziness is seen with loss of clarity of diaphragm and heart.
- In **Staphylococcal pneumonia**, later in disease more homogeneous opacification of lung fields occur.
- Ground-glass appearance is also seen in infracardiac total anomalous pulmonary venous connection (**TAPVC**).
- Ground-glass haziness is also seen in alveolar proteineosis, diffuse pulmonary hemorrhage, eosinophilic pneumonia, and Wegener's granulomatosis.

Differential Diagnosis of Bilateral Upper Lobe Fibrosis
- TB (including atypical mycobacterial infections)
- Sarcoidosis
- Histoplasmosis
- Allergic bronchopulmonary aspergillosis
- Chronic extrinsic allergic alveolitis
- Progressive massive fibrosis
- Ankylosing spondylitis.

Airbronchogram Sign
Parenchymal lung consolidation may result in visualization of the intrapulmonary bronchi, which are otherwise not visible on normal chest radiograph. This occurs because the air within their lumens will then stand out in contrast to the surrounding opaque lung, known as **airbronchogram**.

Differential Diagnosis of Airbronchogram Sign
- Normal person with phase of long exposure
- Consolidation

- Atelectasis (except in obstructive type)
- Alveolar cell carcinoma
- Pulmonary alveolar microlithiasis
- Pulmonary edema
- Pulmonary infarction (temporary)
- Pulmonary lymphoma of alveolar type
- Pulmonary hemorrhage
- Aspiration
- Sarcoidosis.

Silhouette Sign

Described by Felson and Felson (1950), the **"silhouette sign"** is loss of interface by adjacent disease and permits localization of lesion on film.

Diaphragm, cardiac and aortic outlines, which are normally seen as adjacent lung is aerated, and difference in radiodensity is demonstrated.

When aerated alveolar spaces are replaced by fluid/soft tissue, there is no longer a difference in radiodensity between that part of lung and adjacent structures. Thus, the silhouette is lost and **"silhouette sign"** is seen.

Conversely if border is retained and abnormality is superimposed, the lesion must be lying either anteriorly or posteriorly.

Obliteration of these borders may occur with pleural, mediastinal or pulmonary pathology.

Structure of silhouetted	Pathology
Right heart border	Right middle lobe pathology
Left heart border	Lingular lobe pathology
Aortic knuckle	Apicoposterior segment of LU
Right aortic border	Right middle lobe
Hemidiaphragm	Basal segments of lower lobe

ROLE OF CXR IN THORACIC TRAUMA

- Rib fractures
- *Pulmonary contusion* is the result of hemorrhagic exudation into the alveoli and interstitial space and appears as patchy, nonsegmental opacity/consolidation. Shadow appears within the first few hours of

penetrating or nonpenetrating trauma, usually improves in 2 days, and clears in 3–4 days. They are hence invariably managed conservatively.
- *Pulmonary lacerations* as a result of nonpenetrating trauma may appear as round thin-walled cystic spaces.
- *Pulmonary hematomas* are often multiple.

Emphysema

It is an increase beyond the normal size of the air spaces distal to the terminal bronchioles with dilatation and destruction of their walls.

Types of Emphysema

- *Panacinar/pan lobular emphysema:* Destruction of the entire lung distal to terminal bronchiole. Basal predominance seen classically associated with Alpha 1-antitrypsin deficiency.
- *Centriacinar/centrilobular:* Associated with smoking selective dilatation and destruction of respiratory bronchioles, i.e. central portion of the lobule only affected upper zones more severely involved than bases.
- *Paraseptal type:* Seen as isolated phenomenon in young adult involving periphery of secondary lobules, usually in lung periphery. Hence often marginated by interlobular septa and strikingly scan in subpleural location.
- *Paracicatricial/irregular type:* Distension and destruction of terminal airspaces adjacent to fibrotic lesions, most commonly seen in pulmonary tuberculosis.
- Compensatory emphysema
- *Emphysematous bulla:* An emphysematous space with a diameter more than 1cm in distended status and its wall made up of compressed surrounding lung or pleura.
- Obstructive emphysema/hyperinflation.

CXR in Emphysema

- Hyperinflated lung fields
- Low-posed and flat diaphragm
- Tubular heart
- 'Inverted mustache' sign
- Peripheral pruning with change in vessel caliber
- Barrel chest (AP diameter > side to side)

- Retrosternal air space >2.5 cm
- Saber sheath trachea.

Note: High-resolution computed tomography (HRCT) thorax is best investigation for diagnosis and characterization of emphysema.

PEDIATRIC CHEST

The lung is derived from two major embryologic sources: The lung bud of the primitive foregut (during the early part of the fourth week of fetal life) and the pulmonary vascular anlage of the sixth embryonic arch. During the fifth week, the lung bud becomes completely separated from the esophagus, which also develops from the primitive foregut. Failure of complete separation is responsible for the development of *congenital tracheoesophageal fistula*. Major developmental anomalies, such as *hypoplasia and aplasia* of the airways, vasculature, and supporting structures are especially likely when interference in lung growth occurs during the first 26 days of fetal life. Examples of these anomalies include *sequestration of the lung, arteriovenous malformations, cystic adenomatoid malformation, congenital lobar emphysema, bronchogenic cysts, vascular and bronchial coarctations, and various atresias, stenoses, and fistulas*. After the 26th day of fetal life, injurious stimuli tend to interfere with the normal growth and development of the terminal air sac and usually produce less severe abnormalities. Because the alveoli do not become fully developed until about 8 years of age, injuries before that age interfere with normal growth of the terminal air sac. The 24 million alveoli, normally present at birth, increase to 300 million by about 8 years of age. They also grow. The *McLeod syndrome* is an example of hypoplastic emphysema that results from severe or recurrent lung infections during early childhood that interferes with the normal growth and development of the terminal air sac.

Thymus: X-ray signs of thymic shadow:
- Anterosuperior mediastinal widening without tracheal shift
- Sail sign → a triangular projection to one or both sides of mediastinum
- Mulvay wave sign → wavy or rippled thymic outline due to indentation by costochondral junctions and anterior ends of ribs
- Notch sign → indentation at the junction of thymus with heart.

CONGENITAL LESIONS

Transient Tachypnea of the Newborn (TTN or Neonatal Wet Lung Disease)

- Prematurity, LSCS, maternal DM, breach delivery predisposes
- The most common cause of respiratory distress in newborn

- Occurs within 6 hours of life and peaks at 1st day of life.
- **CXR**
  - Linear opacities
  - Perivascular haze
  - Thickened fissures
  - Interlobular septal thickening (interstitial edema)
  - Symmetric perihilar radiating congestion
  - Mild hyperaeration
  - Small amount of pleural fluid.

Respiratory Distress Syndrome (Hyaline Membrane Disease)

- Predisposing factors: Prematurity, LSCS, diabetic mother.
- M:F = 1.8:1.
- Occurs within 2–5 hours after birth and peaks at 24–48 hours followed by gradual improvement.
- As **Hyaline membrane disease (HMD)** progresses, influx of plasma renders the lungs more radiopaque, reticulogranular shadowing becomes more confluent and ground glass haziness is seen with loss of clarity of diaphragm and heart.
- **CXR**
  - Diffuse granularity of reticulogranular pattern ("groundglass" appearance)
  - Prominent airbronchogram
  - Hypoaeration with volume loss
  - Bilateral symmetrical distribution.

Pulmonary Sequestration

Sequestrated lung is **defined as** "a congenital mass of aberrant pulmonary tissue that has no normal connection with the bronchial tree or with the pulmonary arteries".

It is **usually located** in one of the basal segments of lower lobe. In 98 percent cases intralobar sequestration involves medial parts of left lower lobe. 98 percent of extralobar sequestrations are left sided.

Two varieties of pulmonary sequestration are known: Intra and extralobar type.

Extralobar Sequestration

Extralobar Sequestration (ELS) is the most common variety in neonates and infants, is located between the lower lobe and diaphragm, has its own pleural covering, and other anomalies are common (65%)

in ELS (like pulmonary hypoplasia, horseshoe lung, CCAM, bronchogenic cysts, diaphragmatic hernia and cardiac anomalies).

Intralobar Sequestration

Intralobar sequestration (ILS) diagnosed after adolescence, contained within lung with no separate pleural covering and is intimately connected to adjacent lung.

It is usually supplied by an anomalous artery arising from aorta and its venous drainage is via the azygos system, the pulmonary vein, or IVC. Hence, angiography is **useful for confirmation of the diagnosis**, which shows one or more systemic vessel entering the mass, usually arising from aorta at or below diaphragm.

The **imaging modality of choice for pulmonary sequestration is CECT now**. Doppler ultrasound may, sometimes, demonstrate the vascular connection to the sequestration.

Congenital Diaphragmatic Hernia

- It is the most common intrathoracic fetal anomaly due to absence of closure of pleuroperitoneal canal by 9th week of gestation
- Presents as respiratory distress in neonatal period due to life-threatening deficiency of small airways and alveoli, and scaphoid abdomen.
- *CXR*:
  - Bowel loops in chest.
  - Contralateral mediastinal shift.
  - Complete/partial absence of diaphragm.
  - Absence of stomach/small bowel in abdomen.

It Occurs in Two Locations
1. Posterolateral pleuroperitoneal canal (Bochdalek hernia)—common
2. Anteromedial pleuroperitoneal canal (Morgagni hernia)—rare

Left sided (Bochdalek) hernias are much more frequent than right sided.

- **Bochdalek's hernia** usually causes severe respiratory distress in neonate and is one of the most common congenital anomalies of thorax.
- The neonatal radiograph shows a left sided large intrathoracic mass of soft tissue density and the more characteristic pattern of intrathoracic air-filled loops developing after several hours.

- The differential diagnosis of other cystic appearing intrathoracic masses in newborn is lobar emphysema, CALD, pulmonary sequestration, bronchogenic cyst, etc.
- The diagnosis is frequently now made prenatally at ANC USG or MRI and involves left pleuroperitoneal canal in 75 percent cases.
- On USG, congenital diaphragmatic hernia can be detected as early as at 17th week of gestation.
- Small intestine in 88 percent, stomach in 60 percent, colon in 56 percent, spleen in 45 percent, liver in 51 percent and kidney is in 22 percent chances of herniation into chest in Bochdalek hernia.
- Mediastinal deviation is often seen first and is the **most obvious USG sign** of CDH.
- **Absolute diagnostic ultrasonographic sign** is visualization of peristalsis in chest and paradoxical motion of the abdominal contents on fetal inspiration.
- Supportive signs include mediastinal shift, heart displaced to the side opposite to herniation with only sometimes heart axis being changed, stomach in chest, abdominal circumference lower than fifth percentile for gestational age and polyhydramnios.
- Pulmonary hypertension is the most vital prognostic determinant of CDH.
- Other prognostically vital parameter are degree of lung hypoplasia and time of operative correction.
- The appropriate time to operate a case of CDH is debatable but should certainly be done after 24 to 48 hours of birth.
- In Morgagni hernia, omentum and colon are the most frequent hernial contents. It is known to be associated with trisomy syndromes. It usually presents as opacity at® and cardiophrenic angle in adults, mostly asymptomatic. Thirteen pairs of ribs and non-vertebral anomalies occur in association with a Bochdalek's congenital diaphragmatic hernia.

Congenital Cystic Adenomatoid Lung Malformation

- It is congenital cystic abnormality of lung characterized by a interlobar mass of disorganized pulmonary tissue.
- Presents with respiratory distress and severe cyanosis in first week of life (66%) or within first year of life (90%)
  - Equal frequency in all lobes seen
  - *Three types are known:* microcystic, macrocystic and mixed type.
- CXR:
  - Unilateral expansile mass with well-defined margins (80%)
  - Multiple air/occasionally fluid-filled
  - Compression of adjacent lung cysts

- Contralateral mediastinal shift (87%)
- Hypoplastic ipsilateral lung
- Proper position of abdominal viscera
- Spontaneous pneumothorax (late sign)
- CT scan is confirmatory test in congenital cystic adenomatoid malformation (CCAM).

Congenital Lobar Emphysema (CLE)

- Progressive overinflation of one or multiple lobes, usually of the upper lobes or right middle lobe (left upper lobe → 43 percent, right middle → 32 percent, right upper → 20 percent and lower lobe 5%)
- Thus, location: Let upper lobe (LUL) most common (43%)
- The word emphysema is misnomer as there is no alveolar wall destruction
- The etiology is unknown in many cases but is related to obstruction of the bronchus by a ball valve mechanism.
- Present with respiratory distress (90%) with progressive cyanosis within 6 months of life.
- Male to female ratio is 3:1.
- Associated congenital anomalies (cardiovascular) are seen in 50 percent cases.
- CXR:
    - Hazy mass like opacity immediately following birth
    - Air trapping
    - Hyperlucent expanded lobe after clearing of fluid
    - Contralateral mediastinal shift
    - Widely separated/reduced vascular markings
- CT scans are useful in indeterminate cases
- *Treatment* is by lung resection.

McLeod's (Swyer-James) Syndrome/Unilateral Hyperlucent Lung Syndrome

- Obliterative bronchiolitis resulting from childhood viral infection may occasionally affect one lung and present in adult life as Swyer-James syndrome.
- CXR may show pulmonary hyperinflation, and decreased vascularity in unilateral lung field.
- HRCT is characterized by unilateral lung hypoattenuation, bronchiectasis, and air trapping.

Foregut Duplication Cysts

Bronchogenic Cysts

Bronchogenic cysts are usually solitary asymptomatic mediastinal masses which may present at any age. Typically they are thin-walled with a respiratory or enteric mucosal lining, which often contains cartilage and mucous glands. The cyst contents usually consist of thick mucoid material. The cysts can grow very large without causing symptoms, but they compress surrounding structures.

They are often narrow and displace the trachea and can cause life-threatening airway obstruction. They are usually found beside the trachea or between the trachea and the esophagus.

Cystic duplication of the tracheobronchial free, presently usually as mediastinal mass, but intrapulmonary is also known.

Esophageal Duplication Cyst

Esophageal duplication cyst is round or tubular lesion occurring in the lower posterior mediastinum, which often distort esophagus but only rarely communicate with the esophageal lumen. A chest X-ray may show a right-sided mediastinal mass and *associated vertebral anomalies* like hemivertebra, block vertebra, butterfly vertebra or spina bifida, if present. Proximal esophageal duplication cysts may be associated with tracheal compression and present with upper airway obstruction. While distal esophageal cysts are often asymptomatic and found as an incidental chest X-ray finding. Barium meal will confirm the presence of a smooth extrinsic esophageal filling defect and CT/MRI will demonstrate its cystic nature.

Neuroenteric Cyst

Neuroenteric cyst/esophageal duplication cyst is round or tubular lesion occurring in the lower posterior mediastinum, which often distort esophagus but only rarely communicate with the esophageal lumen. A chest X-ray may show a right-sided mediastinal mass and *associated vertebral anomalies* like hemivertebra, block vertebra, butterfly vertebra or spina bifida, if present. Proximal esophageal duplication cysts may be associated with tracheal compression and present with upper airway obstruction. While distal esophageal cysts are often asymptomatic and found as an incidental chest X-ray finding. Barium meal will confirm the presence of a smooth extrinsic esophageal filling defect and CT/MRI will demonstrate its cystic nature.

FOREIGN BODY ASPIRATION

Due to straighter, broader and short right bronchus with only 25° angle of bifurcation, foreign body aspiration is common on right side. However, the right and left main stem bronchi are same and above said things are not true for children.

Aspiration pneumonitis or aspiration of foreign body **in supine position** usually affects posterior segment of right upper lobe or the foreign body will be lodged into posterior segment bronchus of right upper lobe.

While the foreign body aspirated in upright position will be lodged into superior or apical segment of right lower lobe (gravity dependent areas usually affected).

Specific affection almost invariably in **pulmonary sequestration** includes posterobasal segment of left lower lobe.

PULMONARY INFECTIONS

Bronchopneumonia is multifocal, heterogeneous inflammatory involvement of distal airways, with distribution along vessels is usually absent and volume loss is common with occasional pneumatocele formation.

Lobar pneumonia is usually the localized disease. It spreads rapidly via the **pores of Kohn and canals of Lambert** across segmental boundaries producing a uniform consolidation in lung parenchyma. It spares distal airways.

Staphylococcal Pneumonia

- Infection with *S. aureus* is the most commonly seen in infancy or in older immunocompromised child
- Most commonly seen in infancy or in older immunocompromised child
- Pyoderma, caused by Staph can disseminate or be associated with lung infection
- In acute phase à necrotic, cavitating pneumonias with associated pleural-effusion
- Often multifocal and bilateral
- No lobar predilection
- Bronchopneumonia
- Air bronchogram is unusual
- Characteristic pneumatoceles (thin walled cavities secondary to localized pulmonary destruction)
- Even after clinical resolution of acute illness **ghost cavities** (Pneumatocele) may persist for months on radiograph
- Multiple lung abscesses

- Bronchopleural fistula
- Empyema
- Hydropneumothorax
- Pneumothorax
- In acute phase it may cause a necrotic, cavitating pneumonia and associated pleural effusion
- It is often multifocal and bilateral
- Airbronchogram is unusual
- It leads to pneumatocele formation, which are thin walled cavities secondary to localized pulmonary destruction
- Even after clinical resolution of acute illness, **ghost cavities (pneumatoceles)** may persist for months on radiograph
- Drugs for treatment of VRSA include *Quinupristin, Dalfopristin, Teicoplanin,* and *Linezolid.*

Klebsiella Pneumoniae

- Caused by **Friedlander's bacillus**.
- Typically affects elderly debilitated men.
- Usually causes lobar consolidation, more often right sided, and frequently upper lobar.
- The volume of affected lung may be increased due to copious exudation of fluid producing typical **"Bulging fissure" or "Bow fissure" sign**.
- Cavitation is also known.

Mycoplasma Pneumoniae

Mycoplasma pneumoniae are a major nonbacterial cause of community-acquired pneumonia in patients of 20 to 40 years. The onset is gradual with fever, malaise, headache and sore throat. Early in the course of disease there is a characteristic but nonspecific *rise of the serum cold agglutinins*. The definitive diagnosis is, however, made by detecting a rise in complement fixation titer, a delayed manifestation. Radiological evidence of unilateral lower-lobe involvement beginning at hilum and fanning out to the periphery as a patchy, heterogeneous, frequently segmental, peribronchial consolidation that may progress to become lobar and homogeneous is *the most common and typical pattern* of involvement. CT demonstrates ground glass and homogeneous opacities, centrilobular nodules and bronchovascular thickening. Majority of HIV-infected patients, who develop *P. carinii* pneumonia present with fever, dyspnea, nonproductive cough, weakness and weight loss. The CXR in most patients of PCP demonstrates bilateral, diffuse, symmetrical, and fine to medium reticular opacities. However, *Mycoplasma* may, sometimes, show evidence of bilateral interstitial pattern.

Pulmonary Tuberculosis

Mycobacterium Tuberculosis Infection

Primary TB
- Ghon's complex
- Pleural/pericardial involvement
- Tuberculoma
- Regional adenopathy
- Miliary TB
- Extrapulmonary TB.

Secondary TB (Postprimary TB)
- Acinar consolidation
- Tuberculoma (caseation)
- Cavitation
- Endobronchial spread
- Miliary TB.

Ghon's focus (primary focus of TB) → Often present in mid zone of lung, located peripherally in subpleural region and right side is affected more than left. Associated hilar adenopathy common.

Simon's focus → During early bacillemia, seeding may occur in lung apex.

Puhl's lesion → The most common site of isolated lesion of chronic pulmonary TB is apex of the lung because the blood flow is sluggish at the apex and diffusion is poor.

Ashman's focus → Infraclavicular lesion of chronic pulmonary TB

	TB Primary pulmonary	Secondary/Postprimary reactivation/Reinfection/Adult TB
Inactive	1. Normal radiograph 2. Scarring (any site) + sequelae 3. Calcification (nodes, lung)	1. Normal radiograph 2. Scarring (restricted site) + sequelae 3. Calcification (nodes, lung and pleura)
Active	1. Consolidation (any site) 2. Adenopathy + sequelae 3. Effusion (pleural, pericardial) 4. Miliary TB 5. Other (e.g. bone)	1. Consolidation (restricted site) 2. Endobronchial lesion + sequelae 3. Effusion (pleural, pericardial) 4. Miliary TB 5. Other (e.g. bone)
Indeterminate acivity	1. Tuberculoma	1. Tuberculoma

Restricted site = Apical and posterior segment of upper lobes and superior segment of lower lobes.

Bronchoscopy is important for the diagnosis of tuberculosis (TB) with cultures of BAL fluid producing the most sensitive (over 90%) single test result. In patients with confirmed TB whose prebronchoscopy sputum samples are smear-negative, about half have smear-positive BAL fluid. Transbronchial biopsy (TBBX) is a useful adjunct, because it occasionally reveals the presence of granulomas with mycobacteria in the setting of a smear-negative BAL. BAL is also useful for the diagnosis of nontuberculous mycobacteria, although these organisms can colonize the airway and should be treated only in the appropriate setting.

Mycobacterium Avium Intracellular Complex (MAC) Infection: CXR

- Patchy unilateral/bilateral air-space consolidation
- Small or nodular lesions
- Bronchiectasis
- Cavitations (thick or thin walled)
- Middle lobe syndrome.

Pneumocystis Carinii Pneumonia

Pneumocystis carinii pneumonia (PCP) infection is common in children as in adults.
 The child is usually pyrexial and hypoxemic and may rapidly progress to respiratory failure.
 Pneumothorax may complicate mechanical ventilation due to rupture of pneumatoceles.
The CXR shows progressive bilateral infiltrate evolving to bilateral diffuse airspace opacification.
- In general, CXR in most patients shows bilateral, diffuse, symmetrical, fine to medium reticular opacities.
- These infiltrates may be confined to one to two lobes or segments of lung.
- Sometimes upper lobe predominance may be seen which may be possibly enhanced by use of inhaled (aerosolized) *pentamidine*.
- Unusual radiographic presentation includes:
  - Diffuse or focal miliary nodules
  - Focal airspace consolidation
  - Solitary or multiple well-formed nodules
  - Moderate to thick walled cavitary nodules
  - Normal chest film
  - Pneumatoceles in 10 percent cases (thin walled)
  - Pneumothorax in 5 percent cases with or without bronchopleural fistula

- The radiographic appearance often gets worse during the first three days of therapy, especially with IV trimethoprim (the drug of choice for *P. carinii* infection) probably due to the over-hydration pulmonary edema and due to the inflammatory reaction related to dead and dying parasites.

CXR Feature of *Pneumocystis Carinii* Infection

Bilateral, diffuse, symmetrical, fine to medium reticular opacities. It may be confined to one or two lobes or segments of lung. In some cases infiltrates in upper lobe may predominate and simulate reactive TB, which was possibly a feature enhanced by the use of inhaled pentamidine in past for chemoprophylaxis.

Unusual features include

Diffuse or focal miliary nodules, focal airspace consolidation and moderate to thick walled cavitary nodules and solitary or multiple well-formed nodules. Approximately 5 to 10 percent of patients will have normal chest films at presentation. Pleural fluid and lymphadenopathy are not radiographic features of the infection as such. Pneumatoceles are seen in 10 percent of patients, which are characteristically thin walled, may rapidly increase or decrease in size and over the course of 2 to 3 months resolve gradually. In 5 percent cases spontaneous pneumothorax has been observed which range in size from very small to extremely large, and associated bronchopleural fistulae are common. Radiographic changes generally follow the clinical course of disease and appropriate therapy usually leads to definite radiographic improvement within 10 days.

Summary of PCP
- Common in AIDS patients
- High risk if CD4 counts in HIV positive patients are below 200/mcL
- Patchy bilateral ground-glass opacity
- Central or perihilar distribution characteristic
- Pneumatocele and pneumothorax in 10 percent cases, especially after aerosolized pentamidine therapy
- Interlobular septal thickening (resolving)
- Centrilobular nodules.

Hydatid Disease of Lung

Hydatid disease of lung is the most common site of secondary involvement in children.
- Lower lobes affected in 60 percent cases.
- Calcification of cyst wall is very rare and seen only in 0.7 percent cases.

- When in mediastinum, vertebral erosion in addition to rib erosion may occur with posterior mediastinum being affected in 65 percent cases. May be complicated by bacterial infection after cyst ruptures.

Radiological Signs

- **Meniscus/double arch/moon/crescent sign** due to thin radiolucent crescent in uppermost part of cyst.
- **Combo sign** due to air fluid level inside endocyst and air between pericyst and endocyst.
- Collapsed membranes inside the cyst outlined by air causing **serpent sign**.
- Completely collapsed crumpled cyst membrane floating on the cyst fluid produces **Water Lily sign** of Camelot.
- Cyst-in-cyst sign.

Allergic Bronchopulmonary Aspergillosis

Primary Diagnostic Criteria for Allergic Bronchopulmonary Aspergillosis (ABPA)

- Asthma (84–96%) (Episodes of bronchospasm)
- Roentgenographic transient or fixed pulmonary infiltrates
- Test for *Aspergillus fumigatus* positive (skin)
- Eosinophilia (8–40%)
- Precipitating antibodies to *Aspergillus fumigatus* (70%)
- IgE in serum elevated
- Central (perihilar) bronchiectasis (late manifestation that proves diagnosis)
- Serum specific IgE and IgG *Aspergillus fumigatus* levels elevated.

Secondary Diagnostic Criteria (Less Common)

- *Aspergillus fumigatus* mycelia in sputum
- Expectoration of brown sputum plugs (54%)
- Arthus reaction to *Aspergillus* antigen.
- Fungal ball with 'air crescent' surrounding it (**Air crescent or Monads' sign**) is characteristic of aspergilloma.

Fungal infection is another important source of morbidity in non-HIV immunocompromised hosts. Aspergillus is a common cause of fungal disease in this setting. BAL is reported to be 50 percent to 67 percent sensitive for active Aspergillus infection. *Unfortunately, the presence of fungus on BAL is not specific for active infection because Aspergillus can colonize the airway in immunocompromised hosts.* Consequently, TBBX is often also performed because the presence of tissue invasion on TBBX unequivocally establishes a diagnosis of invasive disease.

Candida Albicans Pneumonia

It may rarely occur in severely immunocompromised/neutropenic patients with leukemia or lymphoma, and lung disease usually develops as a part of hematogenous dissemination, often as a preterminal event. The CXR findings may include *widespread bilateral interstitial or fluffy alveolar infiltrates or lobar segmental consolidation.* The isolation of *Candida* species from bronchoscopic specimens is common because of oropharyngeal and gastrointestinal contamination of BAL specimens. Fortunately, *Candida* pneumonitis is rare even in severely immunocompromised hosts, so unless TBBX confirms tissue invasion, most clinicians do not treat *Candida* present in BAL fluid.

LUNG COLLAPSE

Partial or complete loss of volume of a lung is referred as collapse or atelectasis.

Types:
- Relaxation/passive collapse, e.g. pleural effusion with underlying lung collapse
- Cicatrization collapse, e.g. pulmonary fibrosis
- Adhesive collapse, ARDS, HMD
- Resorption/obstructive collapse, e.g. endobronchial obstruction.

Direct signs of collapse:
- Displacement of interlobar fissures
- Loss of aeration and with obscuration of the adjacent structures
- Crowding of vessels and bronchi.

Indirect signs of collapse:
- Elevation of the hemidiaphragm
- Mediastinal displacement
- Hilar displacement
- Compensatory hyperinflation.

Special Signs of Collapse

- **Rounded atelectasis** → Comet tail sign (vascular shadows seen radiating from opacity)
- **Golden S sign** → Right hilar/central mass with upper lobe collapse seen as convexity at the medial aspect of pulled up major fissure
- **Broncholobar sign** → Lower lobe bronchus is displayed within the opacity of the collapsed left lower lobe
- **Luftsichel sign** → The hyperextended superior segment of the ipsilateral lower lobe accounts for the paramediastinal lucency outlining the medial surface of the collapsed right or left upper lobe.

Following laparotomy it has been established that half of all patients develop some postoperative pulmonary collapse. Volume loss is most often attributed to hypoventilation and retained secretions and seen as **plate-like or discoid atelectasis** especially in LLZ. Subdiaphragmatic pathology may affect LLZ in the form of **Fleischner's plate atelectasis**, i.e. most commonly to be **subphrenic abscess**. However, the subsegmental or plate-like atelectasis as such appears about 24 hours postoperatively and resolves in 2 to 3 days.

Pleural Diseases

Pleural Effusion

- A small amount of free fluid may be undetectable on an erect PA chest film, as it tends initially to collect under the lower lobes of lung. Such small subpulmonary effusions can be demonstrated on lateral decubitus chest radiograph, which has largely been replaced now by newer techniques like USG or CT.
- This view with affected side dependent provides a sensitive means of detecting small quantities of pleural fluid (50–100 mL).
- The posterior and then the lateral costophrenic angles become blunted as the amount of effusion increases, by which time a 200 to 500 mL effusion is present.
- Following this classical signs develop.
- First 300 mL of pleural fluid collection is not visualized on PA view (collected in subpulmonic region first, then spill into posterior costophrenic recess).
- Lateral decubitus views may demonstrate small amount of pleural fluid (as small as 25 mL).
- This view with affected side dependent provides a sensitive means of detecting small quantities of pleural fluid (50–100 mL).

Etiology of Pleural Effusion
Causes of left-sided pleural effusion
- Spontaneous esophageal perforation
- Dissecting aneurysm of aorta
- Traumatic rupture of aorta distal to left subclavian artery
- Transection of distal thoracic duct
- Pancreatic and gastric neoplasm
- Pancreatitis [left sided (68%), right sided (10%), bilateral (22%)].

Causes of right-sided pleural effusion
- Congestive heart failure
- Transection of proximal thoracic duct.

Loculated Pleural Effusion

Fluid can loculate between visceral pleural layers in fissures or between visceral and parietal layers, usually against the chest wall. Fissural interlobar loculation is seen particularly in heart failure and may produce the so-called **phantom tumor/vanishing tumor**.

On lateral view, it is sharply marginated and biconvex and has a tail passing along fissure. A common problem is to differentiate encysted fluid in lower right oblique fissure from middle lobe collapse.

Factors, which favor a collapsed and consolidated middle lobe rather than an effusion, include nonhomogeneity, a straight or concave border in **lateral view**, wedge-like outline with base reaching the sternum and absence of minor fissure.

Fluid loculated against chest-wall, viewed tangentially appears as a localized homogeneous opacity, convex to the lung and sharp edged, with a rather low profile that tails off against chest wall. Enface it has features typical of pleural shadow, with one-edge sharp and other fading off. Extrapleural sign is positive, i.e. the opacity is pleural based with obtuse angle between the medial margin and chest wall on PA CXR.

Pneumothorax

Spontaneous pneumothorax is the most common, and it occurs most commonly due to rupture of *subpleural blebs*.

CXR

- Sharp white visceral pleural line
- Radiolucent pleural space devoid of lung markings
- Underlying collapse of lung

- A large pneumothorax may, sometimes, lead to complete relaxation and retraction of the lung, with some mediastinal shift towards the normal side, which increases on inspiration.

Tension pneumothorax
- Massive displacement of mediastinum
- Kinking of the great vessels
- Ipsilateral lung squashed against the mediastinum, or herniated across the midline
- Depressed or inverted ipsilateral dome of diaphragm.

BRONCHIECTASIS, INDUSTRIAL AND INTERSTITIAL LUNG DISEASES

Radiographic Features of Bronchiectasis

- 'Bunch of grapes' appearance ⎫
- 'Gloved fingered' appearance ⎭ X-ray signs
- 'Ring' shadows ⎫
- 'Tram track' appearance ⎭ X-ray signs
- Signet ring sign on HRCT.

Silicosis

Silicosis occurs due to inhalation of SiO_2.

CXR
- Multiple small (miliary) nodules in mid and upper zones
- Enlargement of hilar nodes with peripheral eggshell calcification
- Presence of nodal calcification may allow differentiating it from CWP
- Aggregation of nodules with formation of larger conglomerate areas of progressive massive fibrosis is hallmark of complicated silicosis
- *Snowstorm appearance* on CXR is characteristic of it.

Incidence of pulmonary TB is higher in patient with silicosis.
Caplan's syndrome is silicosis with RA.

Asbestosis

It is characterized by specific pleural and parenchymal changes (thoracic changes) and some extrathoracic changes.

Pleural Changes

- **The most common radiological feature of asbestos** exposure is the pleural plaque, which is well-defined soft tissue sheet originating on the parietal pleural. The extent of the plaques is related to the severity of exposure. There is a latent period of over 10 years between exposure and plaque development, and calcification within the plaques is rarely seen less than 20 years after exposure. The lesions are usually bilateral, lying in middle and lower zones and over the diaphragm. When calcified they form a **'holly leaf' pattern** with sharp, often angulated outlines.
- Diffuse pleural thickening especially in bases
- Pleural effusions
- Malignant mesothelioma
- Pseudotumor
- Bronchogenic carcinoma.

Pulmonary Changes

The radiological features are similar to those of fibrosing alveolitis.
- Unlike CWP, UZ are spared even in smokers (100 times the rate in nonsmokers).
- Pulmonary pseudotumor can be a feature, which characteristically shows distortion of pulmonary vasculature producing a 'Comet tail' appearance on plain X-ray, and CT.
- 'Comet tail' appearance is also seen in Round atelectasis.

Extrathoracic changes: Peritoneal mesothelioma and laryngeal carcinoma.

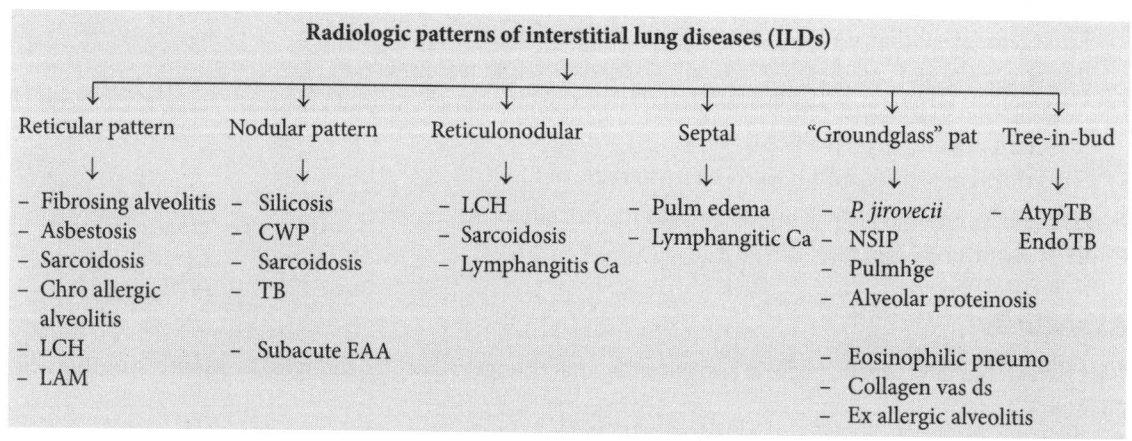

Lymphangiitis Carcinomatosa

It is permeation of pulmonary lymphatics by neoplastic cells.
The most common tumors that spread in this manner are:
- Bronchogenic carcinoma
- Carcinoma breast
- Pancreatic cancer
- Carcinoma stomach
- Carcinoma colon, and
- Carcinoma prostate.

It may be segmental, lobar, unilateral or bilateral.

CXR
- Fine reticulonodular shadowing (more often bilateral and symmetrical)
- Thickened septal lines
- Subpleural edema seen as thickening of fissures
- Pleural effusion.

HRCT
- Nodular shadow scattered throughout the lung parenchyma
- Nonuniform, nodular, thickening of interlobular septa and irregular thickening of bronchovascular bundles
- Patchy air space shadowing
- Acini subtended by thickened interlobular septa are aerated normally
- The abnormalities may involve all zones of both lungs or they may be centrally or peripherally predominant
- Hilar node enlargement is seen only in few patients.

Lymphangioleiomyomatosis

It is characterized by the presence of abnormal smooth muscle proliferation of pulmonary interstitium, particularly in bronchioles, vessels and lymphatics.

It is a rare disease seen exclusively in females, especially of childbearing age group.

CXR
- Bilateral reticular pattern with ring shadows and normal or increased lung volume
- Chylous pleural effusion
- Recurrent pneumothorax.

HRCT

Numerous thin-walled randomly distributed cysts throughout the lungs with normal intervening parenchyma and zonal predilection (virtually diagnostic/pathognomonic feature).

Caplan's Syndrome

Pneumoconiosis with multiple lung nodules with rheumatoid arthritis in coalmine workers with the rheumatoid disease constitute Caplan's syndrome.

Wegener's Granulomatosis

- Mean age of set is approximately 40 years.
- It is characterized by granulomatous vasculitis of upper and lower respiratory tracts (85-90% patients) with glomerulonephritis (77% cases).
- Proteinuria, hematuria with RBC casts can occur.
- CNS involvement is seen in 23 percent cases only.
- Eye involvement may be seen in 50 percent cases.
- Characteristic cavitating lung nodules of varying size (mm to cm) occur without zonal predilection.
- The majority of patients with Wegener's granulomatosis develop nodules that are of varying size from few mm to several cm and have no zonal predilection.
- On CT, a feeding vessel leading to nodules and air bronchogram on it may be seen. Linear bands, spiculations and pleural tags may also be seen in the relation.
- Cavitation is characteristic of it.
- Consolidation and groundglass opacities are also recognized features.

Sjögren's Syndrome

- It is chronic autoimmune inflammatory disease characterized by a triad of dry mouth, dry eyes and arthritis.
- It occurs (60%) in association with other collagen vascular disease, especially rheumatoid arthritis; however, in contrast to latter, there is marked female predominance of pulmonary manifestations.
- Interstitial fibrosis similar to cryptogenic fibrosing alveolitis mainly affecting lower zones and occurrence of lymphocytic interstitial pneumonitis is seen.
- Skin nodules are not seen.

Sarcoidosis

Staging of sarcoidosis according to its appearance on CXR:
Stage I: Lymphadenopathy
Stage II: Lymphadenopathy with parenchyma opacity
Stage III: Parenchymal opacity alone.

Lymphadenopathy

- Encountered in 70 to 80 percent patients
- Bilateral, symmetrical hilar and paratracheal
- Tracheobronchial and bronchopulmonary nodes also affected
- AP windows node enlargement also common
- Only in 1 to 5 percent lymphadenopathy is asymmetrical
- 'Eggshell' calcification can occur
- In 90 percent cases lymphadenopathy disappears within 6 to 12 months.

> **Differential Diagnosis of "Eggshell nodal" Calcification**
> *Common causes*: Sarcoidosis, silicosis
> *Uncommon causes*: Histoplasmosis, lymphoma (postirradiation), blastomycosis, amyloidosis.

Parenchymal Changes

About 50 to 70 percent of patients show parenchymal changes.
These are of three types:
1. Reversible changes
2. Irreversible (fibrotic) changes
3. Mixed.

Reversible

- Encountered in 70 to 80 percent patients
- 2 to 4 mm (5 mm) opacities
- Sometimes aggregate to give ground glass opacities
- Bilateral symmetrical involvement
- Mid and upper zonal predominance.

Irreversible
- Encountered in 10 to 20 percent patients
- Patchy airspace consolidation
- Usually multiple
- Peribronchovascular regions of MMZZ and UZ predominantly affect
- Eighty percent of patients with consolidation have nodal enlargement.

Mixed
Multiple bilateral nodules 10 to 40 mm size.

Complications of Fibrosing Stage
- Traction bronchiectasis/Bullae
- Cor pulmonale
- Mycetoma
- Pneumothorax.

HRCT features
- 1 to 5 mm nodules in perilymphatic fashion predominantly along bronchovascular bundles subpleurally
- Airspace consolidation
- Airway wall thickening
- Patchy ground-glass opacities
- UZ, MZ fibrosis
- Pleural effusions and thickening are unusual. The prevalence of effusions in only about 2 percent and their presence should raise doubts about diagnosis of sarcoidosis
- Bronchial stenosis and airflow obstruction can rarely occur.

In sarcoidosis granulomas, are without necrosis.

Causes of nonsarcoid granulomas, i.e. granulomas with necrotic area are:
- TB
- Gumma
- Cryptococcosis
- Histoplasmosis
- Coccidioidomycosis
- Nocardiasis
- Foreign body granulomas
- Histiocytosis

- Vasculitides
- Chronic granulomatous disease
- Extrinsic allergic alveolitis.

Summary

Rheumatoid arthritis	Lung nodules
Scleroderma	Progressive pulmonary fibrosis
SLE	'Shrinking lung' syndrome
Wegener's granulomatosis	Cavitating lung lesions
Sarcoidosis	Bilateral symmetrical hilar adenopathy
	Parenchymal, interstitial and pleural changes
Goodpasture's syndrome	Diffuse pulmonary hemorrhage
Sjögren's syndrome	Interstitial fibrosis similar to cryptogenic fibrosing alveolitis mainly affecting lower zones and lymphocytic interstitial pneumonitis.

Hypersensitivity Pneumonitis

A wide variety of respirable organic dusts are capable of causing restrictive pulmonary impairment and systemic manifestations. These reactions may be manifested in the lung as either a diffuse interstitial pneumonitis or the syndrome of pulmonary infiltrates with eosinophilia (PIE). The chest radiograph frequently shows bilateral peripheral alveolar infiltrates that may be migratory. "Reverse batwing" pattern is well-recognized CXR feature (resembling *photonegative pulmonary edema*). But when the reaction is of diffuse type, features overlap with those of Diffuse Alveolar Damage, and the differences may be largely semantic.

Important facts	
HRCT	Disease
Reticular pattern	– Many ILDs
Multiple cysts	– Lymphangioleiomyomatosis (LAM)
	– Pulmonary histiocytosis
Lepidote growth	– Bronchoalveolar cancer
Crazy paving	– Alveolar proteinosis > silicosis
"Tree-in-bud" appearance	– Endobronchial TB and
	– Atypical mycobacterial TB

NEOPLASMS

Solitary Pulmonary Nodule

A solitary pulmonary nodule (SPN) is any pulmonary or pleural sharply defined discrete nearly circular radiopacity of <3 cm but >2 cm diameter.

It is called mass when the diameter exceeds 3 cm.

Characterization of SPN

Properties	Benign	Malignant
Size	<2 cm	>3 cm
Doubling time	Longer (18 months)	1–6 months
Margin/Edge	Smooth, well-defined	Irregular, spiculated or notched
Contour	Sharply marginated	Lobulated
Cavitation	Thin, smooth walled	Thick, irregular walled
Calcification	Central, solid, laminated 'popcorn' like (hamartoma)	Peripheral, diffuse, amorphous, rarely punctate
Fat (intranodular)	Seen in hamartoma	—
Internal attenuation	Homogeneous	Bubble like areas of low attenuation.
Pseudocavitation with airbronchogram	Bronchoalveolar carcinoma and lymphoma show significant enhancement on CECT.	
Satellite lesions	99 percent inflammatory lesions show it (TB)	Only 1 percent
Bone destruction	No	Yes
PET scan	<2.5 SUV	>2.5 SUV

About 40 percent of SPN are malignant. A lateral film is often necessary to confirm that a lesion is intrapulmonary. Typically an acute angle with the lung whereas extrapleural and mediastinal masses form obtuse angle. Lung markings (bronchovascular) are not seen through an intrapulmonary mass. A search for associated abnormalities such as effusions, lobar collapse, septal lines and lymphadenopathy should also be made. Tumors smaller than 10 mm cannot be seen on a plain film and often appear as a 'Smudge' shadow rather than a nodule/mass.

Causes of calcifying malignant lung lesions **include, carcinoid (33%), lung cancer (6%), metastases from chondrosarcoma and mucinous adenocarcinoma metastases.**

Morphological features of a solitary pulmonary nodule (SPN) or mass suggesting whether malignant or benign are:

Features	Benign	Malignant
Size	<2 cm	>3 cm
Margin/edge and contour	Smooth, well-defined	Lobulated, spiculated ("Corona radiata") and "Pleural tail"
Cavitation	Thin smooth walled	Thick, irregular walled
Calcification	Peripheral	Diffuse, amorphous
Satellite lesion	Absent	Present
Pseudocavitation and airbronchogram	—	Bronchoalveolar carcinoma or lymphoma
Intranodular fat	Hamartoma	—
Attenuation	Homogeneous	Heterogeneous

Except for complications like pneumothorax in 5 to 30 percent cases, pleural collection in 15 percent cases and rarely self-limiting hemorrhage, transthoracic fine needle aspiration biopsy remains the investigation of choice for solitary pulmonary nodules (SPN) with up to 91 percent sensitivity and 95 to 100 percent for 10 to 15 mm sized malignancies.

PET is another *noninvasive* method to distinguish benign from malignant focal pulmonary abnormalities. It can provide biochemical information about lesions that are indeterminate by conventional imaging methods. 18F-2-deoxy-D-glucose (FDG), a D-glucose analog, is the most commonly used radionuclide. *Increased glucose metabolism by malignant lesions results in increased uptake, trapping and accumulation of FDG, which permits differentiation from most benign abnormalities.* It accurately excludes malignancy in pulmonary nodules as small as 1 cm.

Investigation for SPN	Sensitivity	Specificity	Accuracy
Transthoracic fine needle aspiration biopsy	95–100 percent	91 percent	—
PET (FDG) scan	92–100 percent	52–100 percent	94 percent
CECT	98 percent	73 percent	85 percent
HRCT	—	—	—
MRI	—	—	—

Pulmonary Hamartomas

- The most common benign lung tumor.
- These are benign lung neoplasms with average age of presentation being 40 to 45 years.

- They consist of masses of cartilage with clefts lined by bronchial epithelium, which may contain large collections of fat.

Malignant transformations are either nonexistent/extremely rare.

Carney's triad: Pulmonary chondromas
Gastric leiomyosarcoma
Extra-adrenal paragangliomas
90 percent are peripheral in location.

CXR: Spherical or slightly lobulated well-defined nodule (<4 cm size) with normal surrounding lung, 'popcorn' calcification and frequency of calcification increases with the size of lesion.

CT: *Popcorn calcification* is virtually diagnostic (only DD is a Chondrosarcoma) and central fat density if present also establishes the diagnosis.

Lung Carcinoma

Features	Adenocarcinoma	Squamous	Small cell	Large cell
Percent	50 percent	30–35 percent	15 percent	<5 percent
Sex	Most common Bro. Ca. of female	—	—	—
Smokers	—	Strong association	Strong association	Strong association
Location	Almost invariably peripheral, frequent in scars, upper lobar distribution	Central (2/3) SPN (1/3)	90 percent central	Large peripheral
Metastasis	Early mets, low	Lowest mets	High mets	Early mets
Growth rate	Slow GR	Slowest	Rapid	Rapid
Malignant potential	Intermediate	Least	High	Internal
Pancoast tumor (Chest wall invasion)	—	Most common	—	—
Calcification	1 percent	+	—	—
Cavitation	—	+	—	—
Paraneoplastic syndrome	—	—	Most common	—
Lung to lung metastasis	Most common	—	—	—
Mediastinal adenopathy	+/−	—	—	+
Scar cancer	—	+	—	—

Small cell tumors of lung have the *fastest rate of growth*, usually disseminate at the time of presentation, are *usually central* and are typically *associated with mediastinal and hilar adenopathy*, but rarely cavitate while non-small cell tumors, especially the adenocarcinomas usually arise peripherally, sometimes in fibrotic lung and cavitate less often but squamous cell carcinoma arise centrally, gross relatively slowly and cavitate often. Small cell carcinoma of the lung is a more common cause of paraneoplastic syndromes, particularly the *Eaton Lambert* syndrome of myasthenic myopathy and hypercortisolism due to ectopic ACTH production.

- A peripheral pulmonary mass on chest X-ray is a common presentation of lung cancer.
- Few features can also differentiate between a benign and a malignant pulmonary nodule.
- Malignant tumors are usually larger at the time of presentation, have poorly defined, lobulated, spiculated or umbilicated margins, may cavitate with thick walls with irregular nodular inner margin, may have associated bone destruction and asymmetrical pleural thickening.
- Benign lesion like folded lung or diffuse calcification in a nodule can be easily diagnosed on CT thus excluding malignancy.
- Currently low dose spiral CT is used screening for lung cancer effectively.
- Sputum cytology and bronchoscopic biopsies or washings usually provide assessment of endobronchial pathologies and the cell type of central tumors, if any, but peripheral tumors may require percutaneous biopsy.

AJCC-UICC Classification of regional lymph nodes
- Highest mediastinal nodes
- Upper paratracheal nodes
- Prevascular and retrotracheal nodes
- Lower paratracheal nodes
- Subaortic (aortopulmonary window) nodes
- Para-aortic (ascending aorta or phrenic) nodes
- Subcarinal nodes
- Paresophageal nodes
- Pulmonary ligament nodes
- Hilar nodes
- Interlobar nodes
- Lobar nodes
- Segmental nodes
- Subsegmental nodes.

TNM Staging for Lung Cancer

Nx = Regional nodes cannot be assessed
N0 = No demonstrable metastasis to regional nodes
N1 = Metastasis to nodes in peribronchial or ipsilateral hilar region or both
N2 = Metastasis to ipsilateral mediastinal nodes and subcarinal nodes
N3 = Metastasis to contralateral mediastinal nodes, contralateral hilar nodes, ipsilateral or contralateral scalene or supraclavicular nodes

Peribronchial nodes include interlobar, lobar, segmental, and subsegmental nodes.
Thus, involvement of peribronchial or interlobar nodes indicates N1 stage.

Pancoast Tumor

It includes bronchogenic ca, usually squamous cell type, affecting left lung apex, eroding ribs (1st and 2nd) involving brachial plexus and sympathetic chain (Horner's syndrome). MRI is optimal modality to demonstrate the extent of superior sulcus tumor.

Destructed rib lesions occur most commonly in osteomyelitis or neoplastic diseases. Osteomyelitis is uncommon and may be caused by direct spreads from lung and pleural spaces (actinomycosis) or may be hematogenous (*Staphylococcal* or TB). The only other condition that commonly spreads from lung to rib is bronchial Ca including the pancoast or superior sulcus tumor.

Bronchial Artery Embolization

It is a well-accepted and effective form of treatment for massive and/or recurrent hemoptysis.

Patients most commonly treated by bronchial artery embolization (BAE) are those with **chronic TB, bronchiectasis, and mycetoma** as the longstanding pulmonary inflammation in these patients results in the development of hypertrophied systemic arteries that can be selectively catheterized and occluded. It rarely employed for management of bleeding from malignant disease.

In the great majority of patients, hemoptysis originates from systemic rather than pulmonary arteries and the bronchial vessels are almost universally involved and hence should be the first to be evaluated and embolized.

There is considerable variation in the way in which bronchial arteries arise from thoracic aorta but the most common is one main right artery from a common intercostobronchial trunk at T5 level, and two left bronchial arteries arising a little lower.

While evaluating it is vital to remember that virtually any systemic artery in the chest (from intercostal, inferior phrenic, internal mammary, thyrocervical trunk, costocervical and subscapular vessels and other branches of subclavian and axillary arteries) can contribute to bronchial circulation and be a source of continued hemoptysis after successful embolization of the bronchial arteries, and may even be the sole supply to the lesion responsible for hemoptysis.

The pulmonary arteries are culpable in 5 to 10 percent of patients of chronic disorder like TB with **Rasmussen aneurysm** formation. Rasmussen aneurysm is pulmonary artery branch aneurysm seen in a branch traversing the tubercular cavity.

The adrenals are commonly involved in patients with lung and breast carcinoma on one or both sides by metastases.

CT survey of liver is frequently made in these patients, and the adrenals should *always* be carefully imaged during such examinations. On MRI surveys unilateral or bilateral adrenal masses can also be readily identified. **They are best shown as high-signal lesions on T_2 weighted MR images**.

Although with adrenal metastases, the primary is usually in lung and breast, melanoma, renal and gastrointestinal secondaries and secondary lymhomatous involvement are well known.

MEDIASTINUM

Anatomists divide the mediastinum into four parts. The mediastinum is divided into superior and inferior compartments by an imaginary line traversing the manubriosternal joint and the lower surface of the fourth thoracic vertebra. The inferior compartment is further subdivided into three parts: the middle mediastinum, which contains the pericardium and its contents as well as the major vessels and airways; the anterior mediastinum, which lies anterior to the middle mediastinum and posterior to the sternum; and the posterior mediastinum, which lies posterior to the middle mediastinum and anterior to the thoracic vertebral column. A popular modification of this method divides the entire mediastinum into anterior, middle, and posterior compartments but does not recognize a separate superior compartment.

Pneumomediastinum

It is characterized by presence of gas in mediastinal tissues outside the esophagus and tracheobronchial tree.

Signs of Pneumomediastinum on CXR

- **The "Continuous diaphragms" sign:** Describes the presence of radiographically visible mediastinal air between the heart and the diaphragm. The air trapped in mediastinum posterior to pericardium (on frontal view).

- **"Ring around artery" sign:** Air surrounding intramediastinal segment of right pulmonary artery (lateral view).
- **"Tubular artery sign":** Air adjacent to major aortic branches.
- **"Streaky lucencies"** of air in mediastinum.
- **"Double bronchial wall" sign:** Clear depiction of bronchial wall by an air next to and within bronchus.
- **"V sign of Naclerio" or extra-pleural sign** is mediastinal air extending laterally between mediastinal pleura, lower thoracic aorta and diaphragm.
- **"Spinnaker sail" or "thymic sail" sign** is seen in children is the mediastinal air outlines the thymus.

Esophageal perforation is the most common cause of pneumomediastinum.

Hamman's sign (mediastinal crunch) is *clinical sign* of pneumomediastinum noted on auscultation.

In **Pneumopericardium** the air is limited to distribution of pericardial reflection and the thick shaggy soft-tissue destiny of fibrous pericardium is separated by air from cardiac density.

Air-fluid level is seen in both pericardial effusion and pleural effusion.

Mediastinal Masses

Anterior mediastinal masses	Middle mediastinal masses	Posterior mediastinal masses
Thymic lesions (Most common)	Lymphadenopathy (Common)	Neurogenic tumor (Most Common)
Teratoma	Foregut cyst	Infectious spondylitis (pyogenic, TB)
Thyroid/parathyroid	Hiatal hernia	Aneurysm of descending aorta
Lymphoma	Aneurysm of arch of aorta	Esophageal varies
Aneurysm of ascending aorta	Esophageal tumor	Hematoma
Cysts: Cystic hygroma, bronchogenic cyst, pseudopancreatic cyst	Carcinoma of trachea	Neuroenteric and bronchogenic cyst
Extralobar sequestration	Pericardial lesions	Extramedullary hematopoiesis
Mesenchymal tumors	Hematoma	
Mediastinal lipomatosis		
Morgagni hernia		
Sternal tumor		

Characterization of Mediastinal Node in Various Diseases

Mediastinal or hilar nodes enlargement >2 cm in their short axis diameter is likely to be due to metastatic carcinoma, malignant lymphoma, sarcoidosis, tuberculosis or fungal infection. Lesser degrees of enlargement can be due to lymph node hyperplasia and pneumoconiosis (e.g. silicosis). Widespread

moderate mediastinal adenopathy is frequent accompaniment of chronic diffuse lung disease and bronchiectasis.
- **Sarcoidosis** is the common cause of intrathoracic lymph node enlargement, the hilar nodes being enlarged in almost all cases. The important diagnostic feature of adenopathy in sarcoidosis is its symmetry.
- Lymph node enlargement due to **malignant lymphoma and leukemia** is *bilateral but asymmetrical*, hilar node enlargement is rare without accompanying mediastinal node enlargement, posterior mediastinal nodes are infrequently involved and paracardiac nodes are rarely involved but become vital as sites of recurrent disease.
- Lymph node enlargement due to **tuberculosis or fungal infection** may affect any of the nodal groups in hila or mediastinum. Dense calcification is frequent both in nodes that stay enlarged and in those that shrink. A low-density center with rim-enhancement of the enlarged node is a useful pointer towards the diagnosis of TB.
- A rare cause of strikingly uniform contrast enhancement (lymphnodes bloom out on ECCT) is **Castleman's disease**.
- Sometimes there is a ring of calcification at the periphery of node—so-called **'eggshell calcification'** that is a particular feature of **sarcoidosis and silicosis**.
- Kikuchi disease is necrotizing lymphadenopathy
- Kumuri disease is nonspecific chronic lymphadenopathy especially in neck forming multiple nodular soft tissue lesions in neck.

Some important X-ray signs in chest diseases

Key signs in chest film pathologies	
Sign	*Disease*
Thumb sign	Epiglottitis
Steeple sign	Croup
Air crescent sign	Aspergilloma
Bulging fissure sign	Klebsiella pneumonia
Golden 'S' sign	Right upper lobe collapse
Stag antlers sign/Hands-up signs/Inverted Mustache sign	Earliest radiological sign of pulmonary venous hypertension

Investigations preference for chest diseases	
Diseases	Investigations of choice
• Congenital heart disease	Transesophageal echocardiography
• Portal hypertension	Color Doppler
• Mitral value disease	Echocardiography with Doppler
• Mediastinal fibrosis	CECT, magnetic resonance imaging
• COPD	Pulmonary function tests
• Obstructive sleep apnea	Sleep apnea study
• Pulmonary fibrosis	HRCT
• Interstitial pneumonitis	Transbronchial or open-lung biopsy >HRCT
• Pulmonary thromboembolic disease	Contrast-enhanced spiral CT (CTA)

Hilum Overlay Sign

When there is a mediastinal mass and you still can see the hilar vessels through this mass, then you know the mass does not arise from the hilum.

This is known as the hilum overlay sign.

Because of the geometry of the mediastinum most of these masses will be located in the anterior mediastinum.

Cervicothoracic Sign

The anterior mediastinum stops at the level of the superior clavicle.

Therefore, when a mass extends above the superior clavicle, it is located either in the neck or in the posterior mediastinum.

When lung tissue comes between the mass and the neck, the mass is probably in the posterior mediastinum.

This is known as the cervicothoracic sign.

Chapter 5

Cardiovascular Radiology

HEART

Cardiac Monitoring

Noninvasive Cardiac Output Monitoring Techniques

- Pulmonary Artery (Swan Ganz) catheter (its tip is kept in main or left pulmonary artery while measuring PCWP)
- Thermodilution technique
- Dynamic echocardiography
- Electrical impedance cardiographic technology (The most recent advance in noninvasive cardiac output monitoring).

Cardiovascular Monitoring Techniques

- Transesophageal echocardiography
- Central venous pressure monitoring
- Pulmonary artery catheterization.

The normal pulmonary artery pressures are:
Systolic → 15–30 mm Hg
Diastolic → 3–12 mm Hg
Mean → 9–16 mm Hg
Mean wedge (PCWP) → 8–12 mm Hg

	Cardiovascular imaging protocols			
	Echocardiography	*Nuclear scan*	*CT*	*MRI*
IV Size/function	Initial modality of choice (Provides ancillary structural and hemodynamic information)	Available from gated SPECT stress imaging	Best resolution Highest cost	Best resolution Highest cost
Valve disease	Initial modality of choice Valve motion and morphology studied. Doppler hemodynamics assessed	—	—	Visualize valve motion Delineate abnormal flow
Pericardial disease	Pericardial effusion	—	Pericardial thickening and calcification	Pericardial thickening and malignancies
Aortic disease	TEE rapid diagnosis Acute dissection of thoracic aorta can be diagnosed rapidly	—	Image entire aorta rapidly Acute dissection of any part of aorta can be diagnosed rapidly Acute aneurysm screening Best for acute aortic dissection, especially when time is a concern as in hemodynamically unstable patient	Image entire aorta in 15-30 minutes Dissection of any part of aorta can be diagnosed with maximum accuracy Aortic aneurysm confirmation and evaluation Best for chronic dissection
Cardiac masses	First/initial investigation to detect: – TTE—large intracardiac masses –TEE—smaller intracardiac masses	—	Extracardiac masses Myocardial masses	Extracardiac masses Myocardial masses
Vascular rings	May sometimes be useful	—	Excellent for screening	Best for diagnosing and demonstrating compression of adjacent airways esophagus

Cardiac Borders on Chest X-rays

- The **left heart border** is formed by the main pulmonary artery and heart.

  The knob-like shadow of the aortic arch in superior mediastinum is formed by the posterior part of arch, which is absent or deformed in coarctation of aorta.

  A small 'nipple' may occasionally be seen projecting laterally from aortic knuckle or knob due to the presence of left superior intercostal vein and this normal nipple should not be misinterpreted as adenopathy (aortopulmonary window). Below the aortic knuckle or knob is a concavity, the pulmonary bay, the floor of which is formed by the main pulmonary artery beyond the pulmonary valve.

  The pulmonary bay may be filled in by PDA.

  Below the pulmonary bay, the left ventricle forms the left heart border.

  Just below pulmonary bay is the left bronchus, below which is the left atrial appendage, not forming a discrete shadow unless enlarged, and below that is the level of right ventricular infundibulum, azygous vein lesion on right side and does not contribute to left heart border.

  However, a coronary, artery aneurysm can cause abnormal bulging of left heart border.
- The right heart border is formed by right artrium and SVC
- **CT ratio**
  - The transverse cardiac diameter is the simplest possible measurement of cardiac size. In 90 percent of normal adult males, it measures less than 15.5 cm; in 90 percent of normal adult females it is less than 12.5 cm. The transverse cardiac diameter is the most accurate in assessing cardiac enlargement when related to patient's height and weight.
  - The upper limit of normal for **cardiothoracic ratio** is generally held to be around 50 percent, though it is 55 percent, for Africans and Asians. In neonates it should be more than 65 percent to call it cardiomegaly.
  - Cardiothoracic ratio may be increased by nonstandard radiographic techniques like poor respiration, supine in or AP view.
  - It may normally exceed 60 percent in neonates and elderly.
- Causes of **gross cardiomegaly** are:
  - Multiple valve disease
  - Pericardial effusion
  - Dilated cardiomyopathy (DCM)
  - Ebstein's anomaly
  - Hyperthyroidism
  - Erythrogenic right ventricular dysplasia
  - Heterotopic cardiac transplant.

Signs of Enlarged Right Ventricle on CXR

- **Right ventricle** has a complex shape. From front it resembles a triangle with base on the diaphragm. At the top is the pulmonary valve, leading to pulmonary artery, supported by an infundibulum separating the pulmonary valve from tricuspid valve. On the left inferior, is its apex.
- **The normal right ventricle makes virtually no contribution to the cardiac silhouette in frontal view**, although infundibulum lies close to left upper heart border.
- In lateral view it forms the front of heart, with lower half normally in contact with back of the sternum. With progressive right ventricular enlargement the area of contact between front surface of heart and the sternum increases. This is the **earliest and most sensitive radiological sign of right ventricular enlargement** but must always be interpreted in relation to the shape of chest.
- In frontal view, right ventricular enlargement causes:
    - An overall increase in the cardiac shadow, which adopts a triangular configuration whose long axis is elongated in a downward direction
    - Elevation of the cardiac apex, which is usually formed by the left ventricle
    - Large main pulmonary artery
    - Abnormal peripheral pulmonary arteries, which may be increased, pruned or decreased.
- The characteristic elevation of the apex of heart or 'Coeur en sabot' or 'boot shaped' heart, the appearance of right ventricular enlargement, is seen in untreated tetralogy of Fallot and in pulmonary atresia with VSD. The large right ventricle probably causes it.
- The right ventricle most commonly becomes enlarged as a result of left ventricular enlargement.

Signs of Left Atrial Enlargement on CXR

Selective left atrial enlargement is the selective chamber enlargement most easily detected on the plain film.

Frontal view (PA view)

- Elevation of left main bronchus (earliest sign on PA view) which, if gross, may lead to splaying of carina (second sign).
- Left atrium on enlargement bulges to right, produces a double shadow seen through the right side of heart (buttressing), until it eventually forms part of right heart border. The distinguishing point is that the right atrial border is limited below by the IVC while the left atrial border passes medially towards the spine before fading.

  A distance between the middle of the double density of heart and the left main stem bronchus of more than 7 cm has been shown to indicate left atrial enlargement in over 90 percent of cases.

- Particularly in rheumatic mitral valve disease, there may be left atrial with specific enlargement of the left atrial appendage, first seen as a straightening of left border below the left main bronchus, then as a discrete bulge on the left, immediately below the pulmonary bay and left main bronchus.
- Rarely, descending aorta may also be displaced to the left, (Bedford sign), i.e. the descending aorta is displaced to left by the enlarged left atrium and gives a smooth curve on the descending aorta.

Smooth indentation on anterior wall of esophagus is one of the early signs of *LA* enlargement on Ba swallow study.

CXR Features of CCF

Features of CCF are basically due to the following phases:

Interstitial pulmonary edema: Invariably precedes alveolar edema. Characterized by: Loss of sharp definition of vascular marking; thickening of interlobular septa, i.e. Kerley B-lines; pulmonary venous pressure 17–20 mm Hg; interlobar fissural thickening poorly defined increased bronchial wall thickness.

Air space edema: Poorly defined patchy acinar opacities; coalescence of acinar consolidation particularly in medial third lung giving "butterfly" or "bat wing" appearance (i.e. consolidated hilum + uninvolved lung cortex).

Flow inversion: Long-standing elevation of LA pressure (as in CCF) causes an increase in arteriovenous reflux; eventually LA enlarges, producing a protective atrial pulmonary vascular reflex vasospasm which narrows the lower lobar vessels and decreases arteriovenous reflux. Thus, upper lobar diversion of vessels is seen in CCF (**"hands-up" sign or Stag-Antler's sign**). Basal oligemia and upper lobar hyperemia.

Flow inversion is never seen in pulmonary edema of renal failure/overhydration/low oncotic pressure.

Generalized oligemia may be a feature

Cardiomegaly : Cardiac enlargement

Pleural effusion: CCF, is transudate, often bilateral. CCF is the most common cause in which the effusion usually accumulates first on right, before becoming bilateral.

Earliest sign of pulmonary venous hypertension (ccf) on chest X-ray is flow inversion/upper lobor diversion/cephalization of blood flow/inverted Mustache sign stag Antler's sign/Hands-up sign.

CXR Features of Mitral Stenosis

- Enlarged left atrium:
  - Double cardiac density seen through right cardiac border (Buttressing)
  - Elevation of left main stem bronchus with splaying of main stem bronchi
  - Displacement of descending aorta to left (**Bedford sign**)
  - Bulge of superiorposterior cardiac border below carina (Lateral view)
  - Esophageal displacement to right and posteriorly
- Dilated left atrial appendage with straightening of left heart border (Rheumatic heart disease)
- Calcification of valve leaflets in severe MS
- Small aorta due to reduced forward cardiac output
- Prominent pulmonary conus (Precapillary hypertension)
- RV hypertrophy and dilatation
- Pulmonary vascular cephalization—redistribution to upper lobes ('Hands-up' sign)
- Interstitial pulmonary edema and alveolar edema
- Pulmonary hemosiderosis (Multiple punctate calcific foci in lungs)
- Ossified nodules.

Valve Motion on Fluoroscopy
The aortic valve is oriented near the horizontal plane and usually overlies the spine, while the mitral valve is more vertically positioned and lies to the left of the spine. However, because the valves have a common insertion, it may be difficult to distinguish calcification of one valve from the other in the frontal view. This can be resolved with fluoroscopy in the same projection, because the motion of the aortic valve during the cardiac cycle is near to the vertical while the *mitral valve* moves more from *side to side*.

Pulmonary Plethora is Pulmonary Overcirculation

- It is indicated by enlargement of central (hilar), lobar and segmental pulmonary arteries.
- On CXR, the diameter of the RIPA or RDPA or RLPA >16 mm is considered as a objective sign of pulmonary plethora.
- Also diameter of RIPA exceeding the diameter of trachea, and the diameter of an en face pulmonary vessel exceeding the diameter of its companion bronchus is also suggestive of plethora.
- The visualization of en face vessels below the level of 10th posterior rib and prominence of vessels below the dome of diaphragm on PA view also suggest pulmonary plethora.

On CXR, cardiac configuration and the lung field vascularity many a time may give an important clue for diagnosis of some congenital heart diseases. Considering the same, following are the typical cardiac configuration seen in the various heart disease:

Increased pulmonary perfusion (Plethora)	*Decreased pulmonary perfusion (Oligemia)*
ASD (Primum and secundum defect)	Tricuspid atresia/stenosis
Anomalous pulmonary venous connection	Ebstein's anomaly
Membranous/bulbar VSD	Pulmonary infundibular/valvular stenosis
PDA	Tetralogy of Fallot (TOF)
Sinus venous defect	Pulmonary artery atresia
Gerbode defect	Peripheral pulmonary artery stenosis
DORV	Persistent truncus (type IV)
Single ventricle	Uncorrected transposition with PVS
Aortopulmonary window	Eisenmenger reaction (lung periphery only)
Persistent truncus arteriosus	
Coronary artery to right heart fistula	
TGA with ASD or VSD	
Endocardial cushion defect	

Specific Cardiac Configurations and Signs

- "Boot-shaped" heart (Cor en boot sabot) → Fallot's tetralogy
- "Egg on Side" heart ("Egg in Cup" heart) → TGA
- "Sitting-duck" heart → Persistent truncus arteriosus
- "Snowman" heart ("Figure of 8"/"Cottage loaf of bread" heart) → Supracardiac TAPVC
- "Ground-glass" appearance → Infracardiac TAPVC
- "Globular" heart with plethoric lung fields → TGA
- "Globular" heart with oligemic lung fields → Tricuspid atresia
- The "Great Hilar Dance" on Fluoroscopy → ASD
- "Stag-Antler" or "Hands-up" sign → CCF
- "Reverse 3" sign → Coarctation of aorta
- "Water-bottle" or "Flask-shaped" or "Money-bag" heart → Pericardial effusion
- "Double aortic knuckle" on CXR → Coarctation of aorta
- Double cardiac density/shadow (Buttressing) → LA enlargement
- Scimitar sign/Scimitar vein/Turkish sword appearance → Congenital venolobar syndrome (TAPVC/PAPVC)

- Cardiac wall calcification → Endomyocardial fibrosis
- "Pop-corn" calcification in center of cardiac silhouette → Calcified aortic valve
- "Square root" sign → Constrictive pericarditis
- "Speckled" appearance (glassy heart) on Echo → Amyloidosis
- "Ground-glass" Ventricular septum → HOCM
- "Spade-like" deformity on Echo → Apical hypertrophic cardiomyopathy
- "Goose-neck" deformity on LV angiography → Primum ASD
- "Four-bump" heart → MS/MR due to enlargement of left atrial appendage
- Dock's sign (Inferior notching of 3rd to 8th ribs) → Coarctation of aorta.

CONGENITAL ANOMALIES

Syndromic Association of Few Cardiac Lesions

- TAR syndrome → VSD
- Syndactyly /polydactyly → VSD
- Trisomy 13-15 → VSD
- Trisomy 17-18 → VSD, PDA
- Down's syndrome → Endocardial cushion defect
- Arachnodactyly → ASD
- Ellis-van Creveld (Chondroectodermal dysplasia) syndrome → ASD, single atrium
- Holt Oram syndrome → ASD (familial)
- Rubella syndrome → PDA/PS
- Turner's syndrome → Coarctation of the aorta, PS, AS
- William's syndrome → Supravalvular aortic stenosis, peripheral pulmonary artery stenosis
- Hurler syndrome → MR/AR
- Marfan syndrome → Incomplete coarctation and ASD, mitral valve prolapse, **Tulip bulb aorta,** Annuloaortic ectasia, fusiform aneurysm of ascending aorta, pulmonary artery aneurysm.

CXR Features Atrial Septal Defect

- The **three types of Atrial Septal Defects (ASD)** include ostium secundum or fossa ovalis defect, sinus venosus defect, and endocardial cushion defects (ECD).
- If the left to right shunt (ASD) produces a shunt ratio greater than 2:1, the heart is obviously enlarged, involving RA and RV.

- There is **no enlargement of the LA**, except in few cases of ECD or Lutembacher syndrome.
- The heart in ASD is sometimes displaced to left.
- The ascending aorta and its arch tends to appear smaller than normal, probably due to the rotation of ascending aorta by enlarged RA and RV, causing sagittal alignment of the aortic arch (**Small aortic knuckle**).
- The central pulmonary arteries are enlarged and there is a variable degree of pulmonary plethora, depending on the size of shunt.

> Septal lines (Kerley B lines) in a patient of ASD should always suggest an associated mitral valve abnormality (ECD or **Lutembacher syndrome**).
> The **"great hilar dance"** sign characterizes ASD on fluoroscopy.
> The **"Goose-neck" deformity** is seen in ASD on cardioangiography.

CXR Signs of VSD

Ventricular septal defect; VSD (muscular type → Maladie de Roger)
- CXR in smaller VSDs can range from normal to mild-or-moderate cardiac enlargement with mild or moderate plethora.
- CXR in large VSDs shows moderate cardiac enlargement with prominence of the main pulmonary artery, the hilar pulmonary arteries, and the peripheral pulmonary arteries.
- CXR in VSD with pulmonary arterial hypertension may be characterized by normal size and shape of cardiac silhouette and unremarkable central pulmonary arteries.

CXR Signs of Eisenmenger Syndrome

The group of patients with cyanotic congenital heart disease with pulmonary arterial hypertension–[PAH] (severe) resulting in a right to left shunt at the arterial, ventricular a pulmonary arterial levels are named as **Eisenmenger syndrome.**

Chest radiograph of such patient characteristically shows:
- Prominence of the pulmonary arterial segment and large right and left main pulmonary arteries and their branches.
- The peripheral lung fields are oligemic due to pruning of peripheral pulmonary arteries.
- Ventricles (right and left) return to normal size.

In a patient with congenital heart disease, development of oligemic lung fields and returning of heart to normal size may be the ominous sign rather than good prognostic signs as these signs entail that patient has developed Eisenmengerization.

Tetralogy of Fallot

- The heart is usually not enlarged at birth in Tetralogy of Fallot (TOF) but may be so if there is a large left-to-right shunt (a pink Fallot) later in life it may enlarge due to biventricular hypoxic failure.
- It is generally said that cynotic heart disease no cardiomegaly is likely to be TOF.
- At birth, heart shape is usually nonspecific but it may later become specific in about 25 percent patients with the classic **'Coeur-en-sabot'/'Boot-shaped' silhouette**.
- The classic 'boot-shaped' heart is due to combination of a deeply concave pulmonary bay and elevation from diaphragm of a slightly angular cardiac apex.
- The peripheral vasculature will show oligemia proportionate to the degree of cyanosis. A 'pink Fallot' will show plethora but the pulmonary bay will remain hollow. Ascending aorta is always enlarged and is typically prominent on plain X-ray.

    In 25 percent cases the aortic arch is on right and the descending aorta crosses to left of spine in lower thorax. In fact, it is the most common cardiac anomaly with which right aortic arch is associated.
- The characteristic elevation of the apex of heart or 'Coeur en sabot' or 'boot shaped' heart, the appearance of right ventricular enlargement, is seen in untreated tetralogy of Fallot and in pulmonary atresia with VSD. The large right ventricle probably causes it.
- The right ventricle most commonly becomes enlarged as a result of left ventricular enlargement.
- Pentalogy of Fallot consists of Tetralogy of Fallot with ASD.

Tricuspid Atresia

- On the plain radiograph the heart is of normal size at birth and only subsequently enlarges if there is good-sized VSD and no pulmonary stenosis, leading to pulmonary plethora.
- Tricuspid atresia has strongly a left dominant ECG and it is the only common cyanotic congenital heart disease with marked left axis ECG due to poorly developed RV.
- "Box-shaped" heart may be seen.

Total Anomalous Pulmonary Venous Connection/Drainage

TAPVC/TAPVD is anomalous connection between pulmonary veins and systemic veins secondary to embryologic failure of common pulmonary vein to join the posterior wall of left atrium.

Types of APVC

Contributes to < 1 percent of congenital cyanotic heart diseases.

Classification Based on Obstruction

- Obstructive: In obstructive TAPVC: Normal sized heart with pulmonary hyperemia (ground glass lungs)
- Nonobstructive (commoner).

Classification Based on Severity

- Total
- Partial.

Classification Based on Anatomy

- Supracardiac
- Cardiac
- Infracardiac
- Mixed.

- Subdiaphragmatic (Type III, 12%)—Drainage into portal vein/IVC/ductus venosus/left gastric vein
- Supradiaphragmatic
    - Supracardiac (Type I, 52%)—Drainage into left brachiocephalic/azygous/SVC
    - Cardiac (Type-II, 12%)—Drainage into coronary sinus/RA
- Mixed radiographic features of TAPVC (esp. the supradiaphragmatic variety) include: Overall heart size notably normal. Dilated SVC and left vertical vein giving **"Figure-of-8 or Snowman"** or **"Cottage-loaf" heart configuration** of cardiac silhouette and pretracheal density on lateral film.
- Increased pulmonary blood flow.

- In supracardiac TAPVC → All pulmonary veins join together to form a common pulmonary vein that drains into left innominate vein or SVC.
- In cardiac TAPVC → All pulmonary veins join together to form a common vein that drains into coronary sinus or enters right atrium directly.
- In infracardiac TAPVC → The common pulmonary vein drains into portal vein.

Partial anomalous pulmonary venous return (PAPVR) is associated with–
- ASD
- Hypogenetic lung as a component of congenital pulmonary venolobar syndromes (Scimitar syndrome). Here part/all of the hypogenetic lung is drained by an anomalous vein, which drains into, most commonly, IVC below right hemidiaphragm (when it drains into left atrium known as **meandering pulmonary vein**). It is featured almost exclusively on right side as a tubular structure paralleling the right heart border in the configuration of a Turkish sword (scimitar) on PA view of X-ray chest. On CECT it is seen as nodular or tubular opacity which opacifies in phase with pulmonary vein.

PULMONARY EDEMA

Abnormal accumulation of fluid in extravascular compartment of the lung constitutes pulmonary edema. Causes of pulmonary edema include:
- Cardiogenic (most common cause)
  - Heart disease: LVF, mitral valve disease, left atrial myxoma. These are associated with cardiomegaly.
    - Pulmonary venous disease, e.g. pulmonary embolism
    - Pericardial disease
  - Drugs, e.g. beta-blocker
- Permeability edema with diffuse alveolar damage = ARDS
- Permeability edema without diffuse alveolar damage, e.g. heroin induced.
- Mixed edema due to increased hydrostatic pressure and permeability changes: For example. neurogenic, reperfusion, air embolism.

Causes of Pulmonary Edema with Cardiomegaly

- Cardiogenic (e.g. mitral stenosis)
- Uremic (with cardiomegaly from pericardial effusions and/or hypertension)

Causes of Pulmonary Edema without Cardiomegaly

- Uremia
- Drugs
- Over-hydration
- Pulmonary hemorrhage
- Acute myocardial infarction/arrhythmia.

Features of Interstitial Pulmonary Edema

- Early loss of definition of subsegmental and segmental vessels
- Mild enlargement of peribronchovascular spaces
- 'Bat-wing' edema (10%)
- Kerley lines
- Subpleural effusions
- Progressive blurring of vessels due to central migration of edema at lobar and hilar levels
- Does not necessarily develop before alveolar pulmonary edema.

In cardiogenic pulmonary edema, ill-defined bilateral patchy acinar opacities/rosettes (fluffy shadows) with coalescent air space consolidation particularly in medial third of lung gives classical **"butterfly" or "bat wing" appearance** (i.e. consolidated hilum + uninvolved lung cortex) on CXR. The central/perihilar distribution is supposed to be due to increased fluid accumulation in central alveoli due to their increased elastin content.

KERLEY LINES

Kerley lines are septal lines seen on chest radiography due to thickened connective septa and not visible normally.

- **Kerley A lines**: Relatively long, fine, linear shadows in upper part of lungs seen radiating from hila and are deep within lung parenchyma. The thickened deep septa correspond to Kerley A lines (**A for Apical zone**).
- **Kerley B lines**: Relatively short, horizontally oriented peripheral lines seen in lower zones of lungs extending, abutting, and perpendicular to pleura in costophrenic (CP) angles. Thickened interlobular septa correspond to Kerley B lines. (**B for Basal zone**).
- **Kerley C lines**: Fine "lace-like" or "spider web like" polygonal opacities distributed primarily in peripheral or subpleural location. They are classically seen in pulmonary fibrosis. Kerley C lines represent visible subpleural lymphatic plexus. (**C for Central zone**).
- **Kerley D lines**: Produced due to criss-crossing of Kerley A and B lines.

As hydrostatic pressure increases (PCWP 17–22 mm Hg) the signs of interstitial edema including Kerley lines (A and B) may be visible. However, once the pressure approaches 25 mm Hg, fluid passes into alveoli, the Kerley lines disappear and alveolar shadowing is seen.

Causes of Septal (Kerley) Lines

- Pulmonary edema and pulmonary venous hypertension
- Pneumoconiosis
- Pulmonary fibrosis
- Interstitial pneumonitis
- Hemosiderin depositions in septa
- Lymphangitic tumor spread (Lymphangitis carcinomatosa)
- Lymphangioleiomyomatosis.

Pulmonary Venous Hypertension (PVH)

It is caused by increased resistance to blood flow in the pulmonary veins, due to obstruction or reduced compliance within the left atrium, at the mitral valve, or within the left ventricle.

It is divided into three grades of severity

Grade I PVH
- Reversal of normal gravity dependent gradient of pulmonary blood flow with diameter of upper lobar vessels greater than that of lower lobe vessels
- Enlargement of right superior pulmonary vein with **loss of hilar angle (lateral concavity of hilum)**
- Loss of visibility of mid and distal portions of right descending pulmonary trunk.

Grade II PVH
- Interstitial pulmonary edema
- Pleural effusion.

Grade III PVH
- Alveolar pulmonary edema with bilateral fluffy alveolar opacities
- Cardiomegaly (left atrial enlargement).

Air embolism (mill-wheel murmur) can be detected by measurement of end tidal CO_2 and pulmonary artery pressure before any clinical signs appear.

PULMONARY EMBOLISM

Modalities Used

- D-dimer assay
- Chest X-ray
- Multislice CECT
- VQ scan
- MRI
- Pulmonary arteriography (DSA).

Pulmonary embolism protocol

- Screening → D-dimer assay.
- Investigation of choices/best/perfect investigation→CT angiography (previously it was VQ sacn)
- Definitive/Gold standard→Catheter angiography.

CXR

Well-established chest X-ray signs

- Focaloligemia **(Westermark's sign)**
- A peripheral wedged-shaped density above the diaphragm **(Hampton's hump)**
- An enlarged right descending pulmonary artery **(Palla's sign)**.

CECT

Computed tomography (CT) of the chest with intravenous contrast is **the principal imaging test** for the diagnosis of PE. Multidetector-row spiral CT acquires all chest images with 1 mm resolution during a short breath hold. This generation of CT scanners can image small peripheral emboli. Sixth-order branches can be visualized with resolution superior to conventional invasive contrast pulmonary angiography. The CT scan also obtains excellent images of the RV and LV and can be used for a risk stratification as well as diagnostic tool. In patients with PE, RV enlargement on chest CT indicates a five-fold increased livelihood of death within the next 30 days compared with PE patients with normal RV size on chest CT.

A normal perfusion scan virtually excludes PE because a pulmonary embolus presents as a segmentally hypoperfused but normally ventilated lung (V/Q mismatch). When there is perfusion defect on a ventilation scan and CXR is normal, one must suspect an embolus.

Although **pulmonary angiography** is supposed to be the **definitive and gold standard** means of diagnosing PE, with the decreasing availability of pulmonary arteriography and increasing use of other noninvasive tests like spiral CT, the exact role of pulmonary arteriography is now less clear and there are **only few indications for it**, especially in absence of spiral CT or MRI, which include:

- When V/Q scan is abnormal but cannot be placed into either high or low probability categories (An indeterminate V/Q scan with high clinical suspicion and risky anticoagulant therapy)
- When the identification of sub-segmental emboli is regarded as vital
- When *in situ* thrombolysis of central pulmonary emboli is contemplated
- Specific diagnosis necessary for proper management.

V-P (Ventilation-perfusion) Scan (Second Line Investigation for Pulmonary Embolism)

In VP Scan, concurrent images of distribution of blood flow and distribution of alveolar ventilation (perfusion and ventilation scan respectively) are obtained following IV injections of **^{99m}Tc labeled macroaggregated albumin**, and inhalation of a radioactive gas (e.g. **Krypton 81 m or Xenon 133**) or aerosol of dispersed ^{99m}Tc labeled DTPA or carbon particles known as 'Technegas'.

- **Mismatched perfusion defected**: Cardinal sign of pulmonary embolism (under perfused part of perfusion scan while ventilation scan normal).
- **Matching defects on VP Scans:** Obstructive airways disease whether chronic or reversible, a result of pulmonary arterial blood flow reduction through unventilated parts of lung due to hypoxic vasoconstriction.
- **Reversed mismatched defect:** Hypoxic vasoconstriction is incomplete, so that there is relatively more perfusion than ventilation. It can be seen in COPD, partial obstruction of bronchus, lobar collapse and pneumonic consolidation or large pleural effusion.
- Any pathological disease that causes complete displacement or total destruction of lung parenchyma will result in **complete matched defects** of both V and P. Thus, a completely matched defect in an area of lung is thought to represent pulmonary infarct or infective lobar consolidation with development of necrosis.

Any embolus has potential to cause pulmonary infarction but surprisingly this is uncommon; some estimates suggest that fewer than 15 percent of all embolic episodes result in true infarction, probably because the lung has an additional blood supply in the form of systemic bronchial arteries which may become hypertrophied in chronic thromboembolic disease.

Chronic pulmonary hypertension occurs in less than 5 percent of patients following acute pulmonary embolism.

Pericardium

Calcification within Heart

Endocardial calcification:	Endomyocardial fibrosis
	Thrombus
Myocardial calcification:	Ventricular aneurysm
	Calcified infarct
	Post-Myocarditis
Pericardial calcification:	Chronic pericarditis (tuberculous, hemopericardium, pyogenic, viral)
	Post-traumatic
	Postoperative
	Post-radiotherapy
	Uremic pericarditis
	Asbestosis
	Hydatid cyst
	Methysergide

PERICARDIAL EFFUSION

Normally the pericardial sac may contain up to 50 mL of serous fluid, which essentially has the same chemical composition as serum.

About 300 mL of rapidly accumulating fluid can cause more symptoms than that of chronic effusion of >1000 mL.

Radiographic Features

- Cardiomegaly (with narrow pedicle), producing classical 'flask-shaped' heart
- Nonchamber specific cardiac enlargement
- 'Rounded or globular' appearance'
- Very clear or distinct or sharp cardiac contour/borders
- In large effusion → Obstruction of venous return to right heart causes decreased flow and pressure through lungs producing characteristic cardiomegaly with clear/**oligemic** rather than congested/plethoric lung fields.

- In later stages, after cardiac decompensation, pulmonary plethora/hyperemia may develop.
- **The epicardial fat pad sign** is positive, when visualized in lateral view on anterior pericardial stripe is thicker than 2 mm. This sign is diagnostic of pericardial thickening or fluid.

An abrupt increase in the dimension of the cardiac silhouette without specific chamber enlargement suggests the diagnosis of pericardial effusion.

Other Characteristic Features of Pericardial Effusion include

- Distinct/sharp cardiac borders
- Development of 'flask' or 'water bottle' or globular cardiac configuration
- Bilateral hilar overlay
- Oligemic lung fields in severe cases
- Epicardial fat pad sign is positive on lateral view where an anterior pericardial stripe is thicker than 2 mm.
- Filling of retrosternal space
- **Echocardiography** is most commonly used method for diagnosing pericardial effusions. It is most effective modality because it is sensitive, specific, simple, noninvasive, can be performed at bed-side, and can identify accompanied cardiac temponade.
- **CT/MRI:** The wide field of view and high spatial and contrast resolution, CT and MRI offer a diagnostic alternative to all patients with difficult or nondiagnostic ECHOs and an overall advantage of characterizing the effusions. Thus **diagnosis of pericardial effusion can be confirmed by CT or MRI** and these techniques are superior to ECHO in detecting loculated pericardial effusions and pericardial thickening.

PERICARDIAL TUMORS

Primary tumors of the heart are rare, and this is also true for pericardial tumors. In contrast, secondary tumors are found. Primary pericardial tumors in an order of decreasing frequency are: mesothelioma, sarcoma, teratoma, fibroma, lipoma, and angioma. Echocardiography often displays the tumor as a mass adjacent to the heart, but the exact localization of the tumor and its relationship to the pericardium can only be shown by CT or best with MRI.

In patients with suspected pericardial or paracardiac tumors, MRI has advantages over CT because it is a multiplanar modality. Coronal or sagittal images may more clearly demonstrate the relationship of tumor, pericardium, and other cardiac structures.

Imaging preferences for vascular pathologies							
Disease	Pulmonary embolism	Renal artery stenosis	Aortic dissection	Vertebral artery dissection	DVT	Chronic abdominal angina (Venous occlusion)	Acute mesenteric ischemia (Arterial)
Screening tool of choice	D-dimer	Doppler/CTA	CTA>TEE	CTA	Doppler (Duplex ultrasound)	Doppler	Doppler
Investigation of choice	CTA	3D-dynamic CEMRA	MRI	MRA	Doppler> MRI	CTA	Angiography (MRA >CTA)
Gold standard investigation	Pulmonary arteriography	Renal arteriography	Aortography	Vertebral angiography	Venography	Angiography	Laparotomy

AORTA

Torus Aorticus

The anterosuperior part of septal wall of the right atrium bulges to a variable degree into the atrial cavity as *torus aorticus*. It is caused by the proximity of right posterior aortic sinus and cusp.

Coarctation of the Aorta

- It is a congenital aortic narrowing in the region of the isthmus and may present in the neonate or remain undetected well into adult life.
- About 80 percent of patients are male.
- Hypertension is common, femoral pulses are usually delayed and weakened compared with the carotid and arm pulses.
- A postductal coarctation of aorta with PDA and reversal of shunt is associated with *differential cyanosis* involving the upper limbs only.
- One of the striking features in older children and adults is **collateral circulation** around the obstruction, the main collateral route being internal mammary arteries with retrograde flow to aorta below the coarctation through the intercostal arteries 3–9, the inferior epigastric arteries, scapular, and various mediastinal arteries.

- Rib notching (bilateral but asymmetric, and best seen on inferior aspects of posterior thirds of the upper ribs, sparing 1st two) usually takes several years to develop, and is caused by pressure erosion of adjacent ribs by enlarged tortuous intercostal arteries. So, rib notching is rare in young children, even in severe coarctation.
- In coarctation of aorta, small inferior notching occurs mainly in the mid-third of posterior rib, and the *first two ribs are spared* since the first and second posterior intercostals arteries arise from the costocervical trunk of the subclavian artery. This contrast with the situation in neurofibromatosis type I in which the inferior notch is often wide, can be anywhere, and may be associated with soft tissue opacity.
- The main collaterals in coarctation of aorta are the internal mammary arteries with retrograde flow to the aorta below the coarctation through the intercostals arteries 3–9, the inferior epigastric arteries, scapular and various mediastinal arteries. It takes years to develop and is rare in children.
- *The two CXR hallmark signs of coarctation of the aorta are:*
  - Rib notching (inferior margin of the 3rd to 8th ribs)
  - Figure 3 sign of the proximal descending aorta.
- Rib notching (inferior) is variably present in 75% of adults, but **uncommon in children**.
- The indentation of the figure 3 sign is indicative of the actual coarctation. The upper arc of the figure 3 sign represents the dilation of the left subclavian artery or aorta immediately proximal to the coarctation. The lower arc is the poststenotic dilation of the aorta distal to the coarctation.
- MRI, angiography and echocardiography can diagnose the coarctation, but **MRI is an elegant** non-invasive modality that will demonstrate a focal narrowing of the aorta +/− collateral vessels indicating the aortic coarctation.

Causes of Inferior Rib Notching

- Aortic coarctation
- Aortic thrombus
- Interrupted aorta
- Aortitis (Takayasu's arteritis)
- Arteritis
- Blalock Taussig shunt
- Atherosclerotic occlusion
- Pulmonary atresia
- Fallot's tetralogy

- Multiple pulmonary arterial stenoses
- Pulmonary/chest wall AV malformation
- Chronic SVC obstruction
- Neurofibromatosis
- Poliomyelitis/quadriplegia/paraplegia
- Hyperparathyroidism
- Thalassemia
- Melnick-Needles syndrome.

Causes of Superior Margin Rib Notching

- Normal variant (isolated defects, projectional)
- Paralytic polio
- Quadriparesis
- Rheumatoid arthritis, SLE, scleroderma
- Coarctation of aorta
- OGI (Osteogenesis imperfecta)
- Marfan syndrome
- Hyperparathyroidism
- Restrictive lung diseases
- Chest drainage tube
- Osteochondroma
- Neural tumor.

Dissection of Aorta

- Spontaneous longitudinal separation of aortic intima and adventitia by circulating blood having gained access to the media of aortic wall splitting it into two.
- Transverse tear in weakened intima (95–97%) is most common pathology.
- Peak age is 60 yrs with M:F = 3:1.

Etiology

- Atherosclerotic lesions of aorta
- Cystic medial necrosis

- Fusiform aortic aneurysm (28%)
- Hypertension (60–90%)
- Marfan syndrome
- Ehlers-Danlos syndrome
- Relapsing polychondritis
- Valvular aortic stenosis/bicuspid aortic valve
- Turner's syndrome
- Behcet disease
- Coarctation of aorta
- Trauma (rare)
- Catheterization
- Aortitis (e.g. SLE)
- Pregnancy
- Cocaine abuse.

Types

Clinical Classification
1. Acute <2 weeks old
2. Chronic >2 weeks old

Stanford classification
Type A (60–70%) = Ascending aorta +/– first 4 cm of arch
Type B (30–40%) = Descending aorta only

Debakey's classification
Type I (29–34%) = Ascending aorta + portion distal to arch
Type II (12–21%) = Ascending aorta only
Type III (50%) = Descending aorta only
Subtype A = Up to diaphragm
Subtype B = Below diaphragm

Location

Most commonly (65%) on anterior and right lateral wall of ascending aorta just distal to aortic valve.

Radiological Investigations

- Chest radiograph:
  1. Calcification sign: Inward displacement of atherosclerotic plaque by > 4–10 mm from entire aortic contour
  2. Widening of superior mediastinum
  3. Left-sided pleural effusion (25%)
  4. Atelectasis of lower lobe.
- 2-D ECHO:
  59 to 85 percent sensitive and 63 to 96 percent specific for type A.
- TEE:
  Up to 99 percent sensitive and 77 to 97 percent specific.
- CECT (Rapid diagnostic tool)
  87 to 94 percent sensitive and 87 to 100 percent specific.
- MRI (most sensitive and specific investigation): 95 to 100 (98.3) percent sensitive and 90 to 100 (97.8) percent specific. It is best or preferred or investigation of choice.

  In ideal situation where all the imaging techniques are readily available, initial assessment with CXR and 2D ECHO should be followed by MRI as MRI gives most confident diagnosis and also gives images best understood by the surgeons.

  If the patient is unstable, TEE or CECT should be done instead of MRI.
- Conventional angiography remains "grid standard" tool.

Dissecting Aneurysm

- *They are intramural hematomas that extend to various levels of the aorta causing encroachment on the aortic lumen and disrupting or extending into the branches of the aorta. Rerupture of the false passage into the true lumen may occur.*
- The process begins as a primary laceration of the aorta through which a false passage develops within the aortic media. Two sites are particularly likely as sites of the primary laceration. One is the *tubular portion of the ascending aorta*. The other is at *the junction of the arch and descending aorta*.
- Dissecting hematomas are often subdivided as done by DeBakey, both as to the site of the primary laceration and as to the extent of the false passage. According to this, the three types of dissecting hematomas are as follows:

Type I: The primary laceration is in the ascending aorta, and the false passage within the media extends along the full length of the aorta.

Type II: The primary laceration is in the ascending aorta, and the false passage extends to about the level of the aortic arch.

Type III: The primary laceration is at the junction of the arch and descending aorta, and the false passage extends distally to the terminal part of the aorta.

Although the chest radiograph findings are neither specific nor diagnostic, they may suggest or support the diagnosis of a dissecting hematoma and lead to further studies such as MRI or CT.

CXR
- Normal CXR in 25 percent cases
- **Calcification sign** (Inward displacement of calcification plaque by >4–10 mm from outer aortic contour) or the calcification in the aortic knuckle, which is separated from the outer margin by more than 1 cm, is said to be suggestive of dissection.
- **'Apical cap' sign** (The mediastinal hematoma may dissect over the lung apices (left more often than right) to produce the apical cap sign in the supine position or to produce widening of the paraspinal line to the right or to the left).
- Localized dilation of aortic knuckle and upper descending aorta, which may give rise to prominent **'Lump' sign**.
- Disparity in size between ascending and descending aorta.
- Irregular wavy contour/ indistinct outline of aorta.
- Lateral projection of aortic knuckle.
- Widening of superior mediastinum.
- Left sided pleural effusion.
- Rightward displacement of trachea.

MRI is more accurate and most comprehensive technique compared to established methods such as echocardiography, CT, or angiography. Although cost-effectiveness of MR imaging has not been established, it has emerged as the *preferred technique in selected areas, including diseases of the aorta, such as aneurysm, dissection, and its precursors, intimal tears and intramural hematoma, congenital and inherited heart diseases, and, in particular, for postoperative follow-up* of aortic repair and cardiac malformations.

Within the past 5 years, MR imaging has emerged as the most accurate method for detecting aortic dissection, at least in hemodynamically stable patients who are suspected of having acute aortic syndrome. MR imaging appears to be the method of choice in stable patients with suspected acute or subacute dissections and is certainly the best method for serial follow-up studies after surgical repair or in chronic cases.

However, as a clinical routine, *TEE is recommended in any emergency department setting for immediate diagnostic evaluation of hemodynamically unstable* and clinically deteriorating patients prior to surgical intervention.

Echocardiography most practical investigation for assessing ventricular function, but now MRI is considered most accurate

Aortic Trauma

The most common location of traumatic aortic rupture surviving to diagnosis is the aortic isthmus (80 to 90%). In this region, the relatively fixed position of the aorta due to tethering by the ligamentum arteriosum combines with forces of rapid deceleration to create a point of shearing stress.

Screening for TAI has traditionally relied on the upright frontal chest radiograph. In recent years, contrast-enhanced spiral CT has been demonstrated to be an effective and efficient means of screening for TAI with sensitivity approaching 100 percent and specificity ranging from 81 percent to 99 percent. Spiral CT is the most sensitive means of detecting mediastinal hemorrhage. Confirmation is better with MRI than CT.

Carotid Imaging

DSA: Intra-arterial carotid angiography can be performed via a catheter placed in the aortic arch or by selective catheterization of common carotid artery as gold standard tool or definitive test.

Irregularity due to atheroma must be differentiated from spasm (due to the presence of a catheter), fibromuscular dysplasia (extensive, regular, concentric corrugations of the artery producing "beaded or pile of plates" appearance, frequently bilateral and rarely extending above skull base), and from spontaneous or iatrogenic dissection (extensive narrowing, with some irregularity and slow flow, often extending up to the level of ophthalmic artery), which can practically best possible with MRI.

Color Doppler: The carotid bifurcation is variable in position but is usually close to the level of the superior border of thyroid cartilage. Contrary to the impression, the view, which shows CCA, ICA and CEA simultaneously, is difficult to obtain. The ICA is typically larger than ECA, has bulbous origin, and has no branches in the neck, in contrast to multiple branches of ECA.

Wave form		Peak systolic velocities
ECA —	Triphaisc, high resistance (little flow in diastole c̄ dicrotic notch +)	< 110 cm/s
ICA —	Biphasic flow, less pulsatile, high flow indiastole	70–100 cm/s
CCA —	Same as ICA (i.e sharp systolic peak with integrade flow during diastole)	70–100 cm/s

Post-traumatic pseudoaneurysms can usually be differentiated from a true carotid aneurysm by locating the characteristic to and fro pulsed Doppler waveforms in the neck of the pseudoaneurysm and identifying the internal variability of color flow ("*yin yang*") that is typically seen in any pseudoaneurysm.

CTA: CT angiography can be used and has advantage of showing calcification, but uses ionizing radiation and iodinated contrast, with risk of contrast reaction more than MR contrast. It can be best for rapid screening of intracranial ICA.

MRA: MRA is a flow-sensitive technique and areas of turbulent or slow flow may remain undetected, artificial loss of flow signal is frequent and creates a flow gap. Nevertheless, it is now tool of choice for all structural problems of carotid.

- **A 'four-vessel' angiogram:** It is performed by injection of contrast into both ICA (CCA if there is atheromatous disease at carotid bifurcation) and at least into one vertebral artery, but if reflux of contrast fails to display contralateral PICA, the contralateral vertebral artery is also catheterized.
- **Note:** Mneumonic: "CF-FC", i.e. cerebral angiography → femoral artery approach; Fluorescein angiography → Cubital vein approach.

Carotid Body Tumors (Potato Tumor/Chemodectoma)

These are one of many of a family of paragangliomas that involve the head and neck. These are usually benign, *well-encapsulated masses located at the carotid bifurcation*. These tumors are *hypervascular* and may be bilateral, frequently producing an audible bruit. Some produce catecholamines that can produce sudden changes of blood pressure postoperatively or after manipulation of the carotid bifurcation vessels. Carotid body tumors arise from the carotid body at the level of the carotid bifurcation. Many extend medially far enough to produce a bulge in the oropharyngeal wall. On an MRA, they appear as vascular masses *producing a characteristic splaying of the internal and external branches of the carotid artery (Lyre's sign)*. Color doppler is the best screening tool for CBT.

Thoracic Outlet Syndrome (a Clinical Diagnosis; Doppler may Aid in Diagnosis)

The thoracic outlet is an anatomic region containing the **first rib**, the **subclavian artery and vein**, the **brachial plexus**, the **clavicle** and the **lung apices**. Actually the subclavian artery and vein and the brachial plexus pass through this small anatomic space that is bordered by the first rib, the clavicle and the anterior and posterior scalene muscles. The subclavian artery leaves the chest via the thoracic outlet, where it passes over the first rib, behind the clavicle and between the anterior and middle scalene muscles. The subclavian vein passes over the first rib, behind the clavicle and anterior to the anterior scalene muscle. The brachial plexus, which innervates the upper extremity, also exits from the thorax via the thoracic outlet between the anterior and middle scalene muscles.

Because of the close confines of the thoracic outlet, the subclavian artery, the subclavian vein, and the brachial plexus are subjected to impingement by the surrounding structures, which in turn generate the upper extremity symptoms leading to thoracic outlet syndrome (TOS).

Etiology of Thoracic Outlet Syndrome

Congenital:
- Cervical rib
- Scalenus anticus syndrome (most common) due to wide/abnormal insertion or hypertrophy of the muscle
- Anomalous 1st rib (unusually straight course with narrowing of costoclavicular space or wide first thoracic rib)
- Costoclavicular syndrome
- Scalenus minimus muscle (rare) extending from transverse process of 7th cervical vertebra to 1st rib with insertion between brachial plexus and subclavian artery.

Acquired:
- Fracture of 1st rib or clavicle (with nonanatomic alignment/exuberant callus)
- Muscular body habitus causing arterial compression in pectoralis minor tunnel (pectoralis minor syndrome)
- Slender body habitus (with long neck and sagging shoulder)
- Supraclavicular tumor/lymphadenopathy.

Subtypes of Thoracic Outlet Syndrome

True Neurogenic TOS: Results from compression of lower trunk of brachial plexus by an anomalous band of tissue (fibrous band) connecting an elongated transverse process of C7 with the first rib or a cervical rib. Neurologic deficits include weakness of intrinsic muscles of hand and decrease sensation on palmer aspect of 4th and 5th digits. EMG and nerve conduction studies confirm the diagnosis. Definitive treatment is surgical division of the anomalous band compressing either the lower trunk of brachial plexus or ventral rami of C8 or T1 nerve roots.

Vascular TOS: Results from compression subclavian artery or vein by a cervical rib resulting in arterial and venous lesions like stenosis, occlusion, poststenotic dilatation, thrombus formation and aneurysmal dilatation. Blood pressure is reduced in affected limb, and signs of emboli may be seen in hand; neurologic signs are absent. Noninvasive color Doppler study or angiography confirms the diagnosis. Treatment is with thrombolysis or anticoagulation with or without embolectomy and surgical excision of the cervical rib compressing the subclavian artery or vein.

Disputed TOS: It accounts for most of the cases. These patients present with subjective arm and hand weakness; paresthesias; arm, shoulder and chest pain and headache. Although sensory symptoms are similar to those seen with neurogenic thoracic outlet syndrome, hand wasting is never found and EMG is normal. Treatment of these patients is often unsuccessful.

Role of Imaging

Bi-directional Doppler study: The role of duplex scanning in diagnosis of TOS is not established; however, it can detect rare cases of vascular TOS by revealing stenosis or aneurysmal or thrombotic changes. It is a sensitive test for detecting compression of subclavian or axillary vessels with provocative positioning like:

- **Adson maneuver (for Scalenus anticus muscle):** Hold deep inspiration while neck is fully extended, fully abduct the arm with the head turned towards opposite side.
- **Hyperabduction maneuver (compression by humeral head or pectoralis minor muscle):** Extremity/radial pulse monitored through range of 180° abduction, complete cessation of flow in one position noted.
- **Costoclavicular maneuver** (compression between clavicle and 1st rib): **Exaggerated military position** with shoulders drawn back and downward.

Photoplethysmography

Angiography: May appear normal or equivocal with the arm in returns position, and Adson maneuver may be necessary to confirm the lesion. Findings one should look for are abnormal course of distal subclavian artery, focal stenosis/occlusion, aneurysm, poststenotic dilation of distal subclavian artery, mural thrombus + distal embolization and venous thrombosis or obstruction.

DAS or MRA can investigate the case in a certain manner and less invasively.

Subclavian Steal Syndrome

In Subclavian Steal Syndrome there occurs reversal of blood flow in the ipsilateral vertebral artery. The vertebral artery passes cranially through the foramina transversarium after arising from subclavian artery and passing from subclavian artery towards C6 and then in upper neck it winds around lateral masses of C1 and finally enters the foramen magnum. When the subclavian artery is occluded in its first part, or severely stenotic, the flow in the ipsilateral vertebral artery is reversed leading to decreased blood supply to part of brain supplied by it (Subclavian steal syndrome).

Imaging of Extracranial Vertebral Artery

Evaluation of the extracranial vertebral artery is the logical extension of the routine carotid examination. However, vertebral arteries are variable in size and course and demonstrate a wide variety of pulsed Doppler waveforms. Ninety percent of vertebral arteries run within the transverse foramina of the cervical spine from C6 upward. However, other vertebral arteries may enter the transverse foramina at higher levels. Size of vertebral arteries is variable, with the left being slightly larger than the right in the majority of cases. Congenital hypoplasia or absence of the vertebral artery is also possible. The overlying transverse processes of the vertebral bodies limit a thorough examination of this vessel, as does the deep location of the origin of the vertebral artery. However, ultrasonography has proven somewhat disappointing in the assessment of vertebral artery stenoses, dissections, or aneurysms. Hence, CTA is best screening tool, MRA is investigation of choice/preferred investigation while DSA is definitive or "gold standard" study for vertebral artery pathologies.

Investigations for Aneurysms in General

- **Angiography: (DSA)**
  It is the **first choice for final confirmation and evaluation of the aneurysm.**
- **CECT:**
  TEE: } Screening tools of choice and preferred in unstable patients
- **MRI (most sensitive and specific investigation):** 95–100 (98.3) percent sensitive and 90–100 (97.8) percent specific. It is best/preferred/diagnostic/investigation of choice.

IMAGING IN PERIPHERAL ARTERIAL DISEASE

The initial studies performed to assess suspected peripheral arterial disease include physiologic measurements of segmental pressures and pressure volume recordings. The ankle/ankle-brachial pressure index (ABI) is a valuable and simple screening test. Use of continuous wave-Doppler to measure the ankle systolic pressure is important. Ankle brachial index (ABI) is ankle systolic pressure divided by branchial systolic pressure. Normal valve for ABI is 1; <0.9 is suggestive of ischemia. Normal valve of TSPI > 0.6. For assessment of arterial disease in diabetic patients TSPI (toe systolic pressure index) should be included.

Color Doppler Ultrasonography (CDU) has become a more efficient and accurate method of screening for peripheral arterial disease, but this technique is not universally advocated for the preoperative assessment of patients with claudication. Examination of the peripheral arterial system requires that the entire course of the artery be evaluated with CDU, looking for areas of aliasing and narrowing, which will then be evaluated by velocity analysis.

MRA: There has been a great deal of excitement generated concerning the use of MRA for assessing the lower extremity arteries and 3D CEMRA is upcoming choice.

All said and done, *angiography* (conventional/digital subtraction) remains gold standard.

Thromboangiitis Obliterans (Buerger's Disease)

It is a type of peripheral vascular disease that characteristically occurs in men in their third or fourth decades. The diagnosis is based primarily on the clinical setting and histologic examination rather than on the arteriographic appearance.

Typically, arteries of 1–3 mm in size are involved and demonstrate chronic inflammation of the vessel wall with intimal thickening and luminal thrombus. Although the inflammatory exudate of round cells involves all layers of the vessel wall, the intimal layer is most involved, and there is a striking preservation of the architecture of the media. The intimal thickening is usually well-demarcated and concentric. Luminal thrombus shows a wide variety in the state of organization but is rarely freshly formed.

Arteriographic characteristics that may be considered typical for thromboangiitis obliterans include the following: *multiple segmental occlusive lesions* in the forearm, hand, leg, and foot; a progressive but regular reduction in the diameter of the arterial tree above the thrombosed segments; and a collateral circulation that is established primarily through the vasa vasorum surrounding the thrombosed segment, giving the typical appearance of *a network of fine "corkscrew" collaterals* accompanying the diseased vessel.

Takayasu's Aortoarteritis (Pulseless Disease/Nonspecific Aortoarteritis)

- It is a primary arteritis of unknown cause, first described by a Japanese ophthalmologist, Takayasu.
- It commonly affects the aorta, the brachiocephalic branches, and pulmonary arteries.
- The *most commonly affected artery* being the subclavian artery.
- It is most common in young Asian women (M:F = 1:10).
- Collateral circulation around the stenosis and occlusions may be seen and this is a rare cause of rib notching.

Deep Venous Thrombosis

Doppler study has shown to be **very sensitive** and cost-effective for detection of acute lower limb thrombus, especially if this involves the vessels above the knee.

Venography (89 percent sensitivity and 97 percent specificity) is the **gold standard and definitive means**. But is invasive and cumbersome.

I-125 labeled fibrinogen study is 90 percent sensitive for calf vein thrombus and 60 to 80 percent for femoral vein thrombus and not sensitive for thrombus in upper vein and pelvis.

VASCULAR RINGS

The aberrant right subclavian artery arises as the last brands of aortic arch; its first part is persistence part of distal right arch, which may be larger than its expected diameter, known as Kommerell's diverticulum. This aberrant vessel **passes obliquely upwards and to right, posterior to esophagus, causing posterior indentation on it**. If the vessel is dilated at this point it makes wide indentation. There is no vascular ring with this anomaly and it is *almost always asymptomatic*.

- *CXR*
    - The plain chest radiograph is important in assessing patients with vascular rings
    - *Right aortic arch* ⇒ indentation of the lower trachea.
    - *Double arches* ⇒ an aortic knuckle can be seen on both sides, the right almost always being larger and higher than the left, and there may then be bilateral indentation of the trachea.
- *Barium swallow*
    - Right-sided indentation of the esophagus ⇒ from **right aortic arch**
    - Posterior indentation ⇒ from a retroesophageal vessel
    - Larger posterior indentation ⇒ Aberrant subclavian artery (with diverticulum) and retroesophageal course of the aorta.

- *Imaging*
  - In young children the elements of the vascular ring can often be identified on echocardiography, particularly with a suprasternal window. MRI with its multiplanar capability is especially useful in older children and adults. In most children, however, angiography may be required to define the anatomy.
- *Rx*
  - Surgery for vascular rings is aimed at dividing the ring at the most suitable point. This may involve just dividing the arterial ligament but in double arch the arch itself has to be divided on the smaller side. The ring usually then springs apart releasing the compression on the trachea and esophagus. Tracheomalacia may cause continuing problems after surgery in both children and adults.

Double Aortic Arch

- Double aortic arch is the most common cause of symptomatic vascular ring in children
- Presentation is usually in the neonatal period with respiratory distress.
- Older children present with stridor or dysphagia.
- The most common pattern is for the ascending aorta to divide in front of the trachea, the right and left anterior arches passing upwards on each side to give off common carotid and subclavian branches. The larger right element then crosses to the left behind the esophagus to join the left descending aorta and so forms a tight vascular ring.

DYSPHAGIA LUSORIA

- Several vascular anomalies may produce dysphagia by compression of the esophagus.
  - Classically this is due to → an aberrant right subclavian artery (arteria lusoria).
- However, esophagus is more commonly compressed by vascular rings, such as a double aortic arch.

- Double aortic arch is the only complete vascular ring and always necessitates surgical repair. Patients with a double aortic arch present with predominant airway symptoms (stridor, respiratory distress, and cough). They also present earlier than the other vascular rings since the aerodigestive tract is completely encircled by the ring, rather than only being partially compressed.
- Aberrant right subclavian artery is seen in a patient with a left aortic and aberrant origin of the right subclavian artery as the last branch from the aortic arch (from the descending thoracic aorta) and results in posterior indentation of the esophgus. This anomaly is the most common vascular

anomaly of the aortic arch system and can be found in 0.5% of humans, although the majority is asymptomatic.
- The pulmonary artery sling is a rare vascular ring that occurs when the left pulmonary artery arises off of the right pulmonary artery and encircles the right main stem bronchus and trachea as it passes between the trachea and esophagus prior to entering the left lung, with esophageal compression anteriorly. Due to the significant compression in these patients, they usually present early in life with respiratory symptoms.
- The right aortic arch with a left ligamentum arteriosum and aberrant left subclavian artery is almost as frequent as the double aortic arch. As this ring does not constrict the trachea and esophagus as much as seen in a double aortic arch, these patients usually present later, usually within the first few years of life. Airway symptoms in these patients are similar to those with a double aortic arch, though these patients also have dysphagia.

- Vascular compression like dysphagia lusoria, aberrant right subclavian artery, right-sided aorta, left atrial enlargement, aortic aneurysm can cause dysphagia.
- MRI with its multiplanar capability is extremely useful.

Right-sided Aortic Arch

There are two common forms of right-sided aortic arch:
- *The first is the so-called mirror-image type, with the brachiocephalic branches being the mirror image of normal.*
    - It is the most usual form of right arch to be found in association with cyanotic heart diseases (25% incidence in tetralogy of Fallot and pulmonary atresia).
- *The second form of right arch is that with an anomalous origin of the left subclavian artery*
    - This is almost the mirror image of the anomalous right subclavian type, in isolation this rarely causes symptoms, but when associated with a left-sided ductus arteriosus forms a vascular ring.
    - In this circumstance the proximal portion of the aberrant vessel usually forms a prominent diverticulum known as the **Kommerell diverticulum**.

Right aortic arch with 'mirror image' branching → is the most common type associated with cyanotic congenital heart disease.
Right aortic arch with an anomalous origin of the left subclavian artery arising from a posterior diverticulum → is the most common type of right aortic arch to occur as an isolated abnormality.

Diagnosing a vascular ring		
Screening tool	Preferred/diagnostic/Investigation of choice	Definitive/"Gold standard"/Tool for evaluation
CTA	MRA	Catheter (Invasive/conventional) angiography DSA

Magnetic resonance imaging chest
The role of MR imaging in the evaluation of respiratory system disease (pulmonary parenchyma) is less well-defined than that of CT.

Fogarty Catheter

The concept of removing embolic material from a blood vessel by means of a balloon catheter was introduced by Fogarty et al (1963).

The transvenous aspiration of pulmonary thrombus using vacuum cup introduced percutaneously through venotomy was described by Greenfield et al (1969).

The Fogarty catheter technique remains the treatment of choice for removing embolic in aortoiliac region, but in smaller arteries, the aspiration of embolic material through a custom designed catheter under fluoroscopic control is a superior method, as it does not require an arteriotomy unlike the Fogarty technique.

Chapter 6

Abdominal Imaging

MODALITIES AVAILABLE FOR ABDOMINAL PATHOLOGIES

- X-ray abdomen (erect view, supine film or left lateral decubitus film)
- Barium and water-soluble iodinated contrast procedures
- Ultrasonography (transabdominal, endoluminal and intraoperative)
- CT scan
- MRI
- Nuclear scans (including PET scan).

\multicolumn{3}{c}{Protocol and summary in general for abdomen radiology}		
Radiological study	*Clinical utility*	*Key comments*
Abdominal radiograph (X-ray abdomen)	– Pneumoperitoneum – Bowel obstruction } Gold standard – Calcification and calculi	– Chest X-ray is the most sensitive X-ray for detecting minimum pneumoperitoneum, although standing X-ray abdomen is standard view done routinely – CT is the most sensitive method to detect air as well as calcification
Barium studies	– Indirectly assess GI pathologies – Initial test of choice to evaluate of case of dysphasia is **barium swallow**	– Barium sulfate is contrast media used – CT and MR enteroclysis are now possible

Contd...

Contd...

	– Enteroclysis (a special study better than BMFT for small bowel) is excellent study for many non-neoplastic lesions small bowel (e.g. malabsorption, intestinal strictures, CD, TB, etc.) – Barium enema is one of the best studies for diagnosing and evaluating colorectal pathologies like UC, CD. Diverticulosis, Hirschprung's disease, colonic polyps, volvulus, etc.	
Water soluble contrast study	– Bowel perforation – TO fistula	– Barium is relatively contraindicated if there is suspected bowel perforation. – Chest X-ray with coiled rubber catheter is highly suggestive of TO fistula with esophageal atresia
Ultrasonography	– Initial test of choice for any case of obstructive jaundice – Initial tests of choice for acute abdomen – Initial test of choice for abdominal trauma (Protocol = FAST) – Excellent for detecting gallstones and other conditions like adenomyomatosis of gallbladder, CHPS. Intussusception, minimal ascites, etc.	– Air and bone obscure imaging with USG as they produce "post-acoustic" shadow – Probe of frequency 3.5-7 MHz is used – EUS/endoluminal sonography due to its high sensitivity is mainly used for ca esophagus and stomach staging, insulinoma, periampullary tumors and terminal bile duct calculi detection
CT	– Blunt abdominal trauma	– Multislice spiral CT is best machine – No "tissue overlap" and rapid diagnosis are key advantages – Air and bone do not create hinderance in CT imaging – It is the "triple phase" CECT usually done for hepatic and pancreatic lesions – Virtual endoviewing is now possible
MRI	– Liver hemangiomas of size < 2.5 cm, especially when triple phase CECT is equivocal. – MRCP is screening tool of choice for	– Due to abdominal wall motion and bowel peristalsis, overall for abdominal pathologies MRI has not achieved the popularity compared to CT

Contd...

Contd...

- primary sclerosing cholangitis, bile duct anomalies, cholangiocarcinomas and dital intrahepatic bile duct lesions.
- MRI with ER coil is supposed to be better than CT or TRUS for assessing the locoregional spread of carcinoma rectum
- It is tool of choice for preoperative staging of cervical, endometrial and prostatic cancer.
- It is excellent tool for anorectal region pathologies.

- However, due to high filed strength MRI machines intraoperative MRI, newer and faster MRI pulse sequences (e.g. HASTE) MRI is gaining its own importance.
- MRI can be supposed to be better than CT for many vessels in abdomen, for some liver lesions, rectal cancer staging, pelvic pathologies (especially the female pelvis) and screening of the biliary tract with MRCP

X-ray appearance	Diagnosis
• 'String of beads' sign	• Small bowel obstruction
• Cupola sign	• Pneumoperitoneum
• Rigler's (double-wall) sign	• Pneumoperitoneum
• Foot-ball sign	• Pneumoperitoneum
• Coffee bean sign	• Sigmoid volvulus (Strangulated bowel obstruction)
• 'Bird of prey' sign	• Sigmoid volvulus
• 'Coiled-spring' appearance	• Intussusception
• 'Claw' sign	• Intussusception
• 'Saw-toothed' appearance	• Diverticulosis
• Hat sign	• Colonic polyp
• 'Apple core' appearance	• Carcinoma colon
• 'Thumb-print' sign	• Ischemic colitis
• Reverse '3' sign of Frostburg	• Carcinoma head of pancreas
• Moulage sign	• Malabsorption (Celiac disease)
• String sign of Kantor	• Crohn's disease
• String sign	• CHPS
• 'Pseudobiloth' appearance and 'Ram's horn' stomach	• Crohn's disease
• – String sign – Fleishner's sign	• Ileocecal TB

Contd...

Contd...

- Inverted umbrella sign
- Widened ileocecal angle
- "Contracted-pulled" cecum
- Amputed cecum
- Bull's eye lesion
- Mucosal granularity

- Leiomyoma (GIST) on Ba
- Liver metastases and hepatic candidiasis on USG
- Earliest sign of ulcerative colitis on Ba enema

IMPORTANT PRELIMINARY CLINICORADIOLOGICALLY TERMS

Chilaiditi's syndrome	A cause of pseudopneumoperitoneum characterized by intestine between liver and diaphragm.
Dietl's crisis	After an attack of acute renal pain a swelling in loin is found-Sometimes later, following the passage of large volume of urine, the pain is relieved and swelling disappears. This is Dietl's crisis, a feature of intermittent hydronephrosis, is seen in PUJ obstruction
Strangury	When the stone is in the intramural ureter, the pain is referred to the tip of the penis. In both sexes there may be strangury
Steinstrasse	Immediately after ESWL, the treated stone may look larger, appear less dense, and margins that are more indistinct. However, the appearance of the stone may have changed very little if it is in a tightly enclosed space, despite fragmentation. The fragments may disperse and conform to the shape of the pelvicalyceal system or ureter. Multiple small stone fragments that columnize in the ureter are common and are known as **Steinstrasse, or "street of stone"**. Ureteral obstruction may occur from a solitary fragment or from Steinstrausse.
Meganblase	Distension of Splenic flexure causing pain due to heavy fatty diet
Meteorism	Abdominal distension 24 to 48 hours after abdominal injury is probably due to retroperitoneal hematoma implicating splanchnic nerves
Mittleschmerz	Pain ovulation with abdominal discomfort at regular intervals usually about 14th day and may be associated with spotting due to estrogen withdrawal

PNEUMOPERITONEUM

The presence of free, intra-abdominal gas almost always indicates perforating viscus, the **most common cause** being perforated peptic ulcer.

About 70 percent of perforated ulcers will demonstrate free gas, a phenomenon that is almost **never seen in** the case of a perforated appendix.

Other causes of pneumoperitoneum
- Blunt/penetrating abdominal trauma
- Typhoid ulcer perforation (Ileal)
- Iatrogenic (e.g. postoperative, laparoscopy, diagnostic)
- Diverticulitis (e.g. ruptured Meckel's diverticulum)
- Necrotizing enterocolitis with perforation
- Inflammatory bowel disease (toxic megacolon)
- Malignant tumors of GIT
- Imperforate anus
- Hirschsprung's disease
- Meconium ileus
- Dissection from pneumomediastinum
- Ruptured urinary bladder
- Perforation of uterus/vagina
- Culdocentesis
- Tubal patency test
- Gas forming peritonitis
- Anterior abdominal wall defect.

Signs of pneumoperitoneum on supine film are
- Football sign (air dome)
- Rigler's double wall sign (visualization of both sides of bowel wall)
- Saddlebag/Mustache Cupola sign (air trapped below the central tendon of diaphragm)
- Doge's cap sign (triangular collection of gas in Morrison's pouch)
- Lucent liver sign
- Inverted 'V' sign (medial and lateral umbilical ligament visualization)
- Visualization of falciform ligament
- Urachus sign
- Right upper quadrant gas (perihepatic, subhepatic, Morrison's pouch)
- Gas in scrotum (in children)
- Tell-tale triangle sign (air seen between bowel loops) on lateral horizontal beam film

The free intra-abdominal gas almost always indicator perforated viscus. The most common cause is perforation of a peptic ulcer.

About 70 percent of perforated ulcers will demonstrate free gas, a phenomenon that is rarely seen in case of a perforated appendix.

As little as 1 ml of free gas can be demonstrated radiographically, either in an erect chest or a left lateral decubitus abdominal radiograph.

If a perforated viscus is suspected, a horizontal ray radiograph, either an erect chest or a decubitus abdomen is mandatory.

Small amount of gas is easily detectable under the right hemidiaphragm on erect radiograph but on the left it can be difficult to distinguish free gas from stomach and colonic gas.

- A left lateral decubitus radiograph will almost always resolve the problem by demonstrating gas between the liver and the abdominal wall and is best view to visualize minimum free gas in abdomen. Radiographic technique is also important, and the patient should remain in position for 5 to 10 minutes before the horizontal ray so as to ensure that the free gas if present has had time to rise to the highest position.
- However, with the advent of CT scan, as minimum as 1 ml of free air can be easily detected on CT scan, especially when viewed under lung window.

Although as little as 1 ml of free gas can be demonstrated radiographically, either in chest PA or a left lateral decubitus abdominal film, CT is superior to plain radiographs in detecting minute quantities of pneumoperitoneum.

CT is most sensitive investigation for detection of free intraperitoneal gas.

Small pockets of free air can be seen over liver and anteriorly in mid-abdomen or peritoneal recesses.

In order not to miss small amounts of free gas, the images should be reviewed on lung window setting. Free air demonstrated in CT can be distinguished from bowel gas due to its nondependent location and lack of haustra or valvulae.

ASCITES

Hellmer's sign (on abdominal radiograph) → ascitic fluid between liver and the lateral abdominal wall may result in the visualization of a lucent band, the fluid being slightly less dense than liver. Blood has a similar density to liver, and a hemoperitoneum does not demonstrate this sign. Earliest radiographic sign is a fluid density within pelvis or 'dog ears' visualized lateral to rectal gas shadow.

Ultrasound and CT are very sensitive for small amounts of peritoneal fluid.

Ultrasound may be more sensitive than CT in detecting a small amount of ascites in the pelvis, particularly in thin patients with unopacified small bowel.

SPLEEN

Calcification in Spleen

The most common cause of splenic calcification is prior granulomatous disease, usually tuberculosis or histoplasmosis. It is said that the presence of numerous granulomas suggests histoplasmosis.

Splenic Trauma

The spleen is the most commonly injured intraperitoneal organ following blunt trauma.

A "left-sided package" resulting from left-sided injury includes free, subcapsular, perisplenic, or intraparenchymal splenic blood, rib fractures, pneumothorax, and renal injury.

Plain AXR Features of Rupture of Spleen

- Obliteration of splenic outline
- Obliteration of psoas shadow
- Indentation on left side of gastric bubble
- Fracture of one or more ribs of left side
- Elevation of left diaphragmatic dome
- Free fluid between gas field intestinal coils causing ground glass abdominal haze.

Splenic Vein Thrombosis

Splenic vein thrombosis, or so-called left-sided or isolated portal hypertension. Splenic vein occlusion usually occurs secondary to chronic pancreatitis, carcinoma of the pancreas, or pancreatic pseudocyst, and less often as a result of abdominal trauma, polycythemia, other coagulopathies, and idiopathic thrombosis. In these cases, gastric varices are fed primarily by the short gastric veins.

The association of gastric and esophageal varices is generally seen in intrahepatic portal obstruction while isolated gastric varices without esophageal varices may indicate splenic vein thrombosis.

Patients with longstanding portal hypertension develop focal deposits of iron particles, called Gamna-Gandy bodies (siderotic nodules), seen as low signal intensity round lesions on T2-weighted MR images.

Hyposplenism

Intestinal ulceration, pneumatosis, neuropathy, hyposplenism, the cavitary mesenteric lymph node syndrome, and the development of a malignant neoplasm are the major complications of celiac disease.

Hypersplenism

It is characterized by increased pooling or destruction of the corpuscular elements of the blood by the spleen. Hypersplenism may be seen in many disorders, including cirrhosis with portal hypertension; hematologic abnormalities such as idiopathic thrombocytopenic purpura, thalassemia major, and hereditary spherocytosis; and diffuse splenic infiltration from primary malignancies such as leukemia and lymphoma. Signs of hypersplenism include splenomegaly, thrombocytopenia, leukopenia, and anemia, and symptoms may include abdominal discomfort, pain, respiratory distress, and early satiety. Surgical removal or transcatheter ablation of splenic parenchyma is often performed for the management of hypersplenism.

Neoplasms of Spleen

Hemangiomas are the most common noncystic benign splenic lesions.

Primary splenic neoplasms are rarely encountered, except for *hematopoietic malignancies*. Primary neoplasms of spleen are exceedingly rare, among which angiosarcoma of spleen is most common.

Lymphoma is the malignancy most commonly involving the spleen.

Secondaries in spleen are most common from lymphoma. Tumors that commonly metastasize to the spleen include melanoma, ovary, breast, colon, lung, and prostate. *Melanoma* is the most common nonlymphoma metastasis.

ESOPHAGUS

Barium Swallow Study

The esophagus is a muscular tube, 20 to 24 cm in length, lined by *stratified squamous epithelium*. The outer half of the esophageal wall is composed of muscle arranged in an outer longitudinal and an adjacent inner circular layer. The musculature is striated in the proximal one-third of the esophagus and smooth in the remainder.

Despite widespread application of endoscopy, barium studies still remain the primary imaging technique in suspected esophageal disorders, especially in cases of dysphagia.

> A ***clinical clue*** that is often used to differentiate mechanical from functional obstruction is: Dysphagia for solid food only or a progression from dysphagia from solid food only to also include liquids suggests a worsening mechanical obstruction, such as a neoplasm or stricture. Motor disorders, on the other hand, usually present from the outset with dysphagia for both solids and liquids.

Barium studies are simple to perform, inexpensive and highly sensitive. Endoscopy will often be required after a barium swallow, especially for biopsy purposes. It is helpful that barium studies precede endoscopy. This particularly applies to high dysphagia when an unsuspected pharyngeal pouch can be readily entered and perforated with scope. Also esophagoscopy is less good at identifying motility disorders.

Barium Study Feature of Few Esophageal Diseases

- *Tertiary esophageal contractions* (presbyesophagus, diffuse esophageal spasm, neuromuscular diseases)
  - "Yo-Yo" motion of barium
  - "Corkscrew" appearance (scalloped configuration of barium column)
  - "Rosary-bead/Shish kebab" configuration (compartmentalization of barium column)
- *Feline esophagus* (transient contraction of longitudinally oriented muscularis mucosa)
  - Normal variant
  - Gastroesophageal reflux disease
- *Double-barrel esophagus*
  - Dissecting intramural hematoma
  - Mallory-Weiss tear
  - Intramural abscess
  - Intraluminal diverticulum
- *Candidal esophagitis*
  - 'Cobble stone' mucosa
  - Shaggy/fuzzy contour of the esophagus with small diffuse superficial ulcers
  - Plaques
  - Thickened mucosal folds
- *Cytomegalovirus esophagitis*
  - Giant ovoid flat ulcers (vasculitis of submucosal vessels)
  - Gastroesophageal junction with adjacent part of stomach is commonly affected.
- *Herpes esophagitis*
  - Discrete superficial punctate/linear serpentine/stellate/diamond shaped ulcers
- *Scleroderma*
  - The smooth muscle (distal two-thirds) of the esophagus including the LES is involved
  - Dilated aperistaltic esophagus with patulous gastroesophageal junction and free GER
  - Sliding hiatus hernia
  - Esophageal shortening as the disease progresses
  - *Hidebound* esophagus

Involvement (feeble or absent peristalsis in) of the *distal two-thirds,* i.e. smooth-muscle portion of the esophagus occurs characteristically in scleroderma but may be found also in other connective tissue disorders, esophagitis, presbyesophagus, alcoholism, diabetes, idiopathic intestinal pseudo-obstruction, myxedema, anticholinergic medication, and variants of achalasia.

Tracheoesophageal Fistula

The above findings suggest a clinical diagnosis of tracheoesophageal fistula, which usually occurs in association with esophageal atresia but may also occur as an isolated anomaly. Plain radiography may show air in esophagus and stomach (most common variety being upper end of esophagus, being blind, and lower end connected to trachea). Actually, contrast study of esophagus (*water soluble low-osmolarity nonionic iodinated contrast agent is ideal*) confirms the diagnosis. If simple swallow doesn't show the fistula, modification may be required in the form of contrast injection into NG tube with patient prone and as the tube (Rubber) is withdrawn the fistula is seen.

Esophageal Varices

Varices are seen as serpiginous (*worm-like*) filling defects in the regular contour of esophagus in barium studies.

Barium studies have largely been replaced by endoscopy.

Endoscopic Grading of Esophageal Varices

- *Grade I (F1):* Varices can be depressed by endoscope
- *Grade II (F2):* Varices cannot be depressed by endoscope
- *Grade III (F3):* Varices are confluent around the circumference of esophagus

Hiatus Hernia

Examination of hiatal requires the patient to be placed in **prone/oblique position** on a horizontal table and given a bolus of barium to swallow so there is maximal distension of hiatal segment.

When looking for reflux during barium studies, the usual technique is to have the patient in a supine horizontal position and then slowly to lift left side off the couch while screening continuously.

Barium swallow findings
- Epiphrenic bulge
- >4 longitudinal coarse thick gastric folds above gastroesophageal junction or in the suprahiatal pouch

- Distance between B ring and hiatal margin >2 cm
- Peristalsis causes above hiatus

Antomic landmarks
- A ring – Muscular fold
- B ring – Muscular fold/GE ring
- Z line – Junction of columnae and squamous epithelium

Hiatus hernia

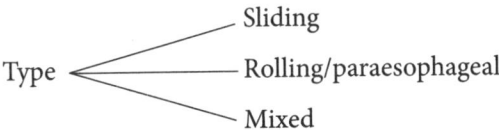

- Sliding hiatus hernia (Ba features)
  - Stomach above hiatus >2 cm
  - 3 or more folds of stomach seen
  - Diameter of hiatus >3 cm

     reflux esophagitis – ulcer at GE function
                    ↓
            Barrett's esophagus (10%)
                    ↓
            Adenocarcinoma (15%)

  - Schatzki ring
- Paraesophageal hernia
  - Cardia below diaphragm, fundus herniates
  - Associated with volvulus of stomach.

Esophageal Motility Disorders

- Primary: Achalasia
             Diffuse esophageal spasm
             Presbyesophagus
             Nutcracker esophagus

- Secondary:
    Congenital TO fistulae
    Intestinal pseudo-obstruction
    Connective tissue disorders
    Neuromuscular disease
    Chemical/physical injuries
    Metabolic and endocrine disorders

> Esophageal manometry is considered the "gold standard" for the evaluation of esophageal motility.

Diffuse Esophageal Spasm

Compartmentalization of esophagus by numerous tertiary contractions, i.e. episodes of pronounced abnormal motility occurs without cause, causing severe chest pain. The intermittent nature of the disorders makes it difficult to diagnose by Barium studies; 24 hours. Manometry is required. The tertiary contractions are nonpropulsive, uncoordinated and nonperistaltic and hence seen as intermitted 'riggles' along the wall of esophagus, as multiple simultaneous contraction rings, or as a segmented barium column producing a "corkscrew," "rosary bead," or "curling" appearance.

Nutcracker Esophagus

It is a nonspecific esophageal motor disorder (NSEMD) characterized by abnormally high amplitude contractions measured manometrically in the distal esophagus in patients who have chest pain or dysphagia. Normal peristalsis is preserved. There are no associated radiographic abnormalities as peristalsis is normal. Isolated LES dysfunction and presbyesophagus are other NSEMD.

Achalasia Cardia

It is a motility disorder of esophagus, probably due to degeneration of myenteric plexus in gastroesophageal junction region, resulting in failure of relaxation of the gastroesophageal junction.

It is defined by the **manometric triad** of aperistalsis of the esophageal body, incomplete, impaired relaxation of the LES to less than 50 percent of the basal LES pressure, and hypertension of the resting lower esophageal sphincter

Clinical features include increasing dysphagia, weight loss, chest pain, repeated attacks of aspiration pneumonia (when esophagus becomes dilated and fills with food debris). However, dysphagia is by far the most common presentation (>90% of patients) and is usually slowly progressive over years and affects both solids and liquids.

CXR may reveal absent fundic bubble, areas of aspiration pneumonitis in lung fields and mediastinal air fluid level.

Earliest change seen on **barium study** is defective distal peristalsis associated with a slight narrowing at G-E junction.

Features

- Megaesophagus/sigmoid esophagus
- "Bird beak" deformity
- Absence of primary peristalsis below level of cricopharyngeus
- Hurst phenomenon (temporary transit through cardia when hydrostatic pressure of barium column is above toxic LES pressure)
- Vigorous achalasia (numerous tertiary contractions in nondilated distal esophagus of early achalasia).

Apart from pneumatic dilatation of affected segment, **Heller's operation** is surgical treatment for achalasia.

> **Causes of "Secondary" Achalasia**
> Intrinsic and extrinsic neoplasm involving the gastroesophageal junction, paraneoplastic syndromes in patients with malignancy but no discernible tumor at the gastroesophageal junction.
> Chagas' disease
> Intestinal pseudo-obstruction
> Eosinophilic gastroenteritis
> Postvagotomy effect.

Dysphagia Lusoria

- Dysphagia due to vascular rings is known as dysphagia lusoria.
- Abnormalities of the great vessels can contract the structures in mediastinum, namely the trachea and esophagus.
- Many vascular rings can be explained by the persistence of failure to regress of parts of the aortic arch system during embryonic development.
- Barium swallow, bronchoscopy, or angiographies are investigations to diagnose but angiography is diagnostic.
- Impressions and displacement of esophagus from vascular causes may be congenital or acquired. Congenital lesions like aberrant right subclavian artery (0.5%) and right-sided aortic arch with

aberrant left subclavian artery may rarely cause esophageal symptoms (dysphagia lusoria) and are often demonstrated as chance findings.
- The **aberrant right subclavian artery** arises as the last branch of aortic arch; its first part is persistent part of distal right arch, which may be larger than its expected diameter, known as **Kommerell's diverticulum**. This aberrant vessel passes obliquely upwards and to right, posterior to esophagus, causing posterior indentation on it. If the vessel is dilated at this point it makes wide indentation. There is no vascular ring with this anomaly and it is almost always asymptomatic.
- **Aberrant left subclavian artery from right** aortic arch is the last branch and passes upwards and to left behind esophagus. A vascular ring is usually formed by arterial depth joins the left pulmonary artery to the left subclavian artery, which occasionally may cause significant esophageal compression. MRI is excellent modality to demonstrate the vascular rings.
- Treatment is indicated for the relief of symptoms and is usually directed at dividing the nondominant avascular component of the rings.

Benign Esophageal Tumors

Leiomyomas are the most common benign tumors of the esophagus, accounting for more than 50 percent of lesions.

Radiographically, these submucosal, i.e. intramural lesions are seen as broad-based, smooth filling defects with intact mucosa and well-defined margins on barium-swallow examination. An abrupt, but not acute, angle with the normal esophageal wall is seen when the lesion is viewed in profile.

Carcinoma Esophagus

Predisposing Factors Associated with Esophageal Malignancy

- Achalasia
- Asbestosis
- Barrett esophagus
- Celiac disease
- Ionizing radiation
- Lye stricture
- Oral and pharyngeal carcinoma
- Plummer-Vinson syndrome
- Tylosis palmaris and plantaris

- Tannins, alcohol, tobacco exposure
- Cancer of the esophagus is three to four times more common in males than in females
- It is twice as common in non-whites as in whites.

Squamous cell carcinoma accounts for 95 percent of the malignant lesions of the esophagus. Adenocarcinomas are far less common. The great preponderance of these (59 to 86%) appears to arise from the metaplastic columnar epithelium of the barrett esophagus.

Radiological Features

- Any stricture, mass lesion, ulcer, or mucosal irregularity of the esophagus must be viewed with suspicion of cancer. The classic radiologic patterns of esophageal carcinoma are annular constrictive, polypoid, infiltrative, and ulcerative.
- The most frequent presentation, the annular carcinoma or *"apple core lesion,"* has sharp overhanging edges proximally and distally.
- *"Rat-tail" esophagus*, shouldering sign are other common features.
- Role of CT in esophageal disease is mainly confined to *cancer staging*.
- Endoscopic USG only overcomes limitation of CT in assessing esophagus cancer and stage in early disease.

STOMACH

Congenital Hypertrophic Pyloric Stenosis (CHPS)

It is the most common acquired obstruction of the young infant.

It is more common in males and develops usually between the third and sixth weeks of life.

The clinical *triad* of projectile vomiting, visible gastric peristaltic waves, and a palpable pyloric mass are frequently diagnostic.

Increased incidence in firstborn male child with M:F ratio 4:1.

Inherited as dominant polygenic trait.

Manifestations

- Usual age of presentation is 3–6 weeks of life with nonbilious projectile vomiting
- Palpable olive-shaped epigastric mass
- Nasogastric aspirate >10 mL
- Positive family history
- Hypochloremic, hypokalemic metabolic alkalosis

Upper GI Imaging (Barium Study)

Precaution
- Empty stomach via nasogastric tube before study
- Remove contrast at the end of study.

Barium study features of CHPS
- Elongation and narrowing of pyloric canal (2 to 4 cm length)
- Passing of small barium streak through pyloric canal seen as a string of barium known as **string sign**.
- Crowding of muscle folds in pyloric canal known as **double/triple track sign**.
- Transient triangular tent-like cleft/niche in mid-portion of pyloric canal with apex pointing inferiorly; seen due to mucosal belonging between 2 separated hypertrophied muscle bundles on greater curvature side within pyloric canal, known as **diamond sign/twinning recess**.
- Outpouching along lesser curvature due to disruption of antral peristalsis, known as **pyloric teat/teat sign**.
- Mass impression upon antrum with streak of barium pointing toward pyloric channel, known as **beak sign/antral beaking**.
- Indentation of the base of duodenal bulb known as **Umbrella/Kirkland/Mushroom sign**.
- Gastric hyperperistaltic waves known as **caterpillar sign**.
- Gastric distension with fluid.

Ultrasound (Investigation of Choice)

- *Target sign*: Hypoechoic ring and hypertrophied pyloric muscle around echogenic mucosa centrally (transverse scan).
- *Elongated pyloric with thickened muscle*:
  - Pyloric muscle wall thickness 2.5–3 mm
  - Pyloric volume >1.4 cm^3
  - Pyloric length >1.2 cm
  - Pyloric transverse diameter 13 to 16 mm with pyloric channel closed.
- Cervix sign (indentation of muscle mass on fluid filled antrum on longitudinal scan)
- Antral nipple sign (redundant pyloric canal mucosa protruding into gastric antrum)
- Exaggerated peristaltic waves
- Delayed gastric emptying of fluid into duodenum and increased residue in stomach.

D/D

- Infantile pylorospasm (muscle thickness 1.5–2 mm) resolves in several days. It can be effectively treated with metoclopramide.
- Milk allergy/gastritis
- Gastric diaphragm
- Duodenal obstruction due to midgut volvulus ('whirlpool sign' on USG and corkscrew appearance or Ba meal).

Peptic Ulcer Disease

When erosions are over 5 mm in diameter, it is conventional that they be called ulcers.

Features	Benign ulcer	Malignant ulcer
Incidence	95 percent	5 percent
Location	Distal stomach and the lesser curvature (distally) (Posterior wall > anterior wall)	Fundus and prox half of greater curvature
Ba studies		
(Enface)	Round or oval, sometimes tear-drop like or with linear contour (collection of barium on dependent wall)	Irregular
(End on)	Ring shadow with barium coating edge of the ulcer crater (ulcer on nondependent wall or is not filled with barium)	
	Radiating folds are smooth and symmetrical and reach/continue to the edge of ulcer crater (good sign of benignancy)	Distorted mucosal folds and these folds *do not reach up to the edge* of ulcer (due to surrounding desmoplastic reaction)
In profile	'Ulcer Niche' (Project beyond lumen of stomach)	Absent
	'Hampton's Line' a pencil-thin line of lucency seen crossing the base of the ulcer (due to preserved gastric mucosa with undermining of more vulnerable submucosa)-*virtually diagnostic*	**Carman's meniscus sign** (It is diagnostic of ulcerative carcinoma of stomach).
	Ulcer collar (a thicker smooth)	Kirklin complex

Hampton's line → Benign gastric ulcer/peptic ulcer
Carman's meniscus sign → Malignant gastric ulcer

Duodenal ulcers are most common in first part of duodenum.

Anterior wall ulcers tend to perforate while posterior duodenal wall ulcers tend to bleed, occasionally by eroding gastroduodenal artery.

When ulcers occur on anterior as well as posterior walls of duodenum, commonly in first part they are known as "*Kissing ulcers*".

"Pseudokidney" Sign

Stomach on endoscopic ultrasound has wall-thickness of 3 mm and around 4 to 5 mm on transabdominal ultrasound.

It has five layers similar to that of esophagus except for 5th layer, where the adventitial layer of esophagus is replaced by serosa and subserosa in stomach, which are classically seen on endoluminal/endoscopic USG (**"gut signature" sign**).

On CT scan the normal wall thickness of stomach is up to 4 mm.

Stomach wall thickening may be seen as "Pseudokidney" sign on USG.

Pseudokidney sign (sonographic mass of reniform appearance with a central hyperechoic region surrounded by a hyperechoic region) can be seen in the following conditions:
- Ca stomach
- Ca colon
- Intussusception
- Inflammatory bowel disease
- Necrotizing enterocolitis
- Midgut volvulus
- Sigmoid volvulus

Gastric Volvulus

It is seen with diaphragmatic hernias, eventrations, or with the heterotaxia syndromes. Patients present with retching, often violent in nature, but without emesis. Plain films reveal a dilated stomach.

Depending on the direction and plane of torsion, gastric volvulus may be divided into two types:

In organoaxial volvulus, the stomach rotates either anteriorly or posteriorly along its long organic axis. The degree of rotation is variable but usually does not exceed 180 degree. The degree of rotation and the original shape and position of the stomach determine the final configuration of the rotated stomach. A superior 180 degree rotation of a high transverse stomach produces a cranial displacement of the body of the stomach with a reversal of the normal locations of the lesser and greater curvatures. A vertical J-shaped stomach rotates mainly from right to left and produces essentially a mirror-image configuration. Organoaxial torsions are seen mainly in elderly individuals with long histories of neglected hiatal hernias and are only rarely associated with significant symptomatology.

Mesenteroaxial volvulus is a less common torsion that develops about an axis perpendicular to the long axis of the stomach that joins the lesser and greater curvatures. This is called the mesenteric axis because it coincides with the axis of the mesenteric attachments of the lesser and greater omenta. The rotated stomach usually assumes an "upside-down" configuration, with the distal antrum and pylorus located cranial to the fundus and proximal stomach. This type of volvulus is more commonly associated with severe obstruction and strangulation. It is seen in children and later in life, often associated with diaphragmatic traumatic hernias.

- A **total or complete volvulus** is defined as a gastric rotation of at least 180 degree. Segmental, partial rotations and mixed forms occur often, making exact classification difficult.
- Ba meal and CECT are diagnostic studies.

Gastric Diverticulum

The gastric diverticulum is a solitary, blind outpouching, usually not larger than 3 to 4 cm, that communicates with the gastric lumen.

The great majority of congenital gastric diverticula (75–90%) are located along the posterior wall of the proximal stomach adjacent to the esophagogastric junction.

Gastric Polyps

These are associated with decreased gastric acidity, with chronic gastritis, and with gastric carcinoma. Five histologic types of gastric polyps have been identified:

1. Hyperplastic polyps are the most common, accounting for 75 to 90 percent of gastric polyps. Malignant change is rare.
2. Adenomatous polyps constitute the majority of other gastric polyps and malignant change may occur.
3. Hamartomas are rare gastric lesions. These are the gastric polyps that are seen in the Peutz-Jeghers syndrome.
4. *Retention polyps*: Seen in patients with the Cronkhite-Canada syndrome.
5. Villous tumors are usually sessile but may be pedunculated.

Radiographically, a polyp is discernible as a filling defect that interrupts or displaces the adjacent normal mucosa and gastric folds.

Gastric Leiomyomas and Leiomyosarcomas

- Submucosal tumors of stomach include leiomyomas, the most frequent of the gastric submucosal tumors, as well as neurogenic tumors, fibromas, leiomyoblastomas, lipomas, vascular tumors, and carcinoids.
- Broad based filling defects with the sharply delineated smooth mucosal surface distinguishes this lesion from a carcinoma.
- Ulceration occurs in approximately half of these cases and is small and central in location, giving typical "bull's eye" or "target" appearance on barium studies.
- The tumor may become necrotic, with central liquefaction or hemorrhage, simulating a cyst.
- Leiomyomas and leiomyosarcomas are now better called as GIST.

Gastric Lymphoma

The gastrointestinal tract is the extranodal site most often involved in NHL, and usually the stomach is affected. Primary gastric lymphoma responds to *H. pylori* R_X and 75 percent of gastric MALT lymphomas regress. However, subtotal gastrectomy, followed by combination chemo (CHOP + rituximab) is useful for high grade lymphomas. Role of radiation is not defined.

Gastric Carcinoma

Various types of gastric carcinoma:
- Early gastric cancer
- Polypoid carcinoma
- Ulcerating carcinoma with a mass
- Ulcerating carcinoma presenting as an ulcer
- Scirrhous carcinoma.

By definition *early gastric carcinomas* are confined to the mucosa and the submucosa, irrespective of whether or not regional lymph nodes are involved.

And by definition advanced carcinomas have spread beyond submucosa and have invaded the muscularis propria.

EUs is best for locoregional spread and CECT is best for advanced ca stomach.

Differential Diagnosis of Linitis Plastica

- Scirrhous carcinoma of stomach
- Metastasis from ca breast
- Hodgkin's lymphoma
- Crohn's disease
- Gastric amyloidosis
- Syphilis
- Corrosive gastritis
- Tuberculosis
- Eosinophilic gastritis.

SMALL INTESTINAL

Small Intestinal Imaging

Barium studies of small intestine may be classified into indirect (e.g. small bowel meal, peroral pneumocolon and reflux examinations) and direct (e.g. enteroclysis) techniques.

Enteroclysis (small bowel enema) gives the best mucosal details.

But, USG to some extent and CECT to greater extent are excellent for neoplastic lesions of small bowel.

Malrotation of Gut

It is serious congenital abnormality of GIT as it predisposes to duodenal obstruction and midgut volvulus. There are no specific plain radiographic findings in malrotation. However, on barium study, the **"corkscrew" pattern** of duodenum and jejunum spiraling around mesenteric vessel is pathognomonic for midgut volvulus. Ultrasound may reveal the reverse relation of SMA and SMV (**Whirlpool sign**).

Malabsorption

There are four Radiologic groups of findings in small intestinal malabsorption, related to alteration in:
1. **Peristalsis** → variable peristalsis is hallmark with hypo- and hypertonic segments, overall leading to increased transit time and segmentation of barium.
   However, transit time may be long/short/normal.
   Painless transient intussusception may be seen on fluoroscopy.

2. **Caliber** → dilatation of segments of bowel coils in 80 percent cases (>3 cm).
3. **Secretions** → increased secretions cause dilution of barium and later clumping, segmentation and flocculation of barium.
4. **Mucosa** → edematous mucosa with thickened valvulae conniventes giving 'Cog-wheel' pattern (colonization of jejunum), instead of their normal 'Feathery' pattern; later atrophy occurs and mucosal folds disappear with thinning of bowel wall.

Valvulae conniventes may exhibit five types of appearance:
1. Normal
2. Squared ends
3. Thickening of valvulae
4. Reversed jejunoileai pattern
5. *Absence of valvulae*: "**Moulage sign**" characteristic of sprue.

Parasitic Infestation

Strongyloides Stercoralis

Its habitat is duodenum (as that of *Giardia lamblia*), hence tends to cause duodenitis and duodenal stricture.

Ascaris Lumbricoides

Ascariasis is a cosmopolitan parasitic infection, especially prevalent among poor children in tropical countries with overcrowded slums and inadequate sanitation. *A. lumbricoides* is the largest and most prevalent of the human nematodes, rivaling pinworms, and whipworms.

Also called roundworm, tend to get entangled with each other and hence manifests as small intestinal obstruction.

Larger collection of coiled worms of Ascaris lumbricoides/roundworms (worm balls) giving the "Medusa lock" appearance may be identified on plain abdominal radiographs itself.

The mass of worms is contrasted against the gas in the bowel, usually in a distended segment, resembling a tangled group of thick cords and sometimes producing a "whirlpool" effect.

The worms can be identified in barium studies as single or multiple smooth longitudinal or coiled filling defects, sometimes with a thin central track of barium outlining the worm's intestinal tract.

Ankylostoma Duodenale

Also called hookworm, has hook-like process with which it sucks blood and hence it manifests as iron deficiency anemia.

Trichuriasis

Trichuriasis is an infection of the colon caused by the whipworm Trichuris trichiura.

Neonatal GI Obstruction

- An abdominal radiography in neonate with **hypertrophic pyloric stenosis** shows a distended air-filled stomach with a relative paucity of bowel gas distally.
- Abdominal radiography in **duodenal atresia** demonstrates the classic 'double-bubble' sign with an absence of distal air.
- **Ladd's band**, the abnormal peritoneal bands, passing from the cecum to porta hepatis region, crossing the duodenum are often present in patients with malrotation and may contribute to partial duodenal obstruction but are rarely the sole cause.
- **Midgut volvulus** (Corkscrew appearance).
- **Jejunal or proximal ileum atresia** often show 'triple bubble' appearance on abdominal radiograph and presence of microcolon should raise suspicion of an earlier, more distal atresia (ileal) or presence of further ileal atresia in addition to a proximal lesion.
- **Ileal atresias** are result of *in utero* vascular insults. Abdominal radiographs show multiple dilated loops, sometimes with greater dilatation of one loop but, unlike meconium ileus, multiple air fluid levels are common. Contrast enema will show an unused microcolon.
- In **meconium ileus** or ileal atresia, dilated meconium packed loops of bowel plain radiographs are helpful in that they can define the level of the obstruction and potentially identify bubbly meconium within the dilated distal small bowel ("soap bubble" appearance).

Small Bowel Obstruction

The distal ileum is the site of small bowel obstruction in most patients with normal or equivocal plain abdominal radiographs.

Features	Small bowel	Large bowel
Haustra	Absent	Present
Valvulae conniventes	Present in jejunum	Absent
Number of loops	Many	Few
Distribution of loops	Central	Peripheral
Diameter of loop	Small	Large
Radius of curvature of loop	30–50 mm	50 mm
Solid feces (only reliable sign)	Absent	May be +

X-ray features include
- Erect films show multiple fluid levels and dilated gas-filled loops of small bowel are readily identified on supine film.
- Dilated fluid-filled loops of small bowel may be seen as 'sausage shaped' soft tissue densities.
- **"String of beads sign"** (gas trapped between valvulae conniventes only when very dilated small bowel is almost completely fluid filled and it is virtually diagnostic of small bowel obstruction).
- **"Step-ladder"** appearance in low obstruction (the greater the number of dilated bowel loops, more distal is the site obstruction).
  The **"concertina effect"** in Jejunal obstruction are known features.
- Single/multiple loops of >2.5–3 cm in diameter with three air fluid levels in erect film (**candy-cone appearance**) is a helpful feature.
- Enteroclysis is proving to be reliable for investigating suspected small bowel obstruction and can differentiate postoperative obstruction from ileus.

> CT is now recommended as the technique of choice for the investigation of suspected intestinal obstruction. Small intestinal obstruction is differentiated from paralytic ileus on CT by demonstrating a **transitional zone** between dilated loops of small intestine proximal to the site of obstruction and collapsed loops of small intestine or colon distal to the site of obstruction. With oral gastrografin contrast, CT is excellent also to evaluate cases of recurrent small bowel obstruction.

- USG may show dilated, fluid-filled intestinal loops in abdomen, particularly in closed loop obstruction.
- *Barium study:* Active peristalsis forms bulbous head of barium column in an attempt to overcome obstruction (**"snake head" appearance**) and barium appears in colon after 12 hours.

> The **'string of beads' sign** on abdominal film, due to bubbles of gas trapped between the valvulae conniventes is seen only when very dilated small bowel is almost completely filled with fluid, and is

virtually diagnostic of small bowel obstruction. It is not seen in normal people, after cathartics or following cleansing enemas.

The **'string of beads' sign** is virtually diagnostic of small bowel obstruction.

Strangulating Obstruction

Strangulating obstruction is a mechanical small bowel obstruction of two limbs of a loop by a band or within a hernia, in such a way as to compromise the blood supply by compression of the mesenteric vessels.
- If gangrene occurs, linear gas shadows are seen in the wall of small bowel.

CT scan signs of strangulated obstruction include:
- Wall thickening of affected loop
- High attenuation in bowel wall (due to hemorrhage)
- Gas in bowel wall
- Mesenteric congestion
- Mesenteric hemorrhage

- **String sign** is also a Barium study feature of CHPS characterized by Passing of small barium streak through pyloric canal seen as a string of barium.
- The 'string of beads' sign on abdominal film is diagnostic of SBO.
- String sign of Keantor ⇒ Chronic disease.

- In India (developing countries) most common cause of small intestinal stricture is tuberculosis while in western countries it is Crohn's disease.

Intussusception

- Telescope-like invagination or prolapse of a segment of intestinal tract (intussusceptum = donor loop) into the lumen of the adjacent intestine (intussuscipiens = receiving loop)
- In children, over 95 percent times its is idiopathic, lymphoid hyperplasia following viral gastroenteritis considered
- Most common acute abdomen of early childhood
- *Types:* Ileocolic (75–95%) > ileo ileocolic (9%) > ileoileal > colocolic
- In adults the most common cause is specific, i.e. tumor.

- **Radiological signs include**

  Plain film
  Target sign → soft tissue mass with concentric circular areas of lucency due to the mesenteric fat of intussusceptum.
  Meniscus sign → crescent of gas within colonic lumen that outlines apex of intussusceptum.

  Antegrade barium study
  "Coiled spring" appearance, "beaklike" abrupt narrowing of barium column demonstrating a central channel (barium between the intussusception and surrounding colon produces a "coiled-spring" appearance).
  Pincer sign

  Barium enema
  Meniscus sign → convex intracolic mass
  Coiled spring sign → edematous mucosal folds of returning limb of intussusceptum outlined by barium within lumen of colon.
  Claw sign

  USG (98–100 % sensitive, 88–100 % specific)
  - Investigation of choice today.
  - **"Crescent-in-doughnut/Target/Bull's eye" sign (transverse scan)** → concentric rings of alternating hypoechoic and hyperechoic layers with central hyperechoic mesentery
  - **"Pseudokidney/Sandwich/Hay fork/Hamburger" sign (longitudinal scan)** → hypoechoic layers in each side of echogenic center of mesenteric fat
  - **"Doughnut"**—seen after successful reduction of intussusception.

  CT
  "Multiple concentric rings"
  Three concentric cylinders scan
  Central cylinder = Canal + wall of intussusceptum
  Middle cylinder = Crescent of mesenteric fat
  Outer cylinder = Returning intussusceptum + intussuscipiens

  Signida de dance/empty right iliac fossa/dance sign is clinical sign of ileocolic intussusception.
  Jejunogastric intussusception is reverse intussusception (efferent loop in 75%, afferent loop in 25%) presenting in two forms: acute (high intestinal obstruction, mass in left hypochondrium and hemetemesis) and chronic or intermittent form (self-limiting).

It is seen in operated patients of gastrojejunostomy and gives "coiled-spring" appearance of gastric filling defect.

Abdominal Tuberculosis/TB

TB abdomen includes:
- Intestinal TB
- Tubercular peritonitis
- Tubercular lymphadenopathy
- TB affecting visceral organs.

Intestinal TB

The main types of intestinal TB are ulcerative form (most frequent), hypertrophic form and mixed form.
Location: Ileocecal region > ascending colon > jejunum > appendix > duodenum > stomach > sigmoid > rectum > esophagus.
  i. Ileocecal area:

Barium Enema Features of Ileocecal Tuberculosis

- Early involvement of the ileocecal region manifesting as spasm and edema of the ileocecal valve. Thickening of the lips of the ileocecal valve and/or wide gaping of the valve with narrowing of the terminal ileum ("**Fleischner**" or "**inverted umbrella sign**") are characteristic.
- **Fold thickening and contour irregularity** of the terminal ileum, better appreciated on double contrast study.
- **Conical cecum** or "**Amputed cecum**" shrunken in size and pulled out of the iliac fossa due to contraction and fibrosis of the mesocolon. The hepatic flexure may also be pulled down.
- Loss of normal ileocecal angle and dilated terminal ileum, appearing suspended from a retracted, fibrosed cecum ("**goose neck deformity**").
- **Purse string stenosis**—localized stenosis opposite the ileocecal valve with a rounded off smooth cecum and a dilated terminal ileum.
- **Stierlin's sign** is a manifestation of acute inflammation superimposed on a chronically involved segment and is characterized by lack of barium retention in the inflamed segments of the ileum, cecum and variable length of the ascending colon, with a normal configured column of barium on either side. It appears as a narrowing of the terminal ileum with rapid emptying into a shortened, rigid or obliterated cecum.

- **String sign**—Persistent narrow stream of barium indicating stenosis.
- **Widening of IC angle** is also a common feature.
  - *Colon*:
    i. Segmental colonic involvement
    ii. Diffuse ulcerating colitis + pseudopolyps
    iii. Amputated/Coned/Contracted cecum.
  - *Gastroduodenal*
    i. Simultaneous involvement of pylorus + duodenum → 'Linitus plastic' appearance.
    ii. Linitus plastic may also be a feature of gastric lymphoma and scirrhous carcinoma, eosinophilic gastritis.

Tubercular Peritonitis

- Dry or plastic form
- Wet form (loculated and generalized ascites)
- Mixed form:
  - Ascites
  - Caseous adenopathy
  - Adhesions
  - Omental cake like mass with separation and fixation of bowel loops
  - Omentum, peritoneum and mesentery all may be involved.
- Purulent form (from genitourinary spread).

Tuberculous lymphadenopathy (Pseudomesenteric cyst due to caseation of large nodes; Mesenteric and retroperitoneal node enlargement is specific a feature of MAIC infection).

Tuberculosis of visceral organs

SMALL INTESTINAL NEOPLASMS

Malignant	Benign
Lymphoma	Leiomyomas
Adenocarcinoma	Adenomas
Leiomyosarcoma	Lipomas and angiomas
Secondaries	
Carcinoid	

Enteroclysis is not more widely used because of perceived patient discomfort potentially high radiation dose and extraluminal pathology is not assessable.

USG has a limited role in the diagnosis and management of disorders of the small intestine.

CT (IV + Oral contrast) show the extent of spread of the mass and evaluate sites of neoplastic involvement like abdominal lymph nodes and solid organs, allowing accurate staging at a single examination.

Carcinoid Tumor

- It arises from the neuroectodermal Kulchitsky cells and are a type of APUDoma.
- The most common site of carcinoid tumors is the appendix.
- Carcinoid syndrome, which is characterized by flushing, diarrhea, and cardiac valvular disease, occurs in a small percentage of patients with carcinoid tumors; it is rarely seen with appendiceal carcinoids.
- It occurs when serotonin is released into the systemic circulation.
- The appropriate therapy for a small carcinoid (less than 2 cm) of the appendix is simple appendectomy.
- CECT shows brilliantly enhancing lesion on mesenteric border with gross desmoplastic reaction (mesenteric puckering).

APPENDIX

Acute Appendicitis

In acute appendicitis usually the clinical findings are typical, a prompt diagnosis is made and an abdominal radiograph is not indicated.

In number of patients, however, the clinical features are obscure and diagnosis is difficult or impossible without laparotomy, when radiology, especially USG and CT, play a significant role.

X-ray signs of acute appendicitis are appendicolith (5–60 mm), sentinel loop, widening and blurring of the properitoneal fat lines, right lower quadrant haze due to fluid and edema, scoliosis concave to the right, mass indenting the cecum, blurring of right psoas shadow and gas in appendix (unreliable). Evidence of appendicolith has high positive correlation with acute appendicitis.

Ultrasound and CT show a great potential to improve diagnostic accuracy in patients with suspected appendicitis. **USG signs** include a noncompressible, nonperistaltic, blind-ending tubular structure of diameter 7 mm or greater, a appendicolith casting acoustic shadow, high echogenicity surrounding fat, surrounding fluid or abscess, edema of cecal pole and maximal probe tenderness in RIF. **The main drawback of ultrasound is that, in most cases, a normal appendix is usually not visualized.**

Nevertheless, USG can diagnose a number of conditions that mimic appendicitis clinically (e.g. ectopic pregnancy, ovarian cyst, etc.).

CT signs of appendicitis include an appendix measuring greater than 6 mm in diameter, failure of the appendix to fill with oral contrast medium or air up to its lip, an appendicolith, and enhancement of its wall with IV contrast. Surrounding inflammatory changes include increased fat attenuation, fluid, inflammatory phlegmon, cecal thickening, abscess, extraluminal gas, and lymphadenopathy. An 'arrowhead' sign consists of luminal contrast or air in the cecum pointing towards the obstructed origin of appendix, seen in 30 percent cases. A normal appendix is visualized more frequently on CT, and this is the key advantage of CT over USG. The sensitivity and specificity of CT is achieved up to 100 percent and 95 percent respectively in diagnosing appendicitis while that for ultrasound it is 78 to 98 percent and 85 to 98 percent respectively.

Clinical examination with leukocytosis is gold standard.

COLON AND RECTUM

Hirschsprung's Disease

It is a form of functional bowel obstruction, which is due to failure of caudal migration of neuroblasts in the developing bowel causing the distal large bowel from the point of neuronal arrest to the anus, aganglionic.

Four forms
1. Ultra-short segment disease (rare) → affects only anal canal at the level of internal sphincter
2. Short segment disease (75% cases) → affects only rectosigmoid region
3. Long segment disease → affects variable portion of colon proximal to sigmoid
4. Total aganglionosis coli → affects entire colon and part of terminal ileum.

Neonates of Hirschsprung's disease present with abdominal distension, vomiting and failure to pass meconium. Children who present in childhood later have history of constipation and failure to thrive.

Imaging Features

Abdominal Radiograph

- Typically shows a low bowel obstruction commonly with colonic dilatation out of proportion to small bowel.
- Absence of rectal gas may be seen.

- Pneumoperitonium may be seen in 5 percent cases.
- Intraluminal small bowel calcifications (enteroliths) in long segment disease.

Water Soluble Contrast Medium/Barium Enema
- Most vital film is a lateral view of the rectum during slow filling.
- Cone-shaped **transition zone**, abnormal, i.e. reversal of **rectosigmoid ratio** (normal >1) and irregular/tertiary rectal contractions are diagnostic features.
- The radiological transition zone is commonly found distal to pathological zone.

Rectal biopsy: A section or full thickness rectal biopsy is required for the definitive diagnosis of Hirschsprung's disease.

Anorectal Malformations

Early in its development, the cloaca is divided by a urogenital fold that causes separation of the urinary and gastrointestinal tracts. It is abnormalities of this process that result in anal atresia and resultant fistulas between the proximal rectum and genitourinary tract.

Air reaches in stomach within seconds after birth, enters small bowel within 1 hour, reaches cecum 3–4 hours after birth, and appears in sigmoid colon by 10–11 hours of birth.

- The traditional radiological approach for imperforate anus/anal atresia is inverted lateral radiograph (invertogram) of which a false interpretation film is obtained when the film is taken within first 24 hours of life, when there has been insufficient time for gas to reach the rectum or if infant had not been held prone for sufficient time to allow gas to reach tip of rectal pouch or there is impacted meconium.
- Best X-ray today is Cross Table Lateral View.
- Given a chance, MRI can best evaluate anorectal malformation.

Necrotizing Enterocolitis

- Most common life-threatening emergences of GIT in newborns
- Preterm infants particularly susceptible (Greatest risk factor)
- *Etiology*: *Triad* of intestinal ischemia, oral feedings and pathogenic organisms has been linked to necrotizing enterocolitis (NEC)
- Onset of NEC occurs usually in first 2 weeks but as late as 3 months of age in VLBW babies

- *First signs* are gaseous abdominal distention and gastric retention
- Persistent loop sign may be seen
- Pneumatosis intestinal—*diagnostic* of NEC (Most common in RLQ)
- Gas in portal vein is a *sign of severe* disease
- Gross pneumoperitoneum can occur if perforation occurs
- Post NEC strictures may occur, in splenic flexure in less severe cases
- Risk of NEC is significantly low in infants on exclusive breastfeeding
- Treatment includes cessation of feeding, nasogastric decompression, IV fluids, antibiotic, removal of umbilical catheter if any.

Solitary Rectal Ulcer Syndrome (Most Common an Anterior Wall of Rectum)

The solitary rectal ulcer syndrome is produced mainly by abnormalities of defecation, with discoordination and internal prolapse of the rectal mucosa. This secondarily causes either trauma or ischemia to the rectal mucosa with resultant inflammation and ulceration. The radiographic changes may vary from subtle mucosal irregularities, to frank ulceration, and eventually fibrosis and stricturing. On rare occasions, the inflamed mucosa may even produce a polypoid type of lesion of the rectal mucosa.

Colitis Cystica Profunda

Rare benign condition characterized by submucosal mucus containing cysts lined by normal colonic epithelium.
- Nodular polypoidal/cauliflower lesion less than 2 cm in size.
- Primary disease of young adults.
- Associated with solitary rectal syndrome.
- Most commonly localized to rectum.

Ischemic Colitis

'Thumb-printing' appearance of the submucosal thickening due to edema and hemorrhage with its crescentic margins has been used to describe ischemic colitis, which can sometimes be detected on plain radiographs but in most cases a barium enema is necessary, which is characterized by following features:
- Gross spasm of affected segment
- Linear ulcers
- Mosaic pattern

- 'Thumbprinting' appearance
- Funnelling of the bowel the level of transition from abnormal to normal gut

> Ischemic colitis **most often affects splenic flexure** and proximal descending colon.
>
> Features of **acute mesenteric ischemia or mesenteric thrombosis** causing small bowel infarction include:
> - Gas-filled, slightly dilated loops of small bowel with multiple air-fluid levels
> - Thickened walls of small bowel loops due to submucosal hemorrhage and edema
> - Linear gas streaks (if gangrenous)
> - Free gas (if perforated).

Crohn's Disease (Regional Ileitis)

- Occurs anywhere along gut from mouth to anus
- Terminal ileum is most commonly affected
- Aphthoid/longitudinal/fissuring/rose-thorn ulcers
- Skip lesions
- Transmural involvement (distinguishing feature)
- Perianal fissure and fistulae
- Noncaseating granulomas
- Cobblestone mucosa
- "String sign" of Kantor on barium enema
- Multiple strictures
- Enteroenteric, enterovesical fistulae
- Mesenteric inflammation, phlegmon, fibrofatty proliferation (Omega sign on barium enema)
- Extracolonic manifestations and changes into carcinoma are less common as compare to UC.

Ulcerative Colitis

- Inflammatory bowel disease.
- Rectum is always involved.
- Bloody diarrhea is the most common presentation.
- Double contrast barium enema (DCBE) is the radiological examination of choice to show disease extent and severity.

Instant enema → In UC the large bowel is inflamed and contains no fecal matter, and hence enema study can be done without bowel preparation.

Acute changes:
- *Earliest radiological change* on DCBE is blurring of mucosal lining and a fine mucosal granularity (enface) due to edema.
- Colorectal narrowing and incomplete filling due to spasm and irritability
- Scalloping of the edges of colon, especially the sigmoid colon
- Mucosal stippling due to crypt abscesses (continuous; not transmural)
- 'Collar button' ulcers
- Toxic megacolon
- Pseudopolyps

Chronic changes:
- Shortening and narrowing of colon
- 'Lead pipe' colon
- Loss of haustrations
- Backwash ileitis
- Thickened rectal valve
- Widening of presacral space (normally 1.5 cm at S_4 vertebral level)
- Benign stricture
- Carcinoma of colon/rectum
  - May be associated with HLA B27
  - May also be associated with seronegative spondyloarthropathies and primary sclerosing cholangitis.
  - Treatment: Acetyl salicylic acid, steroids, methotrexate and immunosuppressants.
  - Surgery: Total proctocolectomy with ileostomy/ileoanal pouch.

Type of abnormality	Radiological feature	Ulcerative colitis	Crohn's disease
Mucosal	Granularity	++	±
	Cobble-stoning	–	+
	Aphthoid ulcers	–	++
Configuration of bowel wall	Fissuring ulcers	–	++
	Haustra blunted	++	+
	Gen. narrowing and shortening (hose-pipe)	++	–

Contd...

Contd...

	String sign of Kantor	–	+
	Widened postrectal space	++	±
Distribution of lesions	Transmural	+	–
	Pseudodiverticuli	–	++
	Rectum involved	++	+
	Continuity	++	±
	Skip areas	–	+
	Backwash ileitis	+	–
	Multiple anal fistulas	–	+
Complications	Enteroenteric fistula	–	+
	Perforation	+	–
	Toxic megacolon	+	±
	Carcinoma	+	±

Diverticulosis of Colon

- It is characterized by herniation of mucosa and submucosa through the muscle layers of colonic wall.
- Most common after 7th decade of life.
- 80 percent occur in sigmoid colon.
- Barium enema study may show:
  - "Saw-tooth" sign (crowding and thickening of haustral fold)
  - Bubbly appearance of air containing diverticulae.
  - *En face* view may show circular line/ring shadow/meniscus with sharp outer edge and fuzzy/blurred inner margin or a fluid-barium level or barium pool and is extramural in location with absent Bowler's hat sign as seen in polyps in oblique view.

Sigmoid Volvulus

It is the classical volvulus, occurring mostly in old age or psychiatrically ill or institutionalized people, usually due to twisting of sigmoid loop around mesenteric axis. Redundancy of colon and long mesentery predisposes to recurrent volvulus.

Plain radiograph can clinch the diagnosis in many cases; however, in up to one-third cases it is difficult to differentiate a twisted sigmoid from a distended but non-rotated sigmoid, or from more proximal colonic distention, when Ba enema may be helpful.

The Plain Radiographic Features

- Inverted U shaped massively distended colonic loop
- Ahaustral margins
- Liver overlap sign (ahaustral margin overlapping lower border of liver shadow)
- Left flank overlap sign (ahaustral margin overlapping haustrated, dilated descending colon)
- Pelvic overlap sign (ahaustral margin overlapping the left side of pelvis)
- D_{10} overlap sign (apex of volvulus lying very high in abdomen, above D_{10} level on left side)
- **Apex under left hemidiaphragm**
- Inferior convergence sign on left side of pelvis
- A fluid ratio greater than 2 percent.

Left flank overlap sign, Apex above D_{10}, under the left dome of diaphragm and inferior convergence sign are highly specific (100%) and sensitive signs for sigmoid volvulus.

Ba enema: "Bird of Prey" sign.

R_x: Flatus tube insertion and sigmoidoscopy may be tried. If no relief, surgical correction with sigmoidopexy can be done.

Carcinoma Colon

- Four morphologic forms are known: concentric thickening (annular or tubular), cauliflower growth, ulcerative lesion and stricturous form.
- "Apple core" appearance is classical of **ca colon** on Ba enema (annular form). But CECT is best for staging.

Ca Rectum

Duke's staging of rectal cancer:
A → involvement of colonic wall except for serosa (confined to bowel wall)
B → serosal and perirectal involvement (spread beyond muscularis propria)
C → involvement of perirectal nodes
D → distant spread

TNM staging:
T1 → tumor penetration up to submucosa
T2 → muscularis propria

T3 → perirectal fat/subserosa
T4 → adjacent structures/perforation
N0 → no nodal involvement
N1 → 1-3 perirectal/pericolic nodes
N2 → >4 nodes
N3 → apical node or one along named vascular trunk
M0 → no distant metastasis
M12 → metastasis
Radiological studies help in detection and staging, where:
MRI > TRUS > CECT.

Villous Adenomas

These may spread superficially along the walls of the rectum rather than grow as an exophytic or intraluminal type of growth. Often, these lesions are extensive before being discovered endoscopically or radiographically, and may contain foci of adenocarcinoma within them. On double-contrast barium enema, these lesions produce a "shaggy" appearance over a large portion of the mucosa and are thus termed "carpet lesions". This type of growth is seen mainly in the rectum and the right side of the colon.

Neoplasms of the Anal Canal

These are often staged radiographically. The most common tumor of the anal canal is squamous cell carcinoma. These are more frequently seen in patients who are immunosuppressed, such as transplant recipients, or patients who are human immunodeficiency virus (HIV)-positive. A rare tumor in this region is a cloacogenic carcinoma. These lesions may be demonstrated by double-contrast barium enema, usually presenting as a plaque-like or polypoid lesion of the anal verge. CT or MRI is used to stage these lesions, and rectal ultrasonography may be used to evaluate the depth of invasion. But overall MRI is best.

Gastrointestinal Bleeding

- The sensitivity of angiography for detecting GI bleeding is about 10 to 20 percent less as compared to nuclear imaging
- Angiography can image bleeding at a rate of 0.5 to 1/min
- ^{99m}Tc-RBC scan will image bleeding at rates as low as 0.05 to 0.1 ml/min
- Angiography will detect bleeding only if extravasation is occurring during the injection of contrast.

Uses of Nuclear Scan in GI Diseases
- Gastrointestinal bleeding detection and localization
  Using Tc-99m sulfur colloid
  Using Tc-99m red blood cells
- Inflammatory bowel disease imaging
- Ectopic gastric mucosa imaging
- Gastric emptying half-time determination
- Gastroesophageal reflux imaging and function study
- Esophageal motility function study
- Salivary gland imaging
- *Helicobacter pylori* detection

BLUNT TRAUMA ABDOMEN

- Plain radiographs should include a supine abdominal radiograph or decubitus abdominal radiograph, with right side elevated if perforation is suspected.
- Ultrasound is less sensitive than CT for detection of bowel and visceral injury but has a sure role where CT is unavailable or may be delayed. It is 86 percent sensitive, 99 percent specific and 98 percent accurate. FAST is best protocol for screening blunt abdominal trauma.
- CT is imaging method of choice for evaluation of stable patients with blunt trauma abdomen.
- Diagnostic peritoneal lavage (DPL) cannot quantify amount of hemoperitoneum and results in a 19 to 39 percent rate of nontherapeutic surgeries.

Focused Abdominal Sonogram for Trauma

- Three most commonly used diagnostic techniques are diagnostic peritoneal lavage, USG and CT.
- DPL is nonspecific, can cause iatrogenic and injury and may not detect retroperitoneal injuries, while CT is expensive and time consuming which may also need IV contrast injection and need transporting the patient but USG overcomes most of these disadvantages.
- Focused assessment with sonography for trauma (FAST) examination is a bedside screening tool to identify free intraperitoneal, pleural and pericardial fluid. It is limited ultrasound examination with 6 views.
- The average time to perform a complete FAST examination is 2 to 4 minutes.

Chapter 6 ❖ Abdominal Imaging

Subxiphoid 4-chamber view of the heart	To look for pericardial fluid
Right intercostal oblique view	To look for right pleural effusion
Right coronal view	To look for free fluid in Morrison's pouch and paracolic gutter
Left intercostal oblique view	To look for left pleural effusion, free fluid in subphrenic space
Left coronal view	For left paracolic gutter
Pelvic (Longitudinal/transverse) view	To detect free fluid in cul-de-sac.

X-ray sign	Clinical condition
Thumb sign	Acute epiglottitis
Steeple sign	Croup (Acute laryngotracheobronchitis)
Outpouching from posterior pharyngeal wall just below inferior constrictor on lateral view	Zenker's diverticulum
'Rat-tail' appearance	Carcinoma esophagus
'Bird-beak' esophagus with mega/sigmoid esophagus	Achalasia cardia
Cork-screw/Shish-Kabab esophagus	Diffuse esophageal spasm
	Presbyesophagus
Shaggy esophagus	Candidiasis
Long, tight, and smooth stricture of esophagus	Lye ingestion
String sign	CHPS
Carman's meniscus sign	Malignant gastric ulcer/Ulcerative form of ca stomach
Hampton's line	Benign gastric ulcer
Duodenal stricture	*H. pylori* and *Strongyloides stercoralis*
Double bubble sign	Duodenal atresia
	Ladd's band
	Annular pancreas
Triple bubble sign	Jejunal atresia
Multiple bubble sign	Ileal atresia
Apple peel bowel	Ileal atresia
Frostburg's reverse '3' sign	Carcinoma head of pancreas
Pad's sign	Carcinoma head of pancreas
Cut-off sign of D3	SMA syndrome
Moulage sign	Malabsorption (Celiac sprue)
Whirl-pool sign	Malrotation with midgut volulus
Medusa-lock sign	Roundworm (Ascaris lumbricoides) infestation
String of beads sign	Small bowel obstruction
Mucosal granularity	Earliest sign of ulcerative colitis

Contd...

Contd...

Lead-pipe or pipe-stem colon	Ulcerative colitis
Thumb-print sign	Ischemic colitis
Saw-tooth appearance of colon (Splenic flexure)	Ischemic colitis
Bowler's hat sign	Colonic polyp
'Apple-core' appearance of colon	Carcinoma of colon
Claw sign	Intussusception
Coiled-spring sign	Intussusception
Inverted 'U' or 'V' sign	Sigmoid volvulus
'Bird of prey' sign	Sigmoid volvulus
Transition zone	Hirschprung's disease
'Pseudobilroth' appearance and 'Ram's horn' stomach	Crohn's disease (Regional ileitis)

HEPATOBILIARY SYSTEM

Segmental Liver Anatomy

Functional segmental liver anatomy by **Couinaud and Bismuth** is based on distribution of three major hepatic veins and divides liver into **8 segments**:

Middle hepatic vein
- Divides liver into right and left lobe
- Also separated by main portal vein incisura, the Cantlie line passing through IVC and long axis of gallbladder

Left hepatic vein
- Divides left lobe into medial-lateral sectors

Right hepatic vein
- Divides right lobe into anterior and posterior sectors

Segment I : Caudate lobe
Segment II : Left lateral superior
Segment III : Left lateral inferior
Segment IV : Quadrate lobe
- Left medial superior
- Left medial inferior

Segment V : Right anteroinferior
Segment VI : Right posteroinferior
Segment VII : Right posterosuperior
Segment VIII : Right anterosuperior

Vessel	Ultrasound/Doppler characteristics
Portal vein	Approximately 25% of the flow into the liver is supplied by the hepatic artery, the remainder by the portal vein. The portal vein walls are seen as well-defined parallel reflective thin lines. Normal portal venous flow is **hepatopetal** and is usually **monophasic** with some fluctuation due to respiration and cardiac activity. Thus, when color flow is being used to assess the portal vein, flow into the liver conventionally appear red. Portal vein pulsatility may be seen in thin healthy subjects, in patients with congestive heart failure and in a very few patients with liver disease. The pulse repetition rate (PRF) may need to be ↓ to detect flow in patients with portal hypertension.
Hepatic artery	The hepatic artery can be identified in most patients at the porta hepatis lying between the portal vein and common bile duct. In a small percentage of patients this anatomy may be altered and the hepatic artery may lie anterior to the bile duct. Color flow imaging allows rapid differentiation of bile duct from hepatic artery. In older patients with an ectatic hepatic artery or in patients with a dilated hepatic artery, which can occur in alcoholic hepatitis and cirrhosis, this may prevent misinterpretation of a dilated common duct. The hepatic arterial wave form characteristically has a high diastolic phase due to the low resistance of the hepatic vascular bed.
Hepatic veins	There are usually three hepatic veins—the right, the middle and the left—which drain into the IVC. These may be differentiated from portal vein radicals not only by their anatomical positions and patterns of drainage but also by the lack of reflectivity of the hepatic vein walls. They are best interrogated either by scanning transversely in the epigastrium or by scanning transversely using an intercostal approach. The hepatic veins characteristically have a triphasic wave form which reflects right atrial and inferior vena caval pressures. This results in flow in the hepatic veins being predominately coded blue, i.e. away from the probe on the color Doppler, but with some phases being coded red. Loss of the triphasic wave form of the hepatic vein is seen in patients whose livers have lost compliance, for example in cirrhosis, acute hepatitis and liver transplant rejection.

Budd-Chiari Syndrome (Hepatic Veno-occlusive Disease)

Obstruction of hepatic veins secondary to an obstruction of IVC by a membrane or thrombus, or occlusion of the major hepatic vein branches (usually by thrombus) is known as Budd-Chiari syndrome (**Global segmental hepatic venous outflow obstruction at the level of large hepatic veins or suprahepatic segment of IVC**). It may be idiopathic but has been described in association with oral contraceptive use, Coagulopathies (polycythemia, TTP), and congenital membranes or webs in IVC.
- Primary (congenital-membranous type) is common in Asia.
- Secondary (thrombotic/nonthrombotic) is common in western countries.

Classifications

- *Type I*: Occlusion of IVC +/– hepatic veins
- *Type II*: Occlusion of major hepatic veins +/– IVC
- *Type III*: Occlusion of small centrilobular veins

Clinical Features

Retractable ascites, abdominal pain and tender hepatomegaly are classical clinical features.

These patients may present acutely with hepatomegaly, abdominal pain and ascites as the liver becomes congested and swells up.

Classic imaging appearance (Doppler study) is the absent/reversed/flat flow in hepatic veins and reversed flow in IVC.

"Spider web" pattern of collaterals on IVC/hepatic venography is pathognomonic.

FOCAL HEPATIC LESIONS

Screening = USG
Best = Triple phase CECT ≥ MRI.

Simple Hepatic Cysts

These are developmental with their incidence increasing with age. They may occur in younger patients with polycystic liver disease, ADPKD and (25–33%) von Hippel Lindau disease (usually >10).

It is usually single an echoic lesion with thin well-defined wall, without septae or debris in it with posterior acoustic enhancement.

D/D of Cystic Lesion in Liver

- Cystic metastases (e.g. ovarian cancer)
- Treated liver abscesses
- Hydatid cysts
- Post-traumatic
- Biliary cystadenoma
- Biliary static cyst
- Choledochal cyst

D/D of Bull's Eye Lesions of Liver
- Disseminated candidiasis
- Metastases
- Lymphoma
- Leukemia
- Sarcoidosis
- Septic emboli
- Kaposi sarcoma
- Other opportunistic infections

Cavernous Hemangiomas of Liver

- These are the **most common benign tumors of the liver**, occurring in all age groups but are more common in adults, particularly women.
- On **USG,** these are typically small, less than 3 cm sized, well-defined, and homogeneous and hyperechoic lesions. Mixed echogenicity can, however, be a feature of atypical liver hemangioma.
- Hemangiomas are characterized by very slow blood flow that won't routinely be detected by either **color or duplex doppler**. There are usually incidental findings observed on routinely performed abdominal sonograms and confirmation is costly and unnecessary.
- However, atypical pattern of hemangioma needs an additional imaging technique to confirm the suspicion of hemangioma.
- If the lesion is greater than 2.5 cm in diameter, a **TC-99m RBC study with SPECT** is recommended.
- If the lesion is less than 2.5 cm in diameter, **MRI** is recommended.
  Dynamic **triple-phase contrast enhanced CT scan** with **delayed sections**, although less specific than both hepatic scintigraphy and MRI, can reliably diagnose liver hemangioma and is presently the investigation of choice.
- CECT characteristically shows:
  - Delayed enhancement
  - 'Filling in' of the hemangiomas centripetally
  - Nodular densities of dilated vascular channels in the vicinity.
- If the imaging investigation provides indeterminate results, either percutaneous **biopsy** (USG guided) or follow-up at 3 to 6 months is recommended.

Focal Nodular Hyperplasia

Focal nodular hyperplasia (FNH) is the only liver tumor, which consistently contains functioning RE cells and so shows uptake of labeled colloids. It characteristically shows prolonged retention of IDA on delayed images (Hot-Spot).

Fibrolamellar Carcinoma (FLC)

On CT and MRI delayed enhancement of the **central scar** is a characteristic which results from the presence of vascularized collagenous tissue, in contrast with the central stellate scar seen in **fibrolamellar hepatic carcinoma**.

Hepatic Adenoma

- Hemorrhage or presence of capsule is pointer towards **hepatic adenoma**.
- Increased incidence of liver adenoma is known in glycogen storage disease type 1 (von Gierke's disease) and OC pill users.

Hepatocellular Carcinoma

Vascular invasion is atypical feature of HCC but tends to occur in larger lesions, which can cause portal vein invasion and thrombosis. Doppler study may distinguish tumor from thrombus as presence of arterial signals within the material occluding a portal vein indicates the presence of tumor. However the most sensitive approach for this study is CT in HCTAP phase and biphasic examination. The CT features of portal venous invasion by HCC include arterioportal fistula, periportal streaks of high attenuation, dilatation of main portal vein and its branches and the 'straight line sign', i.e. complete nonenhancement of the affected lobe (seen in HAP phase). Invasion may also be caused by secondaries in liver also.

Liver Metastasis

- Liver is the most common metastatic site after regional lymph nodes.
- Metastases to liver are most common malignant liver lesions.
- *Organ of origin:* Colon (42%), stomach (23%), pancreas (21%), breast (14%), lung (13%).
- Intraoperative USG is the most sensitive imaging modality.
- "Target Lesions" on USG and enhancement in arterial (CECT) phase can be diagnostic.
- Exclusion criteria for metastasectomy
  - Advanced stage of primary tumor

- > 4 metastases
- Extrahepatic disease
- < 30 percent normal liver tissue/function available after resection.
- Currently, intraoperative USG, PETCT fusion scan, MRI and CECT are modalities best and preferred for detection of liver metastases in that order.

Liver Tumors in Children

Type	Age	Alpha fetoprotein	Important comment and radiology
Hemangioma	Neonatal	Normal	Triple phase CECT
Hemangioendothelioma	Neonatal	Normal	MC tumor in infancy
Mesenchymal hamartoma	0–2 years	Normal	Benign/children
Hepatoblastoma	1–5 years	Elevated (highly)	MC in childhood, ↑ AFP
Embryonal sarcoma	6–10 years	Elevated	Rare
Hepatocellular carcinoma	12–15 years	Elevated	Hepatitis B predisposes

GALLBLADDER AND BILIARY APPARATUS

Diagnostic evaluation of the gallbladder

Diagnostic advantages	Diagnostic limitations	Comment
Plain abdominal X-ray: - Low cost - Readily available	- Relatively low yield - Contraindicated in pregnancy - In general, CT is definitely better than X-ray	*Best for:* - Calcified gallstones - Porcelain GB (a premalignant condition) - Emphysematous cholecystitis (*E. coli*) - Limey bile - Gallstone ileus (Rigler's triad)
Ultrasound: - Rapid - Accurate identification of gallstones (>95%) - Simultaneous scanning of GB, liver, bile ducts, pancreas	- Bowel gas - Massive obesity - Ascites	*Procedure of choice for:* - Detection of gall stones - Adenomyomatosis ("Comet tail" artefacts)

Contd...

Contd...

- "Real-time" scanning allows assessment of GB volume, contractility
- Not limited by jaundice, pregnancy
- May detect very small stones

Oral cholecystogram:
Replaced by ultrasonography

Radioisotope scans (HIDA, DIDA, etc):

- Accurate identification of cystic duct obstruction
- Simultaneous assessment of bile ducts

- Contraindicated in
  - pregnancy
  - Sr. bili>6-12 mg/dl
- Cholecystogram of low resolution
- Less sensitive and less specific in chronic cholecystitis.

Indicated for:
- Confirmation of suspected acute cholecystitis; useful in diagnosis of acalculous
- cholecystopathy, especially if given with CCK to assess gallbladder emptying
- Dysfunctional GB

IMAGING IN OBSTRUCTIVE JAUNDICE

The evaluation of the patient of obstructive jaundice can be done by many biochemical test and imaging modalities (Flow chart 6.1) like:

- Plain abdomen radiograph
- Oral cholecystography (OCG)
- Intravenous cholangiography
- Operative cholangiogram
- USG
- CT
- Isotope imaging
- PTC
- ERCP
- MRI, and
- MRCP.

Flow chart 6.1: Algorithm for management of benign obstruction

USG

- USG and/or CT evaluation of these patients is substantially valuable because of their easy availability, noninvasiveness, relative cost-effectiveness and accuracy in defining the level and cause of obstruction in more than 90 percent cases.

- Ultrasound (USG) is usual screening modality in the patients with jaundice. The principal role of USG is to differentiate obstructive from nonobstructive causes of cholestasis.
- It is primary modality for examining the biliary tree also because of its ease of performance in multiple planes (multiplanar scanning). It is the suitable modality in children or during pregnancy, because there is no radiation hazard. However, USG is operator dependent, stomach and bowel gas usually precludes a complete ultrasound examination of pancreas, surgical dressing or wound or an abundance of subcutaneous fat also preclude ultrasound examination in general and even mesenteric fat can be a difficulty for visualizing extrahepatic causes of obstruction.

CECT

If the cause of obstructive jaundice is not evident on USG and stones are not considered the most likely diagnosis, CT is next useful test. Multislice CT is highly accurate for identifying the level and cause of malignant obstruction (equal to MRI) and CT is good for resectability assessment. It is also preferred to detect extrinsic obstruction, but poor at det calculi.

Percutaneous Transhepatic Cholangiography

Invasive way of examining the bile duct system: This procedure is done under local anestheisa by a radiologist. During the exam, a thin needle is inserted through the skin (percutaneous) and through the liver (transhepatic) into a bile duct. Then contast media is injected, and the bile duct system is outlined on X-rays (cholangiography) (Fig. 6.1).

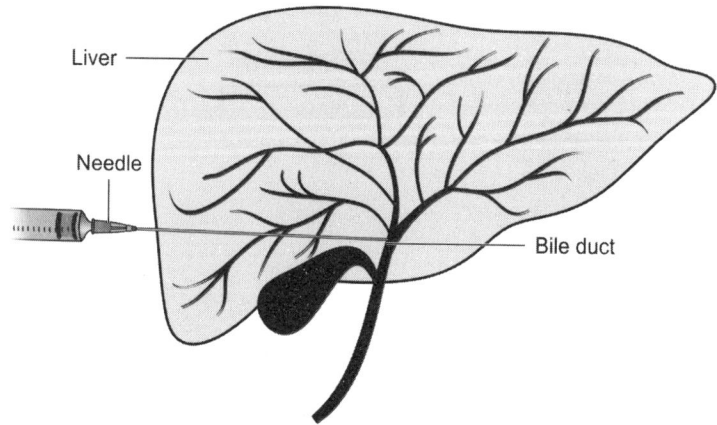

Fig. 6.1: Percutaneous transhepatic cholangiography (PTC)

The indications for percutaneous transhepatic cholangiography (PTC) are:
- To differentiate between hepatocellular and obstructive jaundice when clinical and laboratory examinations are inconclusive.
- To establish the nature and site of suspected obstruction for preoperative planning.
- To evaluate recurrent postoperative jaundice.
- To evaluate preoperatively patients with known biliary fistulas.
- To evaluate the biliary system in cases of congenital atresia.

Contraindications
- Sepsis
- Hypotension, or
- Severe hemorrhagic diathesis.

MRCP

MRCP versus ERCP
In patients with highly suspected pathology in which therapeutic ERCP may have value, there is little value in obtaining an MRCP. Such patients that would benefited from ERCP would include:
- Patients with obstructive jaundice in which ultrasound or CT scan suggests biliary dilatation from either a stone or a mass, where therapeutic remedies such as stone removal or stent placement with cytology aspiration could aid in diagnosis and in improvements in symptoms.
- Biliary dyskinesia in which patients with post cholecystectomy pain syndromes are being considered for sphincter of oddi manometry.
- Recurrent idiopathic pancreatitis in which patients are being considered for pancreatic/common bile duct manometry.
- Patients with pseudocysts in which attempts at endoscopic drainage with 1 of 8.
- Either stents or trans-gastric cyst-gastosotomy are considered.
- Postcholecystectomy bile leaks or surgical bile duct injuries, in which stenting of the bile duct or dilatation of strictures can occur with ERCP.

Examples where MRCP may have added value are in patients with a low probability of correctable pathology as provided with therapeutic ERCP such as:
- Patients with elevated liver function test which have no evidence of hepato-biliary ductal dilatation on abdominal ultrasound nor CT in which the risks of ERCP are especially high. These patients would include those with compromised cardiopulmonary function, patients with known problems with conscious sedation.

- Patients with unexplained abdominal pain in whom a low probability of hepato-biliary pathology such as retained common bile duct stones, cancer, biliary dyskinesia, or idiopathic pancreatitis is suspected by both clinical presentation and previous imaging such as CT and ultrasound.
- Patients with jaundice where there is no evidence of ductal dilatation by US nor CT but CBD dilatation needs to be ruled out.
- As with all new technology, the role of MRCP is still to be defined.

ERCP (Gold Standard Study)

- It has become primary method of direct cholangiography and additionally it offers the ability to examine upper GIT, the papilla of Vater and the pancreatic duct.
- It has developed considerable therapeutic potential and guided biopsies are possible.
- Post-cholecystectomy biliary stricture is important to identify and if ultrasound or other studies suggest that obstruction is low, **ERCP is investigation of choice**.
- Strictures close to the hilum may be well-delineated by ERCP only, but PTC is best.
- Most common complication of ERCP is acute pancreatitis.
- Contraindications to ERCP include Roux-en-Y gastrectomy, acute pancreatitis and pseudocyst of pancreas.

ERCP (Endoscopic Retrograde Cholangiopancreaticography)
It is required in patients with an obstructive pattern of liver function tests or in whom imaging suggests an abnormality of the biliary tract.
- In **chronic pancreatitis**, ERCP has the advantage of providing detailed images of the duct system.
- In chronic pancreatitis, dilatation or multifocal stenosis of main pancreatic duct and its lateral side-branches, intraductal filling defects representing protein plugs, areas of calcification and narrowing of intrapancreatic segment of the CBD. (**"Chain of lake" appearance**).
- When the dorsal and ventral ducts fail to fuse, **Pancreatic divisum** occurs. This anomaly may result in functional stenosis and pancreatitis. ERCP helps in diagnosis.
- ERCP can confirm the diagnosis of **annular pancreas** by demonstrating a segment of pancreas encircling the duodenum. It is an important cause of duodenal obstruction in neonates, apart from duodenal atresia and Ladd's band.

Hepatic Iminodiacetic Acid Scan (HIDA Scan) is a Biliary Scintigraphic Scan

Tc-99m acetanilide iminodiacetic acid analogs are HIDA agents and depending on their lipophilicity, there is a trade-off between renal excretion and hepatic uptake (HIDA is least lipophilic).

Applications and Indications
- Acute cholecystitis (investigation of choice).
- Congenital biliary atresia.
- Biliary leak evaluation.
- Biliary-enteric fistula.
- Chronic GB dysfunction.

Imaging in Cholelithiasis
- *Abdominal plain film* (10–16% sensitive)—20 to 30 percent gallstones may be radiopaque.
- *Oral cholecystography* (65–90% sensitive)—gallstones are seen as filling defect in lumen.
- *CT scan* (80% sensitive) detects hyperdense, calcified gallstones in 60 percent cases while soft calculi in 21 to 24 percent cases are missed.
- *USG* (91–98% sensitive): Gallstones are seen as hyperechoic focus due to echo from anterior surface of gallstone within gallbladder. "Wall-echo-shadow" or "double arch shadow" sign (**WES triad**) may be seen as two echogenic curvilinear parallel lines separated by sonolucent line, i.e. anterior GB wall + bile + stone with acoustic shadow.

Oral Cholecystography
- Graham-Cole was first to perform oral cholecystography (OCG) in 1942.
- Cholecystography used to be the method of choice for demonstrating gallstones but it has been largely replaced by ultrasound, which is simpler, safer, quicker, accurate and without the hazard of ionizing radiations.
- The media in use were sodium ipodate (Biloptin) and calcium ipodate (Solu-iloptin).
- Nowadays it is obsolete and there is probably no useful role for OCG in modern radiology.

RADIOLOGY OF GALLBLADDER AND BILIARY SYSTEM PATHOLOGIES

Gallstone Ileus
- It is a mechanical intestinal obstruction caused by impaction of one or more gallstones in the intestine, usually in the terminal ileum, but rarely in the duodenum or colon.
- Patient most commonly is middle age or elderly female, who often has had recurrent right hypochondriac pain and now the attack is severe and associated with more prolonged vomiting.
- It accounts for about two percent of patients presenting with small bowel obstruction.

- Gas in biliary tree can be recognized by its branching pattern with gas being more prominent centrally.
- Signs of gallstone ileus are:
  - Incomplete or complete small bowel obstruction
  - Gas within the GB and/or bile ducts
  - Abnormal location of a gallstone
  - Change in position of a gallstone
  - Relatively large fluid-gas ratio in distended loops

Gallstone ileus is a mechanical intestinal obstruction caused by impaction of one or more gallstone in the intestine, usually in the terminal ileum but rarely in the duodenum or colon.

It accounts for two percent of small bowel obstruction patients.

The patient, most commonly a middle-aged or elderly woman, often has history of recurrent episodes of pain characteristic of cholecystitis. The most recent attack will have been more severe and associated with more prolonged vomiting than previous episodes.

Radiological Signs of Gallstone Ileus

- Incomplete/complete small bowel obstruction
- Gas in the gallbladder and in the biliary tree branching pattern with gas being more prominent centrally.
- Abnormal location of a gallstone
- Change in the position of a gallstone
- Relatively large fluid: gas ratio in distended loops.

Rigler's Triad of Gallstone Ileus: a+b+c

Causes of Pneumobilia (Gas in the biliary tree) are:
- Physiological due to lax sphincter
- Gallstone fistula (Cholecystoenteric fistula)
- Malignant fistula (Cholecystoenteric fistula)
- Perforated peptic ulcer into bile duct
- Cholangitis (Emphysematous)
- Endoscopic sphincterotomy or following biliary surgery
- Techniques like percutaneous or endoscopic cholangiography.

Acute Cholecystitis

Only about 20 percent of gallstones contain sufficient calcium to be visible on plain radiographs and in normal state also it is very uncommon to identify a normal sized GB on plain radiographs as it is not surrounded by fat and in acute cholecystitis also it may be completely normal or show only borderline dilatation of small or large bowel. Ultrasound is widely used for diagnosing acute cholecystitis with features including thickened wall, associated gallstone, pericholecystic collection and distended GB. Contrast examinations like OCG have now been superseded by scintigraphy (HIDA and P-1P-1DA). Scintigraphy using ^{99m}Tc labeled derivatives of imidoacetic acid (HIDA and PIPIDA) is a simple and highly accurate method for diagnosing it and has a specificity approaching 100 percent. The scan is positive when there is no visualization of GB but prompt visualization of the bile duct and duodenum occurs with a blocked duct.

Features of Cholecystitis on USG

- Cholecystitis produces thickening of gallbladder wall (>2–3 mm)
- In acute cholecystitis, a circumferential lucent zone may be seen in gallbladder wall
- Striated appearance of gallbladder has been described
- In chronic cholecystitis the fibrosis leads to high level echoes and gallbladder is usually small
- Increased vascularity is seen on Doppler study.

Primary Sclerosing Cholangitis

It is a disease of unknown etiology characterized by a fibrosing inflammatory process affecting the intrahepatic and/or extrahepatic ducts and causing progressive cholestasis.

Currently its diagnosis is based on radiological findings.
Ultrasound examination is often normal or inconclusive.
CT may show focal areas of mild duct dilatation peripherally.
Scintigraphy (HIDA) may show multiple focal areas of increased uptake corresponding to dilated ducts.

Direct cholangiography is the **gold standard** investigation to diagnose it and **'pruned tree' appearance** is characteristic finding on cholangiography. However, similar picture is seen in AIDS related cholangiopathy.

AIDS-related Cholangiopathy

AIDS-related cholangiopathy is characterized by cholangitis (irregular thickened was of biliary radicals), papillary stenosis and multifocal extrahepatic biliary apparatus strictures with dilatation of CBD in its entire course. Cholangiography provides the most reliable information characterized by multifocal strictures of intra- and extrahepatic ducts, which, however, mimics the diffuse form of cholangiocarcinoma and is not absolutely diagnostic.

ERCP is the preferred approach because of greater likelihood of success using this method in the absence of intrahepatic duct dilatation.

Stricture in Bile Duct

Trauma (postsurgery), pyogenic or parasitic cholangitis, and sclerosing cholangitis in association with inflammatory bowel disease are the most common causes of biliary strictures. **Postsurgery (cholecystectomy) is the most common cause.**

Acute cholangitis is typically found in patients with obstruction or stone disease. Gram-negative organisms, (*E. coli* is most common) are often responsible. The disease can become quite severe and life-threatening, requiring immediate relief of the obstruction as well as antibiotic therapy.

Carcinoma Gallbladder

Risk Factors for Carcinoma Gallbladder

- Obesity
- Female gender
- Postmenopausal status
- Cigarette smoking
- Chronic *Salmonella typhi* infection
- Exposures to chemicals
- Cholelithiasis
- Porcelain GB
- Chronic cholecystitis
- Gallbladder polyp (adenomatous)
- Primary sclerosing cholangitis

- Congenital biliary anomalies like choledochal cyst
- Inflammatory bowel disease
- Familial polyposis coli.

EHBA

Phenobarbital augmented cholescintigraphy is 90 to 97 percent sensitive, 60 to 94 percent specific and 75 to 90 percent accurate for diagnosis of EHBA. It reveals no visualization of bowel on delayed images at 6 and 24 hrs. It is impossible to differentiate it from neonatal hepatitis in absence of small bowel activity and requires liver biopsy. Liver biopsy has 60–97 percent accuracy. Percutaneous/endoscopic/intraoperative cholangiography may be helpful but not gold standard.

Caroli's Disease

- It is a communicating cavernous ectasia of intrahepatic biliary ducts.
- It is a rare congenital, probably autosomal recessive disorder characterized by segmental saccular intrahepatic ducts.
- Multiple cystic structures converging toward porta hepatis communicating with bile ducts are characteristic features.
- Portal radicals completely surrounded by ciliated bile ducts, called as **'central dot sign'** is diagnostic CT feature.
- However, cholangiography is most diagnostic, featured by **segmental saccular/beaded appearance of intrahepatic bile ducts** extending to periphery of liver.
- It is equivalent to type V choledochal cyst.
- It may present as part of syndrome with congenital hepatic fibrosis and autosomal recessive polycystic kidney disease.
- Patient present in late childhood or early adulthood with cholangitis, rather than in infancy.
- Cholangiocarcinoma can develop later.
- Watson Alagille syndrome is arteriohepatic dysplasia associated with abnormal facies, butterfly vertebra and pulmonic stenosis.

Ultrasound in **Caroli's disease** (type v choledochal cyst characterized by segmental nonobstructive dilatation or ectasia of IHBRs) shows multiple low reflective cystic areas with a **central dot** of high reflection activity representing the portal vein branch surrounded by an ectatic bile duct.

PANCREAS

Radiographic Sign of Acute Pancreatitis

A large number of radiographic features have been described in acute pancreatitis, but these are uncommon and nonspecific hence not of much significance, these include:
- Gas filled dilated duodenal cap and loop
- Sentinel loop sign (single dilated small bowel loop), optimally demonstrated in left lateral decubitus view
- Renal halo sign (the left kidney has surrounding halo due to edema and is displaced down)
- Colonic 'cut-off' sign (dilated transverse colon becomes abruptly gasless in the region of splenic flexure)
- Gasless abdomen due to vomiting
- Dilated loop of other adjacent bowel coils (small bowel, terminal ileum, ascending and transverse colon), paralytic ileus
- Loss of left psoas outline
- Absent right psoas shadow
- Elevated left diaphragm
- Left pleural effusion
- Gas within pancreas, seen as multiple small bubbles giving "**mottled appearance**" or a air-fluid level is diagnostic of pancreatic abscess
- Opaque gallstones
- Pancreatic calcification
- Gastrocolic separation
- Groundglass haze in abdomen due to ascites
- Avascular necrosis and bone infarcts may be rarely seen.

Predict Severe Acute Pancreatitis

Serum markers for diagnosis of pancreatic necrosis, include: macroglobulin complement factor, C3 and C4, and CRP.
Ranson score >3 or APACHE score >8 also indicate severity.
Scoring system for severity of acute pancreatitis by CT (CT Severity Index/CTSI) is as follows: (Balthazar grade).

	CT features	Score
I. Grade		
	Normal gland	0
	Focal/diffuse enlargement	1
	Peripancreatic inflammatory changes	2
	Single peripancreatic fluid collection	3
	2 or more fluid collections or abscess	4
II. Necrosis		
	None	0
	<33%	2
	33–50%	4
	>50%	6

Total CTSI (0-10) = Balthazar Grade (0-4) + CT Scoring (0-6)

Score	Morbidity	Mortality
0–3	8%	3%
4–6	35%	6%
7–10	92%	17%

Computed tomography (CT) also plays an important role in evaluation of extrahepatic biliary tract dilatation and with the advent of newer generation of CT Machines, the resolution of bile ducts, gallbladder, liver parenchyma and peribiliary structures has improved. Imaging of extrahepatic portion of biliary system is usually more successful with CT than with ultrasound because duodenal and colonic gas and mesenteric fat all contribute to the degradation of ultrasound image of CBD.

The common extrinsic cause of biliary obstruction is pancreas. For complete study of pancreas CT is modality of choice for various reasons. Ultrasound is operator dependent, stomach and bowel gas usually precludes a complete ultrasound examination of pancreas, surgical dressing or wound or an abundance of subcutaneous fat also preclude ultrasound examination in general and even mesenteric fat can be a difficulty for visualizing extrahepatic causes of obstruction.

CT will identify the pancreatic head, body and tail including the uncinate process in nearly all patients. Retroperitoneal masses, duodenal lesions and peripancreatic adenopathy as causes of extrahepatic biliary dilatation although may be imaged with either CT or USG, but CT has clear advantage in imaging these cases as bowel gas obscure these regions on USG. The same is true with the area of liver obscured by ribs.

It also helps to assess the possibility of resectability of neoplastic lesions in terms of encasement of vessels, invasion of surrounding tissues and metastatic lesions, as these lesions are likely to benefit from surgical resection. In obese patients or patients with abdominal wounds and bandages also, CT can be investigation of choice. However, it is comparatively expensive and not free from disadvantages like exposure to ionizing radiations. CT plays a relatively minor role in evaluation of some conditions like biliary atresia and primary sclerosing cholangitis, in which radionuclide scan and MRCP/ERCP may be more helpful.

Acute Pancreatitis

CECT is imaging modality of choice for diagnosis and staging (Balthazar CT Severity Index) of acute pancreatitis.

CT features
- Pancreatic edema and loss of or fuzzy (dirty) appearance peripancreatic fat planes with cuffs of fluid around adjacent vessels and thickened fascial planes
- Nonenhancing areas of necrosis
- Nonenhancing localized collection of pus with brightly enhancing wall or rind of inflammatory tissue with gas bubbles
- Nonspecific peripancreatic fluid collection
- Pseudocysts (round to oval collection of pancreatic fluid) with fibrous capsule (with or without complications like infection, hemorrhage, rupture, biliary or pancreatic duct obstruction, or gastrointestinal tract involvement)
- Acute hemorrhage due to vessel erosion or rupture of varices and leakage of arterial aneurysm.
- Edema, necrosis or perforation of adjacent wall of stomach or duodenum.

In **chronic pancreatitis**, atrophy of the gland with dilatation or multifocal stenosis of main pancreatic duct and its lateral side-branches, intraductal filling defects representing protein plugs, areas of calcification and narrowing of intrapancreatic segment of the CBD are characteristic features (**"Chain of lake" appearance**).

Carcinoma Head of Pancreas

- Hypotonic duodenogram, ultrasound (transabdominal, endoscopic and laparoscopic), CT, MRI and ERCP may, under different circumstances, each has a role in the diagnosis of ductal adenocarcinoma (commonest type of pancreatic neoplasm).
- Carcinoma of the head of pancreas frequently causes changes in the duodenal loop (reversed '3' sign of Frostburg) as seen on the duodenogram.

- Transabdominal ultrasound is frequently the first imaging study carried out in these patients as it is inexpensive, widely available and highly accurate in differentiating obstructive from nonobstructive causes of jaundice and even very small pancreatic tumors may be detected.
- CECT is the most effective technique for the diagnosis and staging of potential theoretical advantages over CT and promising results are now emerging.
- ERCP demonstrates a structure and obstruction of pancreatic and common bile ducts and even directly visualizes duodenum and ampulla of Vater and also allows cytological sampling.

Ultrasound, CT, MRI and ERCP, may have a role in diagnosis of pancreatic carcinoma.

In practice, as it is inexpensive and widely available, **USG** is first imaging investigation carried out in patients in the pancreatic carcinoma.

CT with IV contrast (CECT) is the most sensitive and most widely used technique for diagnosis and staging of CA pancreas. Even small sized lesion, perivascular invasion, invasion of adjacent structures; lymph node involved can be assessed to greater extent.

Because the tumor pancreas are less vascular than surrounding normal pancreatic parenchyma, even a smaller lesion is seen as poorly enhanced focal area within the density enhancing normal pancreatic tissue on dynamic contrast enhanced CT.

Role of **MRI** in carcinoma pancreas is emerging.

ERCP is used in many cases as it has ability to visualize directly the duodenum and ampulla of Vater and allow cytological sampling and access for stent insertion, but extraluminal structures are not assessed and it is not sensitive for carcinoma pancreas.

Angiography formerly flayed an important role, that too in assessment of vascular involvement but has been superseded by CT.

Carcinoma head of the pancreas frequently causes changes in the duodenal loop. There may be widening of duodenal loop double contour, irregularity of the inner border, and structuring or distortion of the valvulae conniventes. Barium study of duodenum shows the infrequent but characteristic reversed '3' sign of Frostburg with effacement and distortion of the mucosal pattern on the medial wall of the second part of the duodenum in a patient with carcinoma of head of pancreas.

Periampullary Carcinoma

Double duct sign is dilatation of CBD and pancreatic duct (the CBD is dilated till the terminal end and the main pancreatic duct is also dilated).

It can be seen in:
- Ampullary tumor (Most common)
- Other periampullary tumors

- Store impacted in ampulla of vertex
- Papillary stenosis.

Ampullary Carcinoma

Malignant epithelial neoplasm arising from ampulla of Vater.

Patients present with jaundice, abdominal pain and weight loss with typical history of passing silvery stools.

Classic imaging appearance:
- Lobulated soft tissue mass arising from ampulla of Vater
- "Double duct sign" with obstruction of pancreatic and CBD

    Endoscopic biopsy directs surgical procedure (ERCP)
    Treatment: Local excision vs. Whipple operation.

Pancreatic Cystadenomas (MC Benign Tumor of Pancreas)

Serous = Sunburst calcification
Mucinous = Eggshell calcification

TUMOR LOCALIZATION OF GI NETs (CARCINOIDS AND PANCREATIC ENDOCRINE TUMORS)

- Numerous tumor localization methods are used in both types of NETs, including:
    - Conventional imaging studies:
        i. CT
        ii. MRI
        iii. Transabdominal ultrasound
        iv. Selective angiography
    - Somatostatin receptor scintigraphy (SRS)
    - PET (positron emission tomographic) scanning.
- In PETs, endoscopic ultrasound (EUS) and functional mocalization by measuring venous hormonal gradients are also reported useful.
- Bronchial carcinoids are usually detected by a standard chest radiography and assessed by CT.
- Rectal, duodenal, colonic, and gastric carcinoids are usually detected by GI endoscopy.
- PETs, as well as carcinoid tumors, frequently overexpress high-affinity somatostatin receptors in both their primary tumors and their metastases. Of the five types of somatostatin receptors (SST_{1-5}), radiolabeled octreotide binds with high affinity to SST2 and SST5.

- Interaction with these receptors can be used to localize NETs using [^{111}In-DTPA-D-Phe^1]octreotide and radionuclide scanning (SRS) as well as for treatment of the hormone excess state with octreotide or lanreotide.
- Because of its sensitivity and ability to localize tumor throughout the body, SRS is now the initial imaging modality of choice for localizing both primary and metastatic NETs.
- SRS localizes tumor in 73 to 89 percent of patients with carcinoids and in 56 to 100 percent of patients with PETs, except for insulinomas.
- Insulinomas are usually best localized by intraoperative USG or EUS. EUS is highly sensitive, localizing 77 to 93 percent of insulinomas (occurs almost exclusively within the pancreas).
- EUS is less sensitive for extrapancreatic tumors.

^{18}F-fluoro-DOPA PET in patients with carcinoids or with ^{11}C-5HTP PET in patients with PETs or carcinoids has greater sensitivity than conventional imaging studies or SRS and will likely be used increasingly in the future.

Some important radiological signs

Pancreatic pathology	Important fact
Annular pancreas	Double bubble sign
Chronic pancreatitis	"Chain of lake" appearance of pancreatic duct with intraductal calculi
Ca pancreas	Frostburg's Reverse 3 sign ⎫ Hypotonic duodenographic (Barium) Antral pad sign ⎭ signs "Scrambled egg" appearance (ERCP)
Serous cystadenoma of pancreas	Sunburst calcification in a spongy mass
Mucinous cystadenoma of pancreas	Eggshell clacification in a spongy mass
Insulinoma	– Location: Equally distributed in pancreas – Whipple's triad – 72 hrs fasting levels is "gold standard" and EUS best
Gastrinoma	Pasaro's triangle (Gastrinoma triangle) is most common site. Most common neuroendocrine tumor of pancreas in MEN
Somatostatinoma	SRS (Octreotide labeled radionuclide scan) is investigation of choice. But now likely to be replaced by PET scan
Glucagonoma	Migratory necrolytic erythematous rash
VIPoma	Verner-Morrison syndrome, pancreatic cholera, or WDHA syndrome (watery diarrhea, hypokalemia, and achlorhydria)
Periampullary carcinoma	Double duct sign

Chapter 7

Genitourinary Radiology

Modalities available
- KUB Radiography
- IVU
- Urethrography < RGU
- MCU
- USG and Doppler
- CT
- MRI
- CTU and MRU
- Radionuclide scan
- Retrograde pyelography (not used commonly)
- Nephrostography.

IMAGING KEYS

Definitive diagnosis of patency of renal arteries:	*Contrast angiography*
Chronical renal disease associated with normal or increased kidney size are:	• *Polycystic kidney disease*
	• *Amyloidosis*
	• *Diabetes*
	• *HIV ars. renal disease*
Investigation of bladder – neck obstruction in male is done by:	*Cystourethrography (MCU)*
Investigation of choice after acute renal trauma is:	*CECT*

Contd...

Contd...

Vesicoureteric reflux is best demonstrated:	*Micturating Cystogram*
The dye used for IVP:	*Iohexol (300 mg/kg)*
Isotopes used for scanning kidney:	^{99m}Tc *DMSA/DTPA/MAG$_3$* (DTPA – for GFR, DMSA – for cortex)
Rapid sequence IVP is done in:	*Renovascular hypertension*
Whitaker's test is done to know:	*Ureteropelvic junction obstruction*
Maximum dose of contrast medium administered is:	*600 mg of Iodine/kg body weight in a well hydrated patient*
Choke urethrogram is done for:	*Demonstration of anatomy of urethral stricture*
Internal spermatic venography is an extremely accurate method of demonstrating the location of:	*Undescended testis*
The most accurate method of measuring GFR is by:	^{99m}Tc *DTPA/MAG$_3$ scan*
Renal scarring is best shown by:	DMSA scan

Static renal scans are performed using DMSA, dynamic using DTPA
DTPA is excreted by glomerular filtration, while MAG$_3$ is handled by filtration and tubular secretion.
^{99m}Tc DTPA captopril stress test is used for diagnosis of renovascular hypertension as second line study (MRA is first line).

Bead cystography which measures the posterior urethro vesical angle, is used to evaluate:	*Stress incontinence*

In pregnancy the ureter above the pelvic brim gets dilated, right more than left, this dilation persists for a month after delivery and predisposes to infection.

Combined synchronous video cystometrography (VCMG):	*Indications* Symptoms of outflow obstruction in men below 35 years Urinary incontinence <35 years age Possible outflow obstruction in females Problems following pelvic or plastic surgery Some neuropathic bladder problems
Initial screening test for Renal artery stenosis/ischemic renal disease	*Doppler ultrasonography*
Most sensitive and specific test for diagnosis of RAS:	*MRA*
Most definitive diagnostic procedure for RAS:	*Contrast enhanced arteriography*

Various radiological studies in GUT

Radiological study	Clinical utility	Key comments
KUB X-ray	- Commonly done study for calculus diseases, but is of no vital use compared to CT and IVU - The topography of staghorn calculi is well-assessed with X-ray KUB.	- Noncontrast helical/spiral CT is today the most sensitive and practical technique for a case of ureteric colic - X-ray KUB is of no use for renal infections and tumors
IVU	- Pelvicalyceal anatomy is most reliably assessed by IVU - Best for diagnosing renal TB - Best for diagnosing renal papillary necrosis - Urorenal anomalies - Second line investigation for assessing renal function - Second line investigation for renal and ureteric calculi - Part of FIGO staging for cervical cancer	- IVU is a better term than IVP - DTPA/MAG$_3$ scan is best for assessing renal function - Iohexol (Low osmolar non-ionic iodinated contrast media) is the ideal contrast agent for IVU (Conray is outdated)
USG	- Screening tool for focal renal lesions - Best for diagnosing vesical calculus - Highly sensitive for diagnosing hydronephrosis - Excellent for diagnosing urinoma - USG with renal Doppler is one of the best studies for follow-up of transplanted kidney - USG is tool of choice for follow-up of patients with ADPKD	- Air in bowel interferes with imaging of ureters - It cannot assess renal function - Color Doppler is initial screening tool of choice for renal artery stenosis. But in obese individuals, in patients who do not cooperate with respect to breath-holding its not of much use
CT scan (Multislice helical or spiral CT)	- Ureteric calculi (Noncontrast CT) - Renal and perirenal infections - Renal trauma - Renal tumors: including RCC and oncocytoma (central satellite scar)	- Multislice CT with contrast is the best protocol - Phasic CECT is required for detecting small RCCs - CTA scores over color Doppler as most sensitive and specific test for screening of renal artery stenosis - CT urography is not very popular

Contd...

Contd...		

MRI	– RCC with renal vein and IVC invasion
	– To differentiate bland from tumor thrombus
	– 3D dynamic CE MRA is the most sensitive and specific investigation to detect renal artery stenosis
		– MRU (MR urography is possible today but yet not very popular except for ureteric strictures and congenital anomalies, even for which it is not very cost-effective
		– MRU is possible by two techniques:
		  1. By using heavily T2 weighted turbo spin echo MR sequences
		  2. Gadolinium-enhanced excretory MR urography
		– The main advantage of MRU is no use of ionizing radiation

Nuclear scan	– Assessing renal function (GFR) by MAG_3 or DTPA scan – Renal morphology assessment and detecting renal cortical scars – Iodohippurate is outdated	– DTPA scan is also useful the VUR, PUJO, RAS – The disadvantage of nulcear scans is anatomical delineations is not possible – Captopril enhanced DTPA/MAG_3 renogram is secondline study for renovascular hypertension (RAS)

Intravenous Urography

Main Current Indications

- For assessment of function of the kidney (although scintigraphy is the best)
- Persistent or frank hematuria
- Renal and ureteric calculi (particularly prior to endourological procedures)
- Ureteric fistula
- Ureteric strictures
- Complex urinary tract infection (especially tuberculosis)
- Some urogenital congenital anomalies.

Main Contraindications

- Liver failure with renal failure
- Myelomatosis
- Pregnancy
- Previous of reaction to contrast
- Severally dehydrated patient.

KIDNEYS AND URETERS

Congenital Diseases

Normal Variants of Kidney

- *Persistent fetal lobulation/Dromedary humps*: Lateral kidney bulge, same echogenicity as the cortex
- *Hypertrophied column of Bertin*: Cortical tissue indents the renal sinus
- *Double collecting system*: Sinus divided by a hypertrophied column of Bertin.

	Inherited cystic kidney diseases	
Disease	*Renal abnormalities*	*Extra-renal abnormalities*
Autosomal dominant polycystic kidney disease	Cortical and medullary cysts	Cerebral aneurysms, liver cysts (MC) Pancreatic cysts, colonic diverticuli, and mitral valve prolapse.
Autosomal recessive polycystic kidney disease	Distal tubule and collecting duct cysts (Bilateral large kidneys with multiple radially arranged microcysts)	Hepatic fibrosis: Caroli syndrome
Nephronophthisis I (Juvenile/Adolescent)	Small fibrotic kidneys; medullary cysts	Retinitis pigmentosa
Nephronophthisis II (Infantile)	Large kidneys; widespread cysts	Situs inversus
Nephronophthisis III (Juvenile/Adolescent)	Small fibrotic kidneys; medullary cysts	Retinitis pigmentosa, hepatic fibrosis
Nephronophthisis IV (Juvenile/Adolescent)	Small fibrotic kidneys; medullary cysts	Retinitis pigmentosa
Medullary cystic kidney disease	Small fibrotic kidneys; medullary cysts	Hyperuricemia and gout
Tuberous sclerosis	Renal cystis; angiomyolipomas; renal cell carcinoma	Adenoma sebaceum; CNS hamartomas. Kaenan's tumor, subependymal giant cell astrocytoma
Von Hippel-Lindau disease	Renal cysts; renal cell carcinoma	Retinal angiomas; CNS hemangioblastomas; Pheochromocytomas

Multicystic Dysplastic Kidney

- In MCDK there is no normal overall structural pattern to kidney with loss of lobular organization although small islands of renal tissue are seen microscopically.
- Multicystic dysplastic kidney (MCDK) is nonfunctioning and characterized by an atretic ureter without increased incidence of VUR.
- The MCDK is usually unilateral and if bilateral, it is incompatible with life.
- On US, seen as a small single cyst to large mass containing multiple cysts with largest situated peripherally.

Nephronophthisis (Medullary Cystic Disease of Kidneys)

- Salt-wasting nephropathy causing CRF in adolescents/young adults
- *C/F*: Salt wasting, polyuria, polydipsia hyposthenuria, failure to thrive, growth retardation, uremia, severe anemia, normal sediment, hypertension (only in late phases)
- Bilateral normal/small kidneys with smooth contour
- *Two types*:
  1. Medullary cystic disease (adult onset)
  2. Juvenile nephronophthisis
- *IVP shows*: Poor opacification of collecting system and medullary nephrogram.
- *USG/CT*: Normal or bilaterally small kidneys. Increased parenchymal echogenicity with loss of CM-differentiation. Multiple small corticomedullary or medullary cystic.
  - **Medullary cystic disease and juvenile nephronophthisis** are two different terms for conditions, which differ in inheritance but have similar renal morphology and are radiologically indistinguishable. Both present with slowly progressive renal failure. MCD is autosomal dominant disease and presents up to 4th decade.
  - Ultimate diagnosis can only be made by rectal biopsy.

Medullary Sponge Kidney

'Bunch of flowers' appearance, i.e. thick dense streaks of contrast material radiating from pyramids peripherally "papillary blush" in normal people.

Autosomal Dominant Polycystic Kidney Disease

- It is a bilateral renal cystic disorder which becomes manifest frequently after the 3rd decade of life.
- Gene is located on chromosome number 16 (in 90 % cases) and 4.

- In Autosomal Dominant Polycystic Kidney Disease (ADPKD), there may be associated cysts in the liver (50% of cases), pancreas, spleen, lungs and testis. Other associations are berry aneurysms (which may cause SAH and severe headache), coarctation of aorta, valvular heart disease and colonic polyps. Congenital hepatic and periportal fibrosis is associated with ADPKD.
- Intravenous urography (IVU) typically shows classical stretched appearance of calyces with sometimes spider leg appearance.
- Ultrasonography (USG) typically reveals multiple bilateral (often asymmetrical) noncommunicating cysts of varying sizes, generally scattered throughout the cortex and medulla with normal intervening parenchyma and bilateral enlarged kidneys.
  Ultrasound is 2nd most useful examination.
- CT is best modality for ADPKD especially with complications suspected.
- Timely follow-up of cases is best done with USG.

Horseshoe Kidneys

- When the most medial subdivision of mesonephric bud meets and fuses and the ascent of the kidneys is arrested by the structures arising in the midline (inferior mesenteric artery), it results in a pair of ectopic kidneys that are usually fused at their lower poles, with their junction (isthmus) in front of the L_4 vertebra.
- These kidneys are prone for infection, trauma and nephrolithiasis.
  Other associations include anomalies of Gut, CVS, increased risk of Wilm's tumor, medullary sponge kidneys, Turner's syndrome and Ellis-van Creveld syndrome.
- Intravenous urography (IVU) appearance is characteristic:
  - Kidneys are low lying with their upper poles directing superolaterally
  - Lower pole calyces on both sides being directed inferomedially towards the midline
  - PCS points anteriorly and rarely all or most of the calyces are reversed.
  - Ureters characteristically have **vase-like** curves ('flower vase' ureters).

Vesicoureteral Reflux

- It is retrograde flow of urine from the bladder towards kidney.
- Common in preschool girls
- Eighty percent of children with vesicoureteral reflux (VUR) outgrow the abnormality by puberty.
- Association with acute pyelonephritis as well as sterile reflux with renal scarring in children is well documented.

- Higher grade VUR is treated with ureteral reimplantation surgery as recurrent UTI, subsequent renal scarring, renal failure, hypertension and ESRD can occur if untreated.
- F > M.
- Urinary tract infection (UTI) is its most common presentation.
- A UTI often is the first manifestation of child's underlying anatomic or functional urinary tract abnormality.
- Approximately 30 percent of all children who have bacteriuria and almost 50 percent of those under the age of 3 years show abnormal radiologic studies of the urinary tract. VUR is the most common underlying pathology.
- Radiological investigation is recommended for all children under age of 5 years with UTI, all boys irrespective of age and all girls with pyelonephritis and following 2nd UTI in girls >5 years age.
- Voiding cystourethrogram/Micturating cystourethrogram (VCUG/MCU) investigation of choice for evaluation.
- Renal nuclear scan preferred for follow up.

Megacalycosis

It is nonprogressive, nonobstructive calyceal dilatation with mosaic like arrangement of dilated calyces and faceted appearance.

CALCULUS DISEASE OF KIDNEY

Nephrolithiasis

When a renal calculus is branched, there is no doubt about the diagnosis. An opacity that keeps a constant position relative to the urinary tract during respiration is likely to be a calculus within it. A doubtful opacity can sometimes be shown to be anterior to vertebral bodies on a lateral radiograph and hence outside the urinary tract; such is the finding with calcified mesenteric nodes, gallstones.

Opacities on Plain X-ray, which way be Confused with Renal Calculus

- Calcified mesenteric nodes
- Gallstone or concretion in appendix
- Tablets or foreign bodies in alimentary tract
- Phleboliths
- Ossified tip of 12th rib

- Calcified tuberculous lesion in kidney
- Calcified adrenal.

As distinct from tuberculosis of kidney, TB of bladder is rarely associated with calcification. Bladder calcification is more common in Schistosomiasis. Usually, bladder calcification in schistosomiasis is linear and continuous and occurs chiefly at the bladder base going onto encircle the bladder lumen ('fetal head' like calcification). Lower portions of both ureters are usually involved in schistosomiasis of the bladder. It is unusual for kidney to the directly infected with schistosomiasis; it primarily affects the bladder and lower ureters, with secondary obstructive changes in kidneys.

Composition and calculi	Incidence
Calcium oxalate (Spiculated/lamellated/mulberry stones)	75%
Struvite (magnesium ammonium phosphate/laminated/proteus induced/staghorn)	15%
Calcium phosphate (laminated)	5%
Uric acid	5%
Cystine; xanthine; orotic acid; matrix (mucoprotein or mucopolysaccharide)	Rare

Radiolucent renal calculi are:
- Uric acid stones
- Xanthine stones
- Cystine stones (poorly radiopaque)
- Matrix (mucoprotein) stones.

NECT (Noncontrast spiral/helical CT) is widely used and currently study of choice for renal colic.

It is accurate, less time consuming, no contrast need, 98 percent sensitivity, 97 percent specificity, 100 percent positive predictive value and 97 percent negative predictive value.

Disadvantage: Ionizing radiations and renal function cannot be assessed and indinavir calculi can be missed.

Nephrocalcinosis

- Nephrocalcinosis is deposition of calcium salts in renal parenchyma
- It is of three types:
  1. Medullary (94%)
  2. Cortical (5%)
  3. Chaotic (mixed)

- Causes include:
  - Medullary sponge kidney
  - Alkali excess, Alport's syndrome
  - Renal tubular acidosis
  - Renal medullary/Cortical necrosis
  - Chronic glomerulonephritis
  - Hypercalcemia
  - Hypercalciuria
  - Hyperoxaluria
  - Barter's syndrome
  - Renal tuberculosis.
- Hypokalemia secondary to renal K+ wasting, metabolic alkalosis and normal to low blood pressure are characteristic of **Barter's syndrome**. Medullary nephrocalcinosis secondary to hypercalcemia is frequent. Infants have typical triangular facies prominent eyes and ears. Growth retardation is also seen.
- Medullary nephrocalcinosis is calcifications involving DCT in loops of Henle and constitutes 95 percent of all nephrocalcinosis. Its causes include hypercalciuria due to endocrine cause, milk-alkali syndrome, RTA, hypervitaminosis D, medullary sponge kidney, osseous metastasis, drugs, sarcoidosis, hyperoxaluria, hyperuricosuria, urinary stasis and dystrophic calcification.

FEATURES OF HYDRONEPHROSIS ON IVU

- Large kidney with wasted parenchyma
  - Diminished nephrographic density
  - Moderate to marked widening or dilatation of PC system
- Rim sign—'thin band of radiodensity surrounding calyces' in advanced cases
  - Delayed opacification of collection system
  - Faint nephrogram around the ballooned calyces, may produce 'soap-bubble' appearance.

PAPILLARY NECROSIS ON IVU

- Subtle streak of contrast extending from fornix parallel to long axis of papilla (tracks and horns from calyces)
- Ring shadow of papilla or calyceal ring sign

- 'Egg in a cup' appearance
- Nonspecific features → clubbed, blunt or truncated calices.

RENOVASCULAR HYPERTENSION

- It accounts for 1 to 4 percent of patients with hypertension.
- Atherosclerotic disease is the most common cause of RAS, especially in elderly.
- Majority of patients are > 50 years old (M>F) and common at ostium or within proximal 2 cm of renal artery, and bilateral in 1/3rd cases.
- Fibromuscular dysplasia (medial fibroplasias, medial or fibromuscular hyperplasia, intimal hyperplasia, perimedial fibroplasias) is the most common cause of renovascular hypertension in children and young adults and bilateral in 2/3rd cases.
- Other causes of RAS are arterial dissection, aneurysms, thromboembolism, Buerger's disease, Takayasu's arteritis, neurofibromatosis, postradiation and pheochromocytoma.
- **"String of beads" appearance** of FMD is classically seen on angiography.
- Renal captopril radionuclide scan is a sensitive mean of investigation, but is 2nd line study today.
- However, investigation of choice is MRA.
- CTA (Rapid diagnostic tool) is more specific and sensitive tool than sonography for RAS.

Imaging in Renovascular Hypertension

- **Plain KUB film:** In acute renal artery occlusion, there occurs sudden decrease in size of kidney and the fat space between the kidney and surrounding fascia is increased, seen as increased thickness of the radiolucency surrounding kidney known as **'Renal fascia' sign.**
- **IVU features**
  - Delayed/absent nephrogram (due to feeble perfusion by collaterals)
  - Normal or atrophic kidney without calyceal deformity or abnormality.
  - Ureteral kinking, when retroperitoneal fibrosis/aberrant vessel is the cause.
  - Rim nephrogram.
- **Color Doppler** evaluation of the main renal arteries has limited practical applications as a screening technique. It is very operator dependent, time consuming, it is impossible to visualize the main renal arteries completely in up to 42 percent patients due to presence of bowel gas, obesity, surgical incisions and/or aortic calcification. Tortuosity of the artery may make it impossible to obtain accurate angle corrected velocity.

- However, the development of helical (spiral) CT and now multidetector CT allows volumetric acquisitions to be obtained during single breath hold. It also eliminates respiratory misregistration that often degrades the image quality. Sensitivity and specificity for significant renal artery stenosis with single slice helical/spiral CT are 88 to 97 percent and 83 to 89 percent respectively, compared to catheter angiography.
- **Radionuclide imaging:** Although, IVP and renal scans have been abandoned as screening tests for renovascular hypertension due to their low sensitivity and specificity respectively, recently *captopril renography or captopril enhanced radionuclide renal scan* has been demonstrated to have a very high sensitivity (91%) and specificity (93%) for diagnosing it. However, no anatomic detail other than renal size is provided by the captopril renogram, hence it is 2nd line.
- **Magnetic resonance angiography (MRA)** of renal arteries poses particular problems related to cardiac, respiratory and bowel motion artifacts, overlapping renal veins and IVC, renal vessel tortuosity and complex flow patterns with disparate arterial phase. Contrast and/or time of flight MRA can be, however, used for detecting stenosis of renal artery. Contrast-enhanced MRA has particular advantages overcoming the problems using conventional MRA techniques. 3D CEMRA provides optimum method for its detection and allows the demonstration of small accessory renal arteries and segmental branches. Thus, MRA with gadolinium enhancement (CEMRA) has a sensitivity of 100 percent and a specificity of 93 to 97 percent for detection of proximal renal artery stenosis and best available tool today.
- **Angiography: "String of beads" appearance** of FMD is classically seen on angiography. The catheter or conventional angiographies are "gold standard" or definitive tool.

RENAL INFECTIONS

Renal TB

IVP is Abnormal in 85 to 90 Percent Cases. Distinctive Features of Renal TB (IVU)

- Putty kidney (tuberculous pyonephrosis)
- Autonephrectomy
- Nonfunctioning kidney
- Dystrophic calcification
- "Moth-eaten" calyx smudged papillae (the earliest sign)
- Cavities communicating with collecting system
- Hydrocalycosis with infundibular strictures (most common sign)

- Calyceal truncation
- Phantom calyx/amputed calyx
- Kerr kink (kinking of renal pelvis)
- Parenchymal-calcifications (amorphous/granular/curvilinear/punctate/confluent/toothpaste) involving entire kidney (putty kidney)
- Nephrolithiasis
- Ureteric Tuberculosis →
  - Produces mucosal and wall ulceration, fibrosis, structure and calcification
  - **"Saw-tooth or cork-screw" ureter**
  - Beaded ureter, short, straight, rigid and narrow ureter especially terminal segment
  - Calcification is, however, rare in ureteral tuberculosis and when occurs involves lower segment
- Symmetrical small spastic, and thickened bladder or small multilobular bladder (**thimble bladder**).

Pathognomonic Features of Renal TB

- Lobar caseation
- Lobar calcification
- Focal caliectasis
- Hiked-up pelvis
- Thimble bladder
- Undermined ulcer in bladder.

Xanthogranulomatous Pyelonephritis

- It is chronic suppurative granulomatous infection in chronic renal obstruction.
- It can be focal or diffuse.
- The infecting organism is usually *E. coli* or *Proteus mirabilis*.
- There is marked female preponderance and 10 percent patients are diabetic.
- On IVU there is nonfunctioning kidney, with laminated or branched and fragmented calculi in 80 percent patients.
- CT findings in xanthogranulomatous pyelonephritis (XGP) include loss of CM differentiation with calculi and low attenuation fatty masses replacing the renal parenchyma with some cystic/necrotic foci and perirenal fat stranding.

- While USG reveals calculi with hypoechoic dilated calyces with echogenic rim or hypoechoic masses with low level internal echoes replacing renal parenchyma and loss of CM differentiation. Calcifications are rare.
- If untreated cutaneous and enteric fistula may result from perinephric spread.

RENAL TUMORS

Wilms' Tumor (Nephroblastomas)
- Wilms' tumor is the third most common malignancy in children following leukemia and brain tumors.
- It is the most common pediatric abdominal and renal malignancy.
- The mean age at presentation is 3 years; however, it tends to present at a younger age when bilateral or associated with syndromes.
- Fifty percent of children with Wilms' tumor are younger than 2 years, 75 percent younger than 5 years, and 90 percent younger than 8 years.
- Wilms' tumor is distinctly uncommon in the neonatal period.
- The incidence is equal in males and females.
- Approximately 15 percent of Wilms' tumors are associated with syndromes.
Wilms' tumor is seen in approximately 33 percent of patients with **sporadic aniridia**; 10 percent to 20 percent with **Beckwith-Wiedemann syndrome** (macroglossia, hemihypertrophy, omphalocele, and visceromegaly); and 3 percent with **hemihypertrophy**. It is also of increased incidence in patients with **Drash syndrome (male pseudohermaphroditism, glomerulonephritis, and Wilms' tumor)**. The occurrence of Wilms' tumor with other genitourinary tract anomalies including **horseshoe kidney, hypospadias, cryptorchidism, and ambiguous genitalia** is rare and not of sufficient incidence to be considered an association.
- Nephroblastomatosis if found in a kidney with Wilms' tumor, the other kidney should also be searched for tumor as nephroblastomatosis predisposes to bilateral renal tumor.
Wilms' tumor arises from primitive metanephric blastema in the renal cortex.

Staging
- Stage I Wilms' tumors are limited to the kidney and are completely excised.
- Stage II tumors have extrarenal extension but are also completely excised. Since nephrectomy is indicated for both stage I and stage II disease, visualization of perirenal extension does not change the treatment.

- Stage III tumors have residual postsurgical disease confined to the abdomen. Patients with stage IV disease have hematogenous spread.
- Five to ten percent of patients have bilateral involvement at the time of diagnosis and are classified as stage V, with each side substaged I to IV.
- The most common presentation of Wilms' tumor is as an asymptomatic abdominal mass.
- Ninety percent are palpable. Other possible presenting features include microscopic hematuria, gross hematuria, hypertension, constitutional symptoms, pain, fever, and rarely ascites from venous obstruction. Patients may present with retroperitoneal hemorrhage after mild trauma.
- CT demonstrates a mass that is less dense than normal renal parenchyma. Heterogeneity depends on the degree of intratumoral hemorrhage and necrosis. Calcifications are seen in 10 percent of patients and are curvilinear or amorphous. In contradistinction, calcifications in neuroblastoma are much more common and tend to be more stippled and punctate. Fat within the tumor is rare but can be focal or diffuse. Wilms' tumors enhance less than the normal renal parenchyma. Large tumors compress, distort, and splay the normal renal parenchyma peripherally. Wilms' tumors may be predominantly cystic due to hemorrhage and necrosis. CT can assesses for involvement of lymph nodes, contralateral kidney, vasculature, local extension, and distant metastases. In 10 percent of cases, CT shows decreased function on the side of tumor due to vascular compromise, collecting system compression, or tumor extension.
- On MRI, Wilms' tumors have an elevated T1 and T2 and are therefore of nonspecific decreased signal intensity on T1-weighted images and increased signal intensity on T2-weighted images. MRI shows intratumoral heterogeneity due to hemorrhage, necrosis, or both. MRI is excellent for assessing intravascular extension. A significant drawback of MRI is the greater need for sedation in younger patients compared to CT.
- Angiography is rarely used in the assessment of Wilms' tumors.
- Wilms' tumors are really benign congenital mesoblastic nephroma or fetal mesenchymal hamartoma or mesonephroblastic tumor. Thus, a renal mass in a neonate, which appears as hypoechoic to heterogeneous lesion on USG is most likely to be mesonephroblastic nephroma.

Mesoblastic nephroma is the most common renal neoplasm in first 3 months of life. On USG there are areas of heterogeneous reflectivity, the mass is solid one but there may be hypoechoic areas due to cystic change or necrosis. On neither CT nor US is it possible to reliably distinguish between a mesoblastic nephroma from a Wilms' tumor. It does not metastasize. With complete removal there is an excellent prognosis. These tumors, however, frequently show uptake of ^{99m}Tc-DMSA.

WILMS' TUMOR VERSUS NEUROBLASTOMA

- Finely stippled or amorphous **calcification** is characteristic feature of neuroblastoma seen in up to 50 percent of cases on plain film, while curvilinear calcification is characteristic of Wilm's tumor and seen in up to 10 percent cases only. Neuroblastoma more commonly **crosses midline** than Wilms' tumor and thus mass crossing midline favors neuroblastoma.
- **Intraspinal extension** in the form of widening of intervertebral foramen by tumor extension into the vertebral canal is also seen in neuroblastoma.
- Vascular displacement and encasement rather than invasion is the most useful discriminating feature between neuroblastoma and Wilms' masses when they are especially large. **Invasion of blood** vessels with tumor thrombus is rare with neuroblastoma.
- **Bone metastases** may be seen as submetaphyseal lucencies within long bones and lytic lesions within the skull when leukemia and histiocytosis "X" are important differential diagnosis rather than Wilms' tumor.
- Skeletal secondaries are extremely rare in Wilms' tumor and only occur following lung secondaries.
- A neuroblastoma is **usually solid** with heterogeneous characteristics on USG, CT and MRI. On CT, areas of low attenuation often represent areas of cystic necrosis and hemorrhage. Calcification is seen in over 90 percent cases on CT. Adrenal neuroblastoma, for that matter any adrenal mass, tends to displace the kidney inferiorly and laterally.
- Features suggestive of neuroblastoma include an extrarenal epicenter, irregular shape, irregular margins, calcifications, particularly punctate or stippled, vascular encasement, extension across the midline, and the presence of hepatic or bony metastatic disease in the absence of pulmonary metastatic disease. Features favoring Wilms' tumor include an intrarenal epicenter, round or oval shape, well-defined margins, and vascular displacement or invasion.
- **Neuroblastoma** is commonest extracranial tumor in children and accounts for 6 to 8 percent of pediatric malignancies.
- The median age at diagnosis is 2 years and 2/3rd of these patients have metastases at the time of diagnosis.
- Bone metastases may be seen as submetaphyseal lucencies in long bones, and lytic lesions.
- It occurs most commonly in abdomen, either in sympathetic chain or more commonly in adrenal gland.
- Less common sites are the neck, posterior mediastinum and pelvis.

Paraneoplastic phenomenon, i.e. the opsoclonus-myoclonus syndrome (dancing eye, dancing feet syndrome) can occur.
Peeper syndrome can be seen in these patients with liver metastasis.

- Abdominal and pelvic neuroblastomas are usually form tender and nodular masses.
- Spontaneous regression demonstrated in some stage 4S patients.
- Finely stippled or amorphous calcification is characteristic feature and seen in up to 50 percent of cases on plain film. Intraspinal extension and anterior displacement/encasement of aorta and IVC is characteristic and is the most useful discriminating feature between neuroblastoma and Wilms' tumor.

In contradistinction to Wilms' tumor, invasion of blood vessels with thrombus is rare with neuroblastoma and bone secondaries are more common.

ANGIOMYOLIPOMA (HAMARTOMA)

- It is a renal hamartoma composed of thick walled blood vessels, smooth muscles and fat.
- It is isolated in 80 percent cases and associated with tuberous sclerosis in 20 percent cases.
- Plain AXR may show fat lucency in the renal region.
- The USG may show intensely echogenic mass lesion.
- Contrast-enhanced computed tomography (CECT) shows mass with fat density and highly vascular component.
- Angiography is best investigation for diagnosis, which shows hypervascular mass.

Renal Cell Carcinoma

It is the most common malignant primary tumor of kidney. It is highly vascular tumor.

Robson Staging of RCC

Stage I: Limited to renal capsule
Stage II: Capsule breached with perirenal involvement but limited to Gerota's fascia
Stage IIIa: Tumor extension beyond Gerota's fascia
Stage IIIb: Tumor invasion into renal vein or IVC
Stage IIIc: Regional node involvement
Stage IV: Invasion of adjacent viscera or distant metastases

- The CECT is best study for detection and staging of RCC.
- Renal cell carcinoma (RCC) has a predilection to invade the renal vein at the hilum and extend along it into the IVC and further into right atrium. However MRI is the best technique for defining the extent of venous invasion and the proximal extent of thrombus in IVC, with a very high negative predictive value and accuracy. MRI is superior to CT in differentiating benign from malignant thrombus.

RENAL INJURIES

Incidence

Eight to ten percent of all cases of blunt and penetrating abdominal trauma is constituted by renal injuries

Indication

- Penetrating flank and back trauma =CECT with contrast
- Gross hematuria, but hemodynamically stable or resuscitated patients
- Hemodynamically unstable patient requiring emergency surgery =intraoperative IVU after patient is stabilized
- Microscopic hematoma in the shock = CECT
- Hemodynamically stable patient with microscopic hematoma, but no other indication for CECT
- Hemodynamically stable patient without or with microscopic hematoma with evidence of major flank impact.

BLADDER AND URETHRA

Bladder Diverticuli

These are focal herniations of the urothelium and submucosa through weak sites in the bladder wall.
- Primary/congenital/idiopathic: For example, **Hutch diverticulum** which is located at paraureteral location and has broad neck
- *Secondary diverticuli:* For example, pseudodiverticuli due to bladder outlet obstruction having constricted neck and are usually multiple. They result mostly due to chronic elevation in intravesical pressure and are frequently encountered in male patients above 60 years age. In early stages, multiple small protrusions of the bladder lumen appear between the trabeculae, called sacculations. As they enlarge above 2 cm they become defined as diverticuli. When large, they may produce classical symptom of **double micturition**.

'Tear Drop' Bladder

This appearance results due to compression effect on either side walls of bladder.
- Pelvic lipomatosis
- Bilateral pelvic hematoma
- Rupture of bladder (intraperitoneal)
- Lymphoma.

Ureterocele

Ureterocele is cystic ectasia of subepithelial segment of intravesical part of ureter. Micturating cyslourethrogram (MCU) in children with ureterocele shows a rounded or oval lucent defect near trigone which may, however, be effaced with increased bladder distension and eversion may be seen during micturition.

Intravenous urography (IVU) shows early filling of bulbous terminal ureter (**"cobra head" appearance**) and a radiolucent halo (ureteral wall + adjacent bladder urothelium) giving **"spring onion" appearance**. Thus, ureterocele leads to repeated infection of renal system and has above explained radiological features.

Types

- **Simple Ureterocele** → congenital prolapse of dilated ureter and orifice into the bladder lumen at usual location of trigone and typically is seen with single ureter (orthotopic ureterocele). 30 percent cases are bilateral. M:F = 2:3.
- **Ectopic Ureterocele** → usually seen in upper moiety ureter of duplex PC system with 80 percent incidence.
- **Pseudoureterocele** → no protrusion of ureter into bladder lumen; however, thick irregular halo seen in urinary bladder, e.g. in impacted ureteral calculus (edema in the ureteric wall at the UV junction due to impacted ureteral calculus shows **EDLING SIGN**, i.e. filling defect surrounded by radiolucent halo of edema).
- **Cecoureterocele** → Ureterocele going into bladder outlet and causing outlet obstruction.

Urethral Strictures

Most urethral strictures are caused by trauma or inflammation. Inflammatory strictures most commonly occur at the bulbar urethra, the sites of periurethral glands while traumatic strictures are most commonly seen at bulbomembranous area. Iatrogenic occurs at fixed and narrow sites of urethra like membranous and penoscrotal junction. Voiding cystourethrogram or micturating cystourethrogram demonstrates the prostatic urethra to best advantage, as it is better distended than the membranous and anterior urethra. Retrograde urethrography depicts the membranous and anterior urethra better and is preferred approach for assessing inflammatory lesions and diverticuli. US is able to assess both urethral and periurethral tissues and has shown to be more accurate than conventional urethrography for assessing urethral structures. MRI provides excellent soft tissue contrast and depicts urethra and the periurethral tissues to best advantage.

Posterior Urethral Valves

- Varying degree of chronic urethral obstruction due to fusion and prominence of plicae colliculi, normal concentric folds of urethra.
- Usually, located in posterior urethra just **distal to the level verumontanum**
- It is the most common cause of severe obstructive uropathy in infants and children.
- MCU is gold standard in diagnosis of PUV.

Three types of PUV are described:

Type I

- Most common type
- Anterior fusion of plicae, valves are in the form of two folds with central slit-like orifice.
- Classic imaging appearance (MCU/VCUG) is abrupt transition from dilated posterior urethra to tiny penile urethra at the level of valves, and actual valve may be visible as well-defined linear (radiolucency) filling defect at the transition zone.
- Associated VUR and obstructive bladder changes may be present.

Type II

- Rarest
- Longitudinal folds from veru to bladder neck.

Type III

- Rare
- Disk or windsock like tissue with a pin-hole like eccentric opening in it, resulting in forward ballooning of the valve giving **'wind in the sail' appearance** on oblique view during MCU.
  - Posterior urethral valve is the commonest obstructive uropathy seen in male child and is occasionally diagnosed by ANC ultrasound
  - An MCU is diagnostic for PUV.

Extraperitoneal Bladder Rupture

- It is most **common type of bladder rupture (80%)** after blunt trauma abdomen and is **associated usually with fracture bony pelvis** and posterior urethral injuries. The urine extravasates in perivesical region, first in cave of Retzius, i.e. retropubic space.

- Radiograph may show fracture pelvic bones, pear-shaped bladder density, loss of obturation fat planes, upwards displacement of coils and paralytic ileus.
- **Cystography (gold standard, definitive)** reveals distorted bladder with extravasation of contrast in perivesical space and steaks of contrast into fascial planes giving typical **"sun burst" appearance**.
- US shows **"bladder in bladder" appearance** due to perivesical collection and a rent in bladder wall may also be detected.
- CT cystography is best investigative technique as the exact site and extent of rent, bladder wall contusions, blood clots and surrounding organ injuries can be detected.

In extraperitoneal bladder rupture urine (contrast) dissects through the adjacent fascial planes into the perivesical space of Retzius, the anterior abdominal wall, the inguinal region and upper thigh, the lateral paravesical space, and the presacral space. If there is concurrent disruption of urogenital diaphragm (posterior urethra) and bladder base, urine (contrast) can extend/ extravasate into the perineum and scrotum. Rarely, extravesical urine (contrast) can extend retroperitoneally to the level of kidneys.

In intraperitoneal bladder rupture free intraperitoneal urine (contrast) outline the peritoneal recesses and bowel loops.

PROSTATE AND TESTES

Benign Prostatic Hypertrophy—Radiological Features

- 'Slit-like' elongated and compressed urethra
- Smooth filling defect/ indentation in bladder floor
- Periurethral and subvesical enlargement is very pronounced may produce rounded defect in floor mimicking Foley's balloon.
- Floor of bladder elevated and trigone pushed upwards, with 'J' or 'Fish Hook' deformity of distal ureter.
- Trabeculations and distension of bladder
- Bladder pseudodiverticuli and calculi
- Bilateral hydronephrosis and hydroureter may occur.

Carcinoma Prostate

- Most common noncutaneous cancer in American Men
- Life time risk of developing ca prostate is 18 to 19 percent and increases with age
- *Location:* Peripheral zone 70 percent, transition zone 20 percent and central 10 percent.

- **Spread**: Hematogenous (bone osteoblastic metastasis)/**lymphatic**
- Most important factor affecting prognosis/choice of treatment is presence or absence of extracapsular extension.
- TRUS is most widely used imaging modality for local staging.
- 3D MR spectroscopy (increased choline and decreased citrate levels) ± Endorectal MR imaging increase accuracy in detecting and staging of local and extracapsular extension of prostate carcinoma.
- *Pathologically*: Adults (adenocarcinoma); Children (rhabdomyosarcoma).

Classic Imaging Appearance

T2WI: Decrease signal in a normally high signal peripheral zone

TESTICULAR TUMOR

Ultrasound imaging of the scrotum is the primary imaging method used to evaluate disorders of the testicles, epididymis and scrotum per se.

This study is typically used to:
- Determine whether a mass in the scrotum is cystic or solid.
- Diagnose results of trauma to the scrotal area.
- Diagnose causes of testicular pain or swelling such as inflammation or torsion.
- Evaluate the cause of infertility such as varicocele.
- Look for the location of undescended testis.
- Seminoma is the most common neoplasm in males between ages 15 and 34 years.
- The complications of undescended tests include Trauma, Torsion and Tumor (3Ts).
- Cryptorchidism increases the risk by 10 times with incidence being 5 percent for the abdominal testis and 1.25 percent for inguinal site.
- Testicular tumor <1.5 cm is hypovascular in 86 percent cases and hypervascular >1.6 cm in 95 percent cases (color duplex). Seminoma is the most common tumor in the undescended testis. Usually appears uniformly hypoechoic and confined within tunica albuginea with lobulated confluent nodules.
- Duplex and triplex Doppler US helps greatly to evaluate testicular pathologies.
- MRI and CECT are excellent modalities to detect the para-aortic metastatic lymphadenopathy (which is frequent necrotic and may be sole clinical feature rather than testicular symptoms) from GCT.

SEMINAL VESICLE

Diseases involving the Seminal Vesicles and Vas deferens are rare. Due to their close proximity to the prostate, they are most commonly affected by diseases of the prostate. Secondary tumor invasion is often seen in patients with prostate, bladder, or rectal cancer. Although very rare, primary neoplasms can also occur. Because of the close embryologic relationship with the urinary tract, congenital anomalies of the SV and VD and SV cysts are often associated with other urologic or genital anomalies. TRUS and MRI are commonly used for diagnosing various abnormalities of these organs. Owing to its excellent tissue contrast and multiplanar capability, MR imaging is best for evaluation of these organs.

PENILE IMAGING

- *Modalities available are*
  - Sonography
  - Penile Doppler
  - Penile angiography.
- *Penile Doppler indications*
  - Priapism
  - Trauma
  - Impotence (erectile dysfunction)
  - Revascularization
  - Primary erectile dysfunction
  - Failure of both oral and injectable therapy for erective dysfuction.
- *Penile angiography indications*
  - Erectile dysfunction
  - Priapism.

Spermatic venography is usefully employed in location of undescended testis if this is not identified using cross-sectional imaging. Now for a young man with primary infertility, low volume, fructose negative ejaculate, pathology is most likely to be in seminal vesicles, ejaculatory duct or vas.

Transrectal Ultrasonography (TRUS) is an excellent technique for demonstrating seminal vesicle anatomy and finding ejaculatory duct pathologies.

Chapter 8

Musculoskeletal Radiology

IMAGING PROTOCOLS

Modalities available for musculoskeletal radiology (MSK) radiologic evaluation:

Modalities	Comment	Use (Prototype)
Plain X-ray (Radiograph)	Digital > Conventional	Routine fractures
Ultrasound (not for bone per se)	High frequency probe 7–15 mHz	Screening of rotator cuff tear, popliteal cysts
CT scan (for fine osseous details)	Multislice c̄ 3D Recon	Complex fractures cortical lesions
MRI	STIR, T_1, T_2, Fatsat sequences	The best tool for many lesions
Bone scan (Triple phase)	^{99m}Tc-MDP is ideal agent	Highly sensitive for infection and metastases
Ga-67 ro Indium–111 WBC scan	Indium^{111} > Ga^{67}	Osteomyelitis
PET scan (18 FDG agent of choice)	Better than SPECT	Oncoimaging – FTU and recurrence

Diagnostic imaging techniques for musculoskeletal disorders	
Method	Current indications
Ultrasound	Synovial cysts
	Rotator cuff tears
	Tendon injury
^{99m}Tc scintigraphy	Metastatic bone survey

¹¹¹In-WBC scintigraphy	Evaluation of Paget's disease Acute and chronic osteomyelitis Acute infection Prosthetic infection
⁶⁷Ga scintigraphy	Acute osteomyelitis Acute and chronic infection
Computed tomography	Acute osteomyelitis Herniated intervertebral disk Sacroiliitis Spinal stenosis Spinal trauma Osteoid osteoma Stress fracture
Magnetic resonance imaging	Avascular necrosis Osteomyelitis Intra-articular derangement and soft tissue injury Derangements of axial skeleton and spinal cord Herniated intervertebral disk Pigmented villonodular synovitis Inflammatory and metabolic muscle pathology

MUSCULOSKELETAL RADIOLOGY: DIFFERENTIAL DIAGNOSIS

Delayed Bone Age/Retarded Skeletal Maturity

- Constitutional (familial/IUGR)
- Metabolic (hypopituitarism, hypothyroidism, hypogonadism, Cushing's disease, steroid therapy, diabetes mellitus, rickets, malnutrition, irradiation of brain)
- Systemic (congenital heart disease, renal disease, PEM and anemia, celiac disease, Crohn's disease, ulcerative colitis, BMT)
- Syndromes (trisomies, Turner syndrome, noonan disease, Cornelia de Lange syndrome, Cleidocranial dysplasia, Lesch Nyhan disease, metatropic dwarfism).

Diffuse Osteosclerosis (Increased Bone Density)

- Metastases
- Myelofibrosis
- Melorheostosis
- Mastocytosis

- Metabolic (Fluorosis)
- Hyperparathyroidism with renal osteodystrophy
- Hypervitaminosis
- Hypothyroidism
- Phosphorus poisoning
- Osteopetrosis
- Paget's disease
- Pycnodysostosis
- Sickle cell disease, and tuberous sclerosis.

Patchy Sclerosis of Skeleton
- Mast cell reticulosis/Mastocytosis/Urticaria pigmentosa
- Fluorosis
- Carcinomatosis/Metastasis
- Myelosclerosis
- Lymphoma
- Multiple myeloma.

Lytic Bone Lesion Surrounded by Marked Sclerosis
These are seen by:
- Brodie's Abscess (metaphyseal)
- Osteoblastoma (diaphyseal)
- Osteoid osteoma
- Stress fracture
- Tuberculosis.

Causes of Multilocular Expansile Osteolytic Lesion of Bone
- Aneurysmal bone cyst (diaphyseal)
- Giant cell tumor (epiphyseal)
- Fibrous dysplasia (diaphyseal)
- Simple bone cyst (meta or diaphyseal).

Lytic expansile eccentric lesions include:
   Giant cell tumor
   Fibrous cortical cyst

Condromyxoid fibroma
Aneurysmal bone cyst

Lytic expansile centric lesions include:
Aneurysmal bone cyst
Chordoma
Telangiectatic osteosarcoma
Enchondroma
Hypervascular metastases.

Causes of Multiple Lytic Lesions in Bone

- Metastasis (epiphyseal/diaphyseal)
- Fibrous dysplasia (diaphyseal/epiphyseal)
- Enchondroma (diaphyseal)
- Eosinophilic granuloma (epiphyseal)
- Hyperparathyroidism (Brown tumor)
- Hemangiomas
- Infection (epiphyseal)
- Multiple myeloma (epiphyseal).

Multiple Osteolytic Lesions in Children

- Histiocytosis
- Leukemia
- Metastatic neuroblastoma
- Fibrous dysplasia
- Enchondromatosis
- Multifocal osteomyelitis
- Cystic angiomatosis.

Osteoblastic Bone Lesions

- Bone island
- Osteoma
- Osteoid osteoma

- Osteosarcoma (metaphyseal)
- Parosteal sarcoma
- Metastasis (prostate, breast, lung, bladder, pancreas, stomach, colon, carcinoid and brain)
- Paget's disease
- Myelofibrosis
- Sarcoma
- Mastocytosis.

Mixed Sclerotic and Lytic Lesions

- Osteomyelitis
- Tuberculosis
- Ewing sarcoma (diaphyseal)
- Osteosarcoma
- Metastasis.

Expansile Lytic (Bubbly) Osseous Metastases

- Renal cell carcinoma
- Carcinoma of thyroid (Follicular type)
- Carcinoid tumor
- Osteosarcoma
- Choriocarcinoma
- Islet cell carcinoma of pancreas.

Causes of Lucent Metaphyseal Lines

- Normal variant
- Growth lines
- Leukemia
- Infection (congenital syphilis)
- Neuroblastoma metastasis
- Rickets
- Scurvy.

Causes of Dense Metaphyseal Bands

- Normal variant
- Stress lines
- Heavy metal poisoning
- Healed rickets.

Causes of Cortical Lesions (Especially Lytic) on CT/X-ray

- Osteoid osteoma (sclerotic)
- Fibrous cortical defect
- Chondromyxoid fibroma.

Causes of Lesions with Blood-fluid Levels on MRI

- Aneurysmal bone cyst
- Telangiectatic osteosarcoma
- Hypervitaminosis D
- Hypothyroidism
- Scurvy
- Treated rickets.

D/D of widespread hot spots ("Superscan" appearance)

- Diffuse osteoblastic metastases
- Hyperparathyroidism
- Renal osteodystrophy
- Paget's disease
- Osteomalacia
- Hyperthyroidism
- Myelofibrosis/myelosclerosis
- Aplastic anemia/leukemia
- Systemic mastocytosis
- Waldenstrom's macroglobulinemia (IgM spike and hyperviscosity)

D/D of "cold spots" are seen on bone scan (no osteoblastic activity)

- Multiple myeloma
- Enostosis

- Nonossifying fibroma
- Osteopoikilosis, and
- Fibrous cortical defect.

CONGENITAL SKELETAL ANOMALIES AND SKELETAL DYSPLASIAS

Acro-osteolysis may be seen in

Congenital/Dysplasia	Cleidocranial dysostosis
	Pyknodysostosis
	Idiopathic acro-osteolysis
	Progeria
	Pseudoxanthoma elasticum
Traumatic	Frostbite
	Electrical injuries
Infective	Acute infection of a digit
	Leprosy
Vascular	Scleroderma with Raynaud's phenomenon
	Occlusive vascular disease
Neoplastic	Kaposi sarcoma
	Hodgkin disease
Metabolic	Hyperparathyroidism
Neurotrophic	Tabes dorsalis
	Syringomyelia
	Diabetes mellitus
Poisoning/Drugs	Ergot
	Polyvinyl alcohol
Connective tissue diseases	SLE, RA, Scleroderma
Miscellaneous	Sarcoidosis
	Neurofibromatosis
	Ainhum
	Reticulohistiocytosis
	Psoriasis
	Pityriasis rubra
	Epidermolysis bullosa

Osteopetrosis/Albers Schonberg Disease/Marble Done Disease

Thick sclerotic bones that are structurally weak and brittle characterize it.

Splayed metaphyses and costochondral junctions and fracture even from minor trauma characterize infantile autosomal recessive type.

Adult autosomal dominant type (benign), phenotype I is characterized by diffuse osteosclerosis with cortical thickening and sparing (relatively) of mandible.

While phenotype II is characterized by
- Endobones ("bone within bone" appearance)
- Sandwich vertebrae/Rugger-jersey spine
- Metaphyseal lines
- Longitudinal metaphyseal striations
- Erlenmeyer flask deformity (club-like long bones).

Osteogenesis Imperfecta

- It occurs due to defect/mutation in genes responsible for **type I collagen**.
- It is relatively rare disorder manifested by increased fragility of bones and osteoporosis, dental abnormalities, wormian bones, and lax joints.
- In **osteogenesis imperfecta (OGI) congenita** osteoporosis occurs with short, broad and weak long bones, while in **osteogenesis imperfecta tarda**, which is a benign form, the bones are bowed, thin and gracile.
- There are **four types of OGI** with type I being the most common and mildest form with normal stature and dentigenosis imperfecta in Ib form.
- Type II is the most lethal form.
- All the four forms have autosomal dominant inheritance except type III, which may have AD/AR inheritance.
- In 10 percent, fractures are seen at birth and in 10 percent fractures never occur.

Most fractures occur in young children and are often diaphyseal rather than metaphyseal as in battered baby syndrome in which multiple fractures of long bones, often in various stages of repair may occur.

Fractures are usually transverse and heal with normal callus.

Radiological Features
- Generalized osteoporosis
- Bilateral diaphyseal long bone fractures
- Exuberant callus formation
- Wormian bones
- Platybasia
- Basilar invagination
- Tam O'Shanter skull (typical skull shape due to platybasia)
- Kyphoscoliosis
- 'Codfish' vertebrae
- Calcific 'pop-corn' like lesions in metaphysis
- Severe Protrusio acetabuli.

Battered Baby Syndrome

Caffey (1946) described a syndrome of SDH, associated with multiple fractures of long bones, and often in various stages of repair is now known as battered infant.

Radiographic Findings
- Fracture in different stages of healing.
- Periosteal reaction (particularly in bones of distal forearm or leg).
- Multiple growth recovery lines.
- Injury to skull and ribs.
- Fractures at unusual sites.
- Epiphyseal separators and metaphyseal infarctions.

Melorheostosis (Candle Bone Disease)

It is a nongenetic disease characterized by asymmetrical dense irregular cortical longitudinal hyperostosis of particularly the long bones giving appearance like wax running down the side of a candle ('Molten wax' appearance), vascular anomalies, abnormal pigmentation and muscle contracture and wasting. In osteopoikilosis (spotted bone disease), painless bony discrete sclerotic spots are noted.

Cleidocranial Dysplasia/Dysostosis (CCD)

- Autosomal recessive disease with faulty intramembranous bone ossification
- Large head with small face, abnormal dentition and drooping hypermobile shoulders.

Radiological Features of CCD

Skull
- Platybasia
- Large foramen magnum
- Wormian bones
- Persistent metopic suture
- 'Hot cross bun' skull
- Brachycephaly.

Thorax
- Agenesis or hypoplasia of clavicles
- Small winged scapulae.

Pelvis
- Underdeveloped pelvis
- Coxa valgus early.

Spine
- Biconvex vertebrae
- Hemi vertebrae.

Extremities
- Elongated 2nd metacarpal.

D/D: Pyknodysostosis (confused with CCD because of similar clavicular and skull changes, and pyknodysostosis is also confused with osteopetrosis because generalized increase in bone density, however these patients are not short which differentiate it from CCD).

Multiple Epiphyseal Dysplasia

- Autosomal dominant
- Delayed ossification of epiphyses of the tubular bones
- Delayed ossification of carpus and tarsus
- Short tubular bones of hand and feet and shortening of limbs

- Epiphyseal irregularities
- Only mild irregularity of vertebral endplates
- Mild wedging of vertebral bodies
- Mild acetabular hypoplasia
- Early joint degenerative changes.

Achondroplasia

It is prototype of rhizomelic (disproportionate) dwarfism with autosomal dominant/sporadic (80%) occurrence, caused by defective endochondral bone formation, related to advanced paternal age. Epiphyseal maturation or ossification is unaffected.

Chevron sign is V-shaped deformity of the metaphyses at the wrist due to overtubulation deformity. In achondroplasia the tubular bones are short and wide with the epiphysis deformed by their insertion into V-shaped defects at the metaphyses. The epiphysis thus themselves has V-shaped distal ends with deep intercondylar notches – the 'chevron' sign.

It is also a feature of mucopolysaccharidosis.

Hands, Feet and Limbs
- Rhizomelia (Humeri and femora predominantly affected)
- Trident hands (fingers of equal length and diverge from one another in two pairs) with short stubby fingers
- Chevron sign (V-shaped notch in the growth plates).

Skull and Face
- Depressed nasal bridge with prominent forehead
- Disproportionately large skull.

Pelvis
- Small square shaped iliac bone with 'tombstone' appearance
- Small pelvis with narrow pelvic inlet resembling a 'champagne glass'.

Skull
- Skull changes are mandatory for diagnosis of achondroplasia
- Bullet-nose vertebrae

- Posterior scalloping of vertebrae
- Small funnel shaped foramen magnum.

Chest

- Short ribs with wide anterior ends.

Nail-patella Syndrome (Hereditary Osteo-onychodysplasia or Fong's Syndrome)

- Autosomal dominant inheritance
- Radiologic features
    - Paired posterior **iliac horns (pathognomonic)** – **the Fong lesion**
    - Flared or shortened iliac wings
    - Small or absent patellae
    - Asymmetric femoral condyles
    - Hypoplastic capitellum and medial humeral condyle
- Early death occurs due to renal dysplasia with renal osteodystrophy
- Dysplastic fingernails
- Clinodactyly and joint contracture
- Abnormal iris pigmentation.

Turner's Syndrome

- Short stature, webbing of neck and lymphoedema
- Short 4th metacarpals (positive metacarpal sign)
- Madelung deformity (short ulna with V-shaped angle between distal radius and ulna)
- Flattening of the medial tibial condyle with enlarged adjacent femoral condyle (Blount's disease)
- Osteoporosis
- Scoliosis
- Delayed maturation of skeleton
- Increased carrying angle of elbow (cubitus valgus)
- Renal anomalies like horseshoe kidneys
- Coarctation of aorta
- Streaky ovaries with hypoplastic uterus.

Skeletal Features of Down's Syndrome

- Flaring of iliac wings = "Elephant ears or Mickey Mouse ears" appearance
- Decreased iliac angle and index (<60° iliac index suggests Down's syndrome)
- Sloping acetabula
- 11 pairs of gracile ribs
- Hypersegmentation of manubrium (bifid manubrium)
- Tall squared vertebral bodies, i.e. positive lateral lumbar index
- Attantoaxial subluxation and instability
- Anterior scalloping of vertebral bodies
- Hypertelorism
- Brachycephaly and microcephaly
- Dental abnormalities
- Short hands with clinodactyly of the little finger due to hypoplastic middle phalanx
- Metaphyseal flaring
- Hypoplastic sinuses and facial bones.

Klippel-Feil Syndrome

- Short neck, sometimes webbed
- Low hairline
- Restriction of neck movements due to cervical vertebral fusion
- Congenital genitourinary tract, auditory system, spinal cord, CVS and other musculoskeletal anomalies are associated
- Medial border of scapula, making the scapula equilateral triangle in shape
- Sprengel anomaly (congenital elevation of scapula with inferior poles pointing outwards/laterally away from each other
- Scoliosis and torticolis
- Renal anomalies include duplication, aplasia, horseshoe kidney.

Mucopolysaccharidosis

Types:
MPS I (Hurler's syndrome)
MPS II (Hunter's syndrome; XLR)

MPS III (Sanfilippo syndrome)
MPS IV (Morquio-Brailsford syndrome)
MPS V (Scheie's syndrome)
MPS VI (Maroteaux-Lamy syndrome).

Mucopolysaccharidosis Type I (Hurler Syndrome; Gargoylism)

- Macrocephaly with thick calvarium
- 'J' shaped sella
- Hydrocephalus, leptomeningeal cysts
- Odontoid hypoplasia
- Oar shaped ribs
- 'Hook shaped' vertebral bodies
- Flared iliac wings
- Small, irregular fragmented femoral capital epiphysis
- Coxa valga
- Undertubulation with demineralization
- Short wide phalanges with characteristic proximal pointing of metacarpals (cut corner sign).

Mucopolysaccharidosis Type IV (Morquio-Brailsford Syndrome)

- Normal intelligence
- Short stature
- 'J' shaped sella
- Absent or hypoplastic odontoid peg with cervical instability
- Platyspondyly
- Tongue shaped (anterior central beaking) vertebral bodies (lower thoracic and upper lumbar region)
- Thoracolumbar marked kyphosis
- Joint laxity with knock knees
- Coxa valga
- Progressive disappearance of femoral capital epiphysis
- Flared iliac wings with constricted bases of iliac wings (ape like pelvis)
- As a rule tubular bones are not markedly affected, however, they are short and wide
- Irregular ossification of metaphyses of long bones
- Proximal pointing of 2nd to 5th metacarpals (cut corner sign).

Marfan Syndrome

- Autosomal dominant disease with high penetrance but extremely variable expression
- Etiology is supposed to be the fibrillin gene defect on chromosome 15.
- M:F = 1:1

Metacarpal Index → Averaging the 4 ratios of length of 2nd through 5th metacarpals divided by their respective mid diaphyseal width.
Normal metacarpal index is 5.4 to 8.5.

- *Manifestations*

Musculoskeletal manifestations include: Tall then stature with long limbs, arm span greater than height, muscular hypoplasia and hypotonicity with scarcity of subcutaneous fat.

Skull and spine	Hand and foot	Joints
Dolichocephaly	**Steinberg sign**: Protrusion of thumb beyond confines of clenched fist	Ligamentous laxity
Elongated face	Metacarpal index > 8.8 (male) or 9.4 (female)	Hypermobility
Prominent jaw	Arachnodactyly	Instability
High arched palate	Flexion deformity of 5th finger	Premature osteoarthritis
Scoliosis/Kyphoscoliosis	Pes planus	Patella alta
Ratio of measurement Between + crown and floor > 0.05	Club foot recurvatum	Genu sympphysis and floor
Dural ectasia and posterior	Hallux valgus hip, clavicle	Recurent dislocation of patella, mandible
Increased interpedicular distance	Hammer toes	Slipped capital femoral epiphysis
Expansion of sacral spinal canal and enlargement of sacral foramina	Disproportionate elongation of 1st digit of foot	Protrusio acetabuli
Presacral and lateral sacral meningoceles		
Winged scapulae		

Ocular manifestations
- Bilateral dislocated lens (upward and outward)
- Macrophthalmia
- Glaucoma
- Hypoplasia of iris and ciliary body
- Contracted pupils
- Myopia, retinal detachment
- Strabismus, ptosis
- Blue sclera
- Megalocornea

Cardiovascular manifestations
- Congenital heart disease → incomplete coarctation and ASD, mitral valve prolapse,
- "Tulip bulk aorta"—Symmetrical dilatation of aortic sinuses of Valsalva slightly extending into ascending aorta
- Annuloaortic ectasia
- Fusiform aneurysm of ascending aorta due to cystic medial necrosis
- Pulmonary artery aneurysm

Pulmonary manifestations
- Cystic lung disease
- Recurrent spontaneous pneumothoraces

Abdominal manifestations
- Recurrent biliary obstruction.

Differential Diagnosis

- Homocystinuria (osteoporosis, vascular thrombotic events, inferior and inwards lens dislocation)
- Ehler Danlos syndrome
- Congenital contractual arachnodactyly
- Type III MEN (medullary carcinoma of thyroid, mucosal neuromas, pheochromocytoma, marfanoid habitus).

METABOLIC BONE DISORDERS

Rickets

Faulty mineralization of the bone before the fusion of growth plate, i.e. during endochondral bone growth, is known as rickets.

Clinical features include bone pain, tenderness, irritability, craniotabes, rachitic rosary, bowed legs, swelling of wrists and ankles and delayed dentition.

Location: Metaphyses of long bones subjected to stress are particularly involved (wrist, ankles, knees).

Radiological Features

- Poorly mineralized epiphyseal centers with delayed appearance
- Widening and lengthening of growth plate (zone of provisional calcification affected) is earliest radiographic feature of rickets
- Increased distance between end of shaft and epiphyseal center
- Epiphyseal plates widening and irregularity
- Fraying, splaying and cupping of metaphysis
- Periosteal reaction
- Indistinct cortex with coarse trabeculations
- Metaphyseal spur projecting at right angles to metaphysis in the cortex
- Additional features:
  - Bowing of long bones
  - Genu recurvatum
  - At costochondral junction, epiphyseal widening results in typical 'rachitic rosary'
  - Frontal bossing
  - Scoliosis
  - Slipped capital femoral epiphysis
  - Triradiate configuration of pelvis
  - Basilar invagination.

Fraying and Cupping of Metaphyses

Metaphyseal dysplasias are of many types: Schmid, Jansen's, Pena, Vaandrager and McKusick metaphyseal dysplasia. Metaphyses of long bones are cupped and resemble rickets.

Hypophosphatasia is autosomal recessive congenital disease with low alkaline phosphatase activity causing poor mineralization.

Causes of Cupped and Frayed Metaphyses

- Congenital infections (rubella, syphilis)
- Hypophosphatasia
- Achondroplasia
- Rickets
- Metaphyseal dysplasia
- Scurvy.

Lead Poisoning

- Persistent lead lines
- Bands of increased density at metaphysis of tubular bones
- Bone-in-bone appearance.

Causes of Transverse Lucent Metaphyseal Lines
Normal variant
Growth lines
Rickets and scurvy
Infections like congenital syphilis
Leukemia
Metastases from neuroblastoma

Radiological Features of Scurvy

- Spurs (Pelkan Spur) = Metaphyseal spurs projecting at right angles to axis of shaft
- Subperiosteal hemorrhages = Diaphyseal subperiosteal hematoma with calcification of elevated periosteum is the sure sign of healing (woody-leg)
- Cortical thinning ("pencil-thin" cortex)
- Corner sign of Parke = Subepiphyseal infarction or comminution causing mushrooming or cupping of epiphysis
- Osteoporosis = Characteristically "ground-glass" osteoporosis

- Rarefaction zone of Trummerfield = Metaphyseal radiolucent zone on shaft side.
- White line of Frankel = Metaphyseal zone of provisional/preparatory calcification also seen in lead or phosphorus or bismuth poisoning and in healing rickets.
- Wimberger's sign = Sclerotic ring seen around the low density osteopenic epiphysis.

Imaging Feature of Osteoporosis

- Generalized osteopenia, most prominent in axial skeleton
- Thinning and accentuation of cortices
- Prominence of primary trabeculae with thinning of secondary trabeculae
- Wedge-shaped, biconcave or compressed vertebral bodies
- Insufficiency fracture
- Picture frame vertebrae
- Schmorl's nodes
- Intracortical resorption and tunneling.

Osteomalacia

- It is characterized by defective mineralization of osteoid tissue matrix in mature cortical and cancellous bone.
- Pseudofractures/Looser's zones/Milkman fractures are typical of osteomalacia.
- In osteoporosis equilibrium between the rates of bone formation and bone resorption is lost such that bone resorption predominates resulting in overall loss of bone mass.

Looser's Zones/Looser Lines/Pseudofractures/Osteoid Seams/Increment Fracture/Milkman Syndrome/Umbau Zones

- **Definition**: These are areas of unmineralized woven bone occurring at sites of mechanical stress or nutrient vessel entry (pulsations of the arteries)
- **Common locations**
  - Scapula (lateral and superior border)
  - Medial femoral neck and shaft
  - Pubic and ischial rami
  - Lesser trochanter
  - Ribs and clavicle
  - Ischial tuberosity

- Proximal 1/3rd of ulna and radius
- Phalanges
- Metacarpals and metatarsals.
- They are typically bilateral, symmetrical and at right angles to bone margin.
- 2 to 3 mm stripe of lucency at right angle to cortex (osteoid seams formed within stress induced infarctions–pathognomonic) with nonunion (incomplete union due to mineral deficiency).
- The other features of osteomalacia are decreased bone density with loss of trabeculae and thinning of cortices and blurring of trabecular pattern producing homogeneous groundglass haze.
- **Conditions in which these can be seen**
  - Osteomalacia/rickets (characteristically)
  - Paget's disease
  - Osteogenesis imperfecta
  - Organic renal disease (1%)
  - Fibrous dysplasia
  - Renal tubular dysfunction
  - Congenital hypophosphatasia
  - Congenital hyperphosphatasia
  - Vitamin D deficiency
  - Neurofibromatosis
  - Vitamin A intoxication
  - Cadmium poisoning.
- Focal accumulations of osteoid are seen in compact bone at right angles to long axis; radiographically, these are known as pseudofractures and are distinguishing sign of osteomalacia
- The exact cause of loser's zones is unclear, although they probably represent partial insufficiency fractures, succumbing to vascular pulsations.

Other key imaging features of osteomalacia are: Osteopenia, intracortical resorption (cortical tunneling), coarsened, indistinct trabecular pattern, bowing of bones, true fractures, especially of the femoral neck.

"**Rugger-jersey**" **spine** (resembling the stripes on rugby jerseys) means horizontal sclerosis subjacent to vertebral endplates with intervening normal osseous density. Its causes include hyperparathyroidism (as seen in CRF), myelofibrosis. Thus in CRF or renal osteodystrophy although exact reason for osteosclerosis remains unclear, the presence of excessive osteoid inhibiting octeoclastic activity and excessive increased serum calcium/phosphate product may cause precipitation of osteoid.

- In hyperparathyroidism we get "salt-pepper" appearance of skull, phalangeal resorption, osteopenia, erosions and brown tumor.
- Paget's disease or osteitis deformans is characterized by disordered and exaggerated bone remodeling with features like widening of diploic space of skull with 'cotton-wool' appearance, osteoporosis circumscripta, candle-flame or blade of grass lysis of diaphysis of long bone, (fissure fracture), bubbly destruction of small/flat bones and picture frame and ivory vertebra.

Hyperparathyroidism

Incidence is greatest in middle-aged females.

Parathyroid adenomas account for over 90 percent of cases of hyperparathyroidism.

Key **imaging features** of hyperparathyroidism include:
- **Subperiosteal bone resorption** (an essentially diagnostic/pathognomonic finding): Seen most commonly along the radial aspect of the middle phalanges of the second and third digits and commonly involves phalangeal tufts and the medial metaphysis of the proximal humerus, femur and tibia.
- Bone resorption in other locations (intracortical, endosteal, subchondral, trabecular and subligamentous) characterized by cortical striations, intracortical tunneling and **osteitis fibrosa cystica**, the hallmark of this disorder, seen best in tubular bones of hands.
- **Osteopenia** in vast majority of cases (rarely, osteosclerosis)
- **Brown tumor** represent focal, bone replacing lesions, that occur most often in metaphysis, diaphysis where jaw is known site of involvement manifesting radiologically as radiolucencies. The majority of these lesions heal after removal of the adenoma.
- **Erosions** involving sacroiliac joints, symphysis pubis and ligamentous insertions in addition to resorption of distal or medial end of clavicle and vertebras end plates (aggressive Schmorl's nodes), attributed to **subchondral resorption**.
- Skull may show a characteristic **'pepper pot' pattern** resulting from trabecular resorption and widening and remodeling of the diploic space.
- Erosions of calcaneum and inferior aspect of distal clavicles, attributed to **subligamentous resorption**.
- **Chondrocalcinosis**
- Loss of **lamina dura** of mandible.

In children, metaphyseal changes (like cupping, splaying and fraying, wooly moth-eaten appearance) resembling rickets are common in uremic osteodystrophy (chronic renal failure), which together with cortical erosions can give rise to the so-called **'rotting fence-post'** appearance, particularly at the femoral neck. Otherwise, widening and lengthening of growth plate is earliest radiographic feature of rickets.

Gout

It is a metabolic disorder characterized by hyperuricemia and deposition of **positively birefringent monosodium urate (MSU) crystals** in the form of tophi in periarticular soft tissues including synovium, articular cartilage, joint capsule, ligaments, bursae and even intraosseously.

Primary gout occurs due to enzyme HGPRTase deficiency or increased PPRP synthatase activity or it can be idiopathic (99%).
- Complete HGPRTase deficiency = Lesch-Nyhan syndrome (gout + selfmutilation + mental retardation).
- Partial HGPRTase deficiency = Kelley-Seesgmiller syndrome (gout with nephritis).

Secondary gout is seen in myeloproliferative disorders, blood dyscrasias, Von Gierke disease, CRF, drugs, etc.

Clinical Stages

Asymptomatic hyperuricemia (levels of uric acid correlate with the symptoms)
Acute gouty arthritis—no distinct radiological features except for joint effusion (**earliest sign**), soft tissue swelling and rarely erosions.
Chronic tophaceous gout-characterized by radiological features like
- Absence of osteoporosis
- Absence of joint space involvement (until late in disease)
- Gouty tophi
- Eccentric nonperiarticular erosions with sclerotic rim
- An "overhanging" bony edge along the bony contour (**hallmark**)
- Chondrocalcinosis
- ELBOW= Olecranon bursa 'rising sun' sign
- Knee = Pseudotumor
- Punched out bony lesions
- Intervertebral disk calcification
- Aural calcification

Differential Diagnosis (DD) of Chondrocalcinosis
- Amyloidosis
- Acromegaly

- Diabetes
- Ochronosis
- Gout
- Wilson's disease
- Hemochromatosis
- Hemophilia
- Hypothyroidism
- Hyperparathyroidism (Primary)
- Hypophosphatasia
- Hypomagnesemia (Familial)
- Idiopathic (Aging)
- Pseudogout (CPPD) – characteristic.

Radiographic Picture of Fluorosis

- Generalized increase in bone density (osteosclerosis)
- Cortical thickening
- Osteophytosis
- Ligamentous and musculotendinous attachment ossification/calcification (particularly sacrotuberous ligament)
- Exostosis.

Paget's Disease of Bones

Paget's disease is a chronic skeletal disease characterized by disordered and exaggerated bone remodeling, affecting order individuals.

Sites: (usually polyostotic and asymmetric) Pelvis > lumbar spine > thoracic spine > proximal femur > calvarium > scapula > distal femur > proximal tibia > proximal humerus.

Fibula is virtually never affected.

Radiological features:
- *Skull*:
  - Widened diploic spaces
  - Osteoporosis circumscripta
  - "Cotton wool" appearance (mixed lytic and blastic pattern of thickened calvarium)
  - Basilar impression

- *Long bones*:
  - "Candle flame"/"blade of grass" lysis originating in subarticular site
- *Spine*:
  - "Picture-frame" vertebra,
  - "Bone with bone" appearance
  - "Ivory" vertebra
  - Ossification of spinal ligaments.

BONE INFECTIONS

Osteomyelitis

- In children metaphysis is involved, while in adults epiphysis is involved
- Swelling, with edema and blurring of fat planes become apparent immediately
- Osteoporosis may be visualized within 10 to 14 days of onset of symptoms
- Periosteal reaction starts as edema immediately below the periosteum, and then periosteal ossification occurs but plain radiograph may not show changes until 2 weeks after MRI/USG have demonstrated the abnormality
- **Involucrum** → cloak of laminated/spiculated periosteal reaction or the layer of living bone surrounding the dead bone which forms beneath the elevated periosteum, (develops after 20 days)
- **Sequestra** → detached necrotic cortical bone fragments if surrounded by pus, are not absorbed and remain as sequestra, seen as **more radiopaque densities than the surrounding bone** (develops after 30 days)
- **Cloaca** → are defects in Involucrum or the hole in bone with sclerotic margins or the space in which dead bone resides and also allows the pus and sequestra to escape.

Type of study	Comments
Plain radiographs	- Insensitive, especially in early osteomyelitis
	- May show perfosteal elevation after 10 days, lytic changes after 2–6 weeks.[Q]
Three-phase bone scan (^{99m}Tc-MDP)	- Characteristic finding in osteomyelitis increased uptake in all three phases of scan
	- Highly sensitive (~95%) in acute infection[Q]
^{67}Ga-citrate, ^{111}In-labeled WBCs scans	- ^{111}In-WBCs more specific than gallium but not always available[Q]
	- Lack of consensus over role; often supplanted by MRI when the latter is available
MRI	- As sensitive as ^{99m}Tc-MDP bone scan for acute osteomyelitis (~95%)[Q]
	- High specificity (~87%), with better anatomic detail than nuclear studies

Note: 'Q' as a superscript indicates 'vital indications'

Sclerosing Osteomyelitis of Garre

This is a form of chronic OM in which there is progressive sclerosis without evidence of bone destruction. The bone appears thickened due to periosteal new bone formation and there is loss of corticomedullary differentiation. Garre was principally concerned that the bacteria were found despite the lack of frank pus. We now know that organisms persist for years despite a quiescent illness in keeping with Garre's observation. Bone destruction followed by phases of healing and reaction lead to a mixed pattern that exhibits areas that seem to be aggressively changing and others that are indolent and repairing. Hence the mixed pattern of destruction and bone remodeling that is almost diagnostic of chronic bone infection taken in isolation. The so-called 'sclerosing osteomyelitis of Garre is when there is florid new bone formation and relatively dense bone. CT and MRI are of value in excluding the above conditions which are usually associated with soft-tissue components except for osteoid osteoma. ^{99m}Tc MDP (monodiphosphonate) scintigraphy has high sensitivity but low specificity; 111 In-labelled white cell studies have high specificity but low sensitivity. Radionuclide radiology has a useful screening role in identifying the location and extent of disease but it is not as valuable as MRI. It may have a role in locating occult disease, especially using 111-In labelled white cells or labelled autoantibodies. Gallium is now considered to be a less effective agent.

Brodie's Abscess

- Localized subacute form of osteomyelitis/an intraosseous abscess surrounded by **intense sclerosis**
- Usually found in the cancellous tissue, near the end of a long bone (metaphysis)
- Seen as well-circumscribed area of bone lysis/destruction with surrounding zone of reactive sclerotic rim
- May have a finger-like extension into neighboring bone (tunneling) toward the epiphyseal plate, which, when present, is **pathognomonic** feature
- D/d osteoid osteoma
- Brodie's abscess **typically** enhances on the delayed isotope scan, while osteoid osteoma enhances centrally, both on the blood-pool and delayed scan due to central vascularity (the **double density sign**).
- On MRI, central vascular area of osteoid osteoma exhibits bright signal and enhancement, while necrotic tissue in the Brodie's abscess does not (the **penumbra sign**).

Skeletal Tuberculosis

- It is due to hematogenous spread from a primary site, usually the lungs but at times primary lesion may not be identified.

- Spine is most common site of infection and is present in over 50 percent children, followed by the involvement of large joints of lower extremely like the hip and knee.
- **Shoulder joint (caries sicca)** and bones of the hand and feet **(spina ventosa)** can also be involved. In skeletal tuberculosis single joint affection is the most common pattern.
- **Tuberculous dactylitis (spina ventosa)** involves the short tubular bones of hands and feet with bony expansion; increased bone density with periosteal reaction and soft tissue swelling. The differential diagnosis of tuberculous dactylitis includes sickle cell dactylitis and small round cell neoplasm of childhood.
- The radiographic features of tuberculous arthritis are periarticular osteoporosis and soft tissue swelling with distribution of articular cartilage which progresses more slowly than pyogenic infection. Joint space narrowing is relatively late. Fibrous ankylosis is more common than bony ankylosis except in cases of spinal tuberculosis. Reactive new bone formation is minimal or absent.

Congenital Syphilis

Transplacental transmission cannot occur <16 weeks gestational age
- Diaphyseal periostitis (most common feature)
  - **Saber tibia** (anterior convex bowing of upper 2/3rds of tibia with bone thickening)
  - Bone within bone appearance
- Metaphysitis
  - Metaphyseal irregularities
  - Metaphyseal fractures
  - **Wimberger sign** (symmetrical focal destruction of medial portion of proximal tibial metaphysis, pathognomonic sign)
- Osteitis and osteomyelitis (symmetrical and bilateral involving multiple bones)
- Syphilitic dactylitis
- Skull lesions (frontal bossing due to diffuse thickening of outer table; purely sclerotic or mixed lesions with **"hot cross bun" skull**)
- Spontaneous epiphyseal fractures causing joint immobility due to pain (Parrot's **pseudoparesis**)
- **Hutchinson's triad** (dental abnormalities, interstitial keratitis and 8th nerve deafness)
- Saddle nose, high palate, short maxilla
- Anemia.

Because transplacental transmission of syphilis from the mother does not occur during the first 16 weeks as spirochetes are unable to penetrate the Langhans' layer of the immature placenta, early detection and treatment of infected mothers would effectively prevent this disorder.

Therapy after 16 weeks will usually cure fetal infection in utero.

If treatment is started late the child may show the characteristic lesions of congenital syphilis at birth. A wide variety of symptoms, may be recorded in intrauterine life itself: IUGR; skin lesions (blisters) particularly of the hands and feet; jaundice; snuffles; metaphysitis, diaphysitis (periostitis), epiphysitis.

SKELETAL TRAUMA

Epiphyseal Injuries

Of the fractures peculiar to children, epiphyseal separation is often the most challenging to investigate. Best example of this is at the elbow joint, where epiphyses both appear and fuse in a known sequence.

Epiphyseal injuries are grouped according to the Salter-Harris classification, an important guide to both treatment and prognosis of any particular fracture. Epiphyseal fractures usually occur through the zones of hypertrophic and degenerating cartilage cell columns.

Pneumonic:

- S → **S**eparation of epiphysis
- A → **U**pper fractured (Met**A**physis)
- L → **L**ower fractured (Epiphysis)
- T → **T**ogether (Both fractured)
- ER → **E**piphyseal **R**upture (crush injury).

In type 1 and 2, epiphysis remains intact and these injuries generally have a good prognosis. This contrasts with type 3 and 4, where the epiphysis itself is fractured. Type 5 is a very rare crush injury of physeal cartilage and most serious type. Plain radiography is the sole imaging method required in the majority of epiphyseal injuries. MRI is useful to visualize nonossified growth plate cartilage and in very young children, the unossified.

Epiphyseal Injuries Commonly Occur at the Zone of Cartilage Hypertrophy

Type of fractures		
Type	Bone status	Load
Traumatic	Normal	Single heavy
March/fatigue (stress)	Normal	Repetitive
Insufficiency (stress)	Abnormal (metabolic)	Trivial
Pathological	Abnormal (tumor)	Trivial

Fatigue Stress Fracture

Definition: Normal bone fracture by subjecting it to repetitive stresses

The classic march fracture is seen in military recruits and runners, usually manifested as cortical thickening and periosteal new bone formation along the shafts of the 2nd, 3rd and 4th metatarsals

- Metatarsal fracture → commonly 2nd metatarsal (march fracture)
- Clay shoveler's fracture→ spinous process of lower cervical/upper thoracic spine
- Spondylolysis
- Obturator ring of pelvis
- Tibial shaft and fibula
- Ribs
- Femoral neck
- Sacrum
- Sesamoids of metatarsals.

Insufficiency Stress Fracture

Definition: Fracture of an abnormal bone due to normal physiologic stress

- Calcaneum
- Tibia
- Fibula
- Thoracic vertebrae
- Sacrum
- Ilium
- Pubic bone.

Bohler's, Kite's and Hibb's Angle

In compression fracture of calcaneum the degree of compression can be assessed by use of the Bohler's angle which may normally vary from 20 to 40 degrees.

In the weight-bearing lateral view, the angle formed by the intersection of a line parallel to the inferior border of the talus and a line parallel to the inferior border of the calcaneus (lateral talocalcaneal angle; Kite's angle) is normally 35° to 50°. An angle less than 35° indicates hindfoot equines.

Pes cavus means "hollow foot." It is the term used for the high-arch foot. The significant radiographic measurement of pes cavus is the angle of the longitudinal arch (Hibbs' angle). The angle made by a line parallel to the base of the calcaneus intersects the first metatarsal line. An angle of less than 160° indicates a cavus deformity.

MISCELLANEOUS MUSCULOSKELETAL RADIOLOGY DISEASES

Pigmented Villonodular Synovitis

- Pigmented villonodular synovitis is a benign proliferative disorder of the synovial lining arising in tendon sheaths, bursae and joints.
- If located in a tendon sheath, it is also referred to as giant cell tumor of the tendon sheath.
- MRI detection of hemosiderin is an important indicator of pigmented villonodular synovitis (PVNS). The tumor typically has low signal intensity on T1-weighted and on T2 weighted SE images. It calcium can be excluded radiographically as causing the low signal intensities on the T2-weighted image, the intracapsular soft tissue mass can be diagnosed as PVNS with a high degree of certainty. The tumor enhances on CEMRI.
- Knee joint is most common joint affected by PVNS.

SPONDYLOLISTHESIS

Definition: Slipping or displacement of one vertebral body over another, with respect to lower vertebra

Types
- – Anterolisthesis
  – Retrolisthesis
- Meyerding's classification
  – Type I - 25 percent listhesis
  – Type II - 25 to 50 percent
  – Type III - 50 to 75 percent
  – Type IV - 75 to 100 percent (ptosis)
- – Isthmic (open-arch type) → **most common type** of spondylolisthesis
  – Degenerative (closed arch type or pseudospondylolisthesis)
  – Dysplastic
  – Traumatic
  – Pathologic

Location: L5–S1 or L4–L5 (common).

Radiological Features

X-ray spine AP view
- May show lucency roughly parallel to inferior cortex of pedicle

- Inverted Napoleon's hat or Gendarme's cap sign or Bowline of Brailsford (if anterolisthesis is significant)
- May see single lumbar spine deviated in rotation (without scoliosis).

X-ray spine lateral view
- Clearly demonstrating degree of listhesis.

X-ray spine oblique view
- Optimal view for visualizing (spondylolysis) defect, which appears as **"broken collar or neck" of the Scotty dog** where a linear lucency is seen across the neck of dog (**Scottish terrier sign**).

Scotty dog with Collar or broken neck = spondylolysis
Beheaded scotty dog = spondylolisthesis

OSTEONECROSIS/OSTEOCHONDRITIS

Traumatic avascular necrosis is more common in:
- The head of the femur
- The proximal part of the Scaphoid
- The posterior half of the Talus
- Humeral head → infrequent.

Nontraumatic/idiopathic necrosis of bone/osteonecrosis/osteochondritis: types

Site	Disease
Scaphoid	Preiser disease
Lunate	Kienbock disease (Lunatomalacia)
Navicular	Kohler disease
Head of 2nd, 3rd, 4th, metatarsal	Freiberg's disease
Capitellum	Panner's disease
Medial tibial condyle	Blount's disease
Femoral head	Legg-Calve Perthes disease
Calcaneum	Sever's disease
Tibial tuberosity	Osgood-Schlatter disease (Leander Paes)
Ring-like vertebral epiphysis	Scheuermann's disease
Lower pole of patella	Sinding-Larsen's disease
Blount disease	Medial condyle of tibia
Calve-Kummel-Verneuil disease	Vertebral body epiphysis
Knee	Spontaneous osteonecrosis of knee (SONK)

Osteochondritis Dissecans

- It is the most common cause of loose body in young adult
- It is characterized by partial or complete detachment of fragments of articular cartilage, with or without subchondral bone at particular sites.
- In contradistinction to osteochondral fracture, the separated fragment is avascular, and in contradistinction to avascular necrosis the 'bed' of defect remains vital.
- **Sites of elections** are convex articular surfaces:
  - Medial femoral condyle
  - Capitellum of humerus
  - Trochlear surface of talus
- Twice common in male compared to females
- It occurs characteristically in adolescence and early adults life
- One-third cases are bilateral
- Radiographically a radiolucent ring surrounding the bone fragment is seen on enface view; and the loosening fragment may be seen opposite a pit in the bone when viewed in profile.
- The fragment may become completely separated, may obtain adequate nourishment from synovial fluid and form an intra-articular loose body
- CT is good modality for showing cortical defects and loose bodies, but in the view of entirely cartilaginous loose body MRI should be preferred
- MRI staging of transchondral fractures/osteochondritis dessicans
  Stage I → compression fracture with normal plain radiographs
  Stage II → partially detached osteochondral fragment, fluid deep to fragment, and a discontinuity of fissure in overlying cartilage
  Stage III → the osteochondral defect is detached and loose but remains within the underlying crater
  Stage IV → the defect has become detached and has migrated.

Spontaneous Aseptic Bone Necrosis

- MRI is the most sensitive and accurate means of detecting changes in avascular necrosis.
- With MRI, sensitivity and specificity for aseptic bone necrosis (AVN) approaches 100 percent, while false-negative isotope scans occur early on in the disease.
- Changes at MRI are usually seen in the anterosuperior segment of the femoral head. Radiographs are normal at early stages.
- Steroids and NSAIDs are associated with bone necrosis.

DIFFERENTIAL DIAGNOSIS OF HIP PAIN IN CHILDREN

A wide variety of conditions cause hip pain in children, include:
- Transient synovitis
- Osteomyelitis
- Perthes disease
- Slipped capital femoral epiphysis
- Fracture
- Arthritis are associated with fluid accumulation in the hip joint.

Perthes Disease (Osteochondritis of Femoral Capital Epiphysis/Waldenstrom Legg Calve Perthes Disease/Coxa Plana)

- Age of presentation: 4 to 9 years
- M:F → 4:1
- Age of onset is earlier in girls and prognosis is worse
- Bilateral (but asymmetrical) disease is more common in boys
- No increased familial incidence
- Increased risk of associated congenital anomalies like congenital heart disease, CHPS, hernia, renal anomalies and undescended testes.

Catterall Stages of Perthes Disease

- *Group/stage I:* Initial phase of onset of necrosis of ossific nucleus of femoral epiphysis, characterized by widening of joint space and increased density of nucleus
- *Group/stage II:* Phase of repair which removes the fragmented, crushed necrotic bone
- *Group/stage III:* Healing phase characterized by increase in size and reossification of nucleus
- *Group/stage IV:* Phase of remodeling occurs when the femoral head is completely contained within the acetabulum.

Radiographic Features

Early signs
- Lateral displacement of the femoral head, the **Waldenstrom sign** (prognostic indicator)
- Widening of affected hip joint space is however earliest sign
- Subcortical fissure in the femoral ossific nucleus (frog leg lateral view)
- Reduction in the size of the femoral ossific nucleus of epiphysis

- Increase in density of the femoral ossific nucleus
- Metaphyseal broadening and irregularity
- Sagging rope sign.

Late signs
- Small arch like subcortical radiolucency
- Subcortical fracture
- Femoral head fragmentation
- Femoral neck cysts
- Loose bodies.

Regenerative signs
- Coxa plana
- Coxa magna (remodeling of femoral head to become wider and flatter).

CT Features

Loss of 'asterisk' sign (star-like pattern of crossing trabeculae in the center of femoral head).

MRI Features

- Asterisk or double-line sign (sclerotic nonsignal rim between necrotic and viable bone)
- Hip joint incongruity (lateral femoral head uncovering, labteral inversion, deformed femoral head).

Radionuclide Scan (RNS) Features

In early stage, when no radiological abnormality is yet visible in the child with an avascular lesion, a defect is seen in the femoral head on radionuclide scan. Thus, before any radiographic change become apparent, a RNS may demonstrate photopenia of affected epiphysis. It also gives improved definition of the acetabular roof, femoral capital epiphysis, physis and the greater trochanter.

Transient Synovitis (Toxic Synovitis) of the Hip

It is characterized by:
- May follow upper respiratory tract infection.
- ESR and white blood cell counts are usually normal.
- Ultrasound of the joint reveals widening of the joint space due to anechoic fluid collection.
- The hip is typically held in abduction and external rotation.

DISORDERS OF LYMPHORETICULAR AND HEMOPOIETIC SYSTEM

Radiological Features of Hemophilia

Acute Hemarthrosis

Chronic hemophilic arthropathy
- Changes are most common in **knee** followed by ankles, elbow, wrists, hips and then shoulder
- Osteopenia with coarsening of trabecular pattern
- Epiphyseal enlargement
- Deep intercondylar notch
- Squaring of radial head and patella
- Marginal erosions due to pannus formation
- Growth arrest lines
- Synovial thickening with absolute increase in soft tissue density
- Subchondral cyst formation.

Complications
- Joint deformities
- AVN
- Hemophilic pseudotumor (soft tissue hematoma)
- Degenerative joint disease accelerated
- Ankylosis
- Blood transfusion associated complications.

Radiological Features of Sickle Cell Anemia (SCA)

Marrow hyperplasia
- Generalized osteoporosis
- Widening of diploic spaces and frontal bossing uncommon
- 'Fish-network' appearance in phalanges and ribs due to coarse medullary pattern because of enlarged vascular channels in bone.

Endosteal apposition of bone
- 'Bone within bone' appearance of long bones due to cortical thickening
- In severe cases, medullary cavities may be almost obliterated producing diffuse osteosclerosis, but this does not occur in axial skeleton (an important diagnostic point).

Bone infarcts
- Medullary infarcts (mostly in femoral and humeral heads) with 'snow-cap' sign in shoulder (subarticular area of increased density in humeral head)
- Osteochondritis dessicans to complete collapse of heads
- Diaphysis of long bones, i.e. so called 'intermediate fifths' affected
- Infarcts in vertebral bodies producing characteristic 'h-shaped' vertebrae
- Hands and feet tubular bone infarcts with 'hand-foot' syndrome (sickle cell dactylitis).

Superadded bone infection
- *Salmonella osteomyelitis.*

Soft tissue involvement
- Paravertebral masses
- Hepatosplenomegaly.

Gallstones

Multiple Myeloma

Most common primary malignant neoplasm in adults, which is followed by osteosarcoma.
Age: Usually 5th to 8th decade.

Location
Disseminated form: Vertebrae> ribs > skull > pelvis > long bones
Solitary Plasmacytoma: Vertebrae> pelvis > skull > sternum> ribs.

Radiographic features
- Multiple punched out widespread osteolytic lesions in skull, however, classic 2–3 mm **'rain drop'** circular lytic defects are not always evident
- But mandibular involvement may be helpful indistinguishing it from metastases
- Blown out lesions of skull, long bones (persistent red marrow areas of proximal femora and humeri) and pelvis
- Soft tissue masses adjacent to area of lysis may be seen
- Localized areas of lucency in red marrow areas and generalized osteoporosis are tow cardinal features
- Diffuse osteoporosis can alone cause suspicion of this disease in an elderly patient
- *Spinal myeloma*: Sparing of posterior elements, intervertebral disk spaces and articular surfaces with paraspinal soft tissue mass
- Sclerotic lesions are rare in multiple myeloma
- It is still one of the indications for skeletal survey in today's era of modern imaging.

Bone Scan Features

In multiple myeloma, ^{99m}Tc products do not localize well in the destructive/ lytic lesions (no osteoblastic activity, hence no uptake - *cold spots*). Positive areas of augmented uptake are reported only in 24 percent to 44 percent of patients with radiographically apparent lytic areas. Although the isotope bone scan is far less reliable in multiple myeloma than in metastatic disease, occasionally scan findings will precede roentgen changes. Bone scan is not useful in evaluating multiple myeloma.

Radiological Changes in Leukemia in Childhood

- Diffuse osteopenia/osteoporosis (most common pattern)
- "Leukemic lines"—these are transverse radiolucent metaphyseal bands or thick lines seen just below the epiphyseal growth plate uniformly across the width of metaphysis and these become dense after treatment
- Osteolytic lesions of flat and tubular bones (multiple small) with moth-eaten bony destruction. Lytic lesions distal to knee/elbow in children are suggestive of leukemia rather than metastasis.
- Infrequent but smooth/lamellated sunburst type of periosteal reaction due to periostitis.
- Sutural widening.
- Very rarely metaphyseal osteosclerosis or mixed lesions.

Histiocytosis X

- Bone is the most common site of involvement
- *Three forms of histiocytosis X are known*:
  - Localized histiocytosis (70%), i.e. eosinophilic granuloma
  - Disseminated histiocytosis (30%):
    i. Hand-Schuller-Christian disease (chronic)
    ii. Letterer-Siwe disease (fulminant)
- *Age:* 5 to 10 years most common
- *Location:* Bone (in children) or lung (in adults)
- *Sites:* Flat bones, calvarium > mandible > ribs > pelvis > vertebrae and long bones.
- *Skull:*
  - Diploic space of parietal bone (most common)
  - Round/ovoid punched out lesion with beveled edge (**hole-within-hole appearance**) sharply marginated without the sclerotic rim

- **Geographic skull**
- With "**button sequestrum**"
- With soft tissue mass overlying lesion.
* *Jaw:* Floating tissue mass overlying lesion
* Vertebra plana
* Painful diaphyseal expansile lytic long bone lesions.
* **Eosinophilic granuloma** is the most benign variety of Langerhan's cell histiocytosis.
* *Sites of affection:*
  - *Flat bones:* Calvarium > mandible > ribs > pelvis > vertebrae
  - *Long bones:* It produces solitary collapsed vertebra (most commonly thoracic), i.e. vertebra plana with following characteristics:
    i. Most common cause of vertebra plana in children
    ii. Preserved disk space
    iii. No kyphosis
    iv. Rare involvement of posterior element.

Types of Histiocytosis X

It is a disorder of immune regulation characterized by abnormal proliferation of reticuloendothelial cells.
Three entities considered under it:
1. Letterer-Siwe disease →
   Acute fulminating form
   Toddlers <3 years old affected
   Clinical features: High fever, rash, lymphadenopathy, and hepatosplenomegaly
   Radiological features: Calvarial lytic lesions, rarely irregular lysis in long bone diaphysis with surrounding laminated periosteal new bone.
2. Hand-Schuller-Christian disease →
   Chronic intermittent disease, any time from early childhood through middle age
   Classic triad (rare): Exophthalmos, diabetes insipidus and lytic skull lesions
   Radiologic features: Polyostotic destructive foci in immature skeleton (hallmark)
   Skull—geographic skull, beveled edges, "Hole within-a-hole" appearance
   Long bones: Entire bone may have multiple lytic defects.

3. Eosinophilic granuloma →
   Most common entity
   Least severe form
   Monostotic involvement three times more common than polyostotic (>50 percent involve skull)
   Radiological features:
   Skull—round/oval lytic lesion with beveled edge. Button sequestrum
   Mandible—floating teeth sign
   Spine—thoracic affected mainly, vertebra plana, ghostly appearance of neural arch
   Pelvis—geographic defect
   Long bones—hole-within-a-hole lesion.

BONE TUMORS AND TUMOR-LIKE CONDITIONS

MRI (NMR) in Bone Tumors

MRI is **modality of choice** for diagnosis and evaluation of bone tumors.

Advantages of MRI
- Inherent soft tissue contrast
- No hazard of ionizing radiation
- Flexibility in imaging planes permits advantageous visualization for tumor staging and planning of surgery
- Superb delineation of intra- and extra-osseous extent of tumor
- Relationship between tumor, inflammatory response, blood vessels and important adjacent structures like joints may be very accurately demonstrated, which is important in planning limb-salvaging procedures
- Tumor aggressiveness can also be assessed, especially with IV contrast
- It is also invaluable in monitoring tumor response to neoadjuvant chemotherapy
- Gadolinium enhanced images can help to differentiate between viable tumor, reactive edema and necrosis.

CT scores over MRI only in detection of small foci of calcification and fine osseous details, which many a time are not visualized on MRI.

Bone scan is not fruitful (as there is no osteoblastic activity in the lesions-cold spots).

Skeletal Metastasis

- Bone scintigraphy remains the most cost-effective method for detection of the bony metastatic deposits, although MRI is more sensitive for identification of metastatic disease.
- Any unexplained region of abnormal uptake should be examined by MRI, which is more sensitive than radiography, and more specific than scintigraphy.
- Diffuse osteoblastic metastatic disease, typically from breast or prostate may result in a *'superscan' appearance*. The identification of a 'halo' of high signal intensity around a lesion is a highly specific feature of metastasis on T2W MRI.

Secondaries in Bone

- Bony secondaries are most common bone neoplasms.
- Spine, pelvis and ribs are the most common sites of involvement in metastasis together with the proximal ends of the humeri and femora and, less often, the skull.
- These areas correspond to sites of persistent hematopoiesis in the adults, malignant spread usually occurring by hematogenous route.
- Local spread to lumbar spine and pelvis may be expected from tumors arising in pelvis, notably carcinoma of the cervix.
- Some metastases in bone have a predictable distribution, the majority of renal cell carcinoma metastasize to lumbar spine and pelvis
- **Metastasis distal to the knee and elbow** is rare and usually arises from a primary tumor of bronchus, bladder or colon. (**Pneumonic → BBC**)
- **Osteoblastic bone secondaries usually arise from**
  Prostate carcinoma
  Breast carcinoma
  Lymphoma
  Carcinoid (malignant)
  Brain (medulloblastoma)
  Mucinous adenocarcinoma of GIT
  Bladder carcinoma
  Pancreas carcinoma
  Neuroblastoma.

- **Mixed bone secondaries**
  Breast cancer
  Prostate cancer
  Lymphoma
- **Expansile lytic (bubbly) osseous metastases:**
  Kidney
  Thyroid
  Osteosarcoma
- **Calcifying bone secondaries arise**
  Breast
  Osteosarcoma
  Testicular
  Thyroid
  Ovary
  Mucinous adenocarcinoma of GIT
- **Permeative bone metastasis**
  Burkitt's lymphoma
  Mycosis fungoides
- **Bone metastasis with "sunburst" periosteal reaction arises**
  Prostatic carcinoma
  Retinoblastoma
  GIT malignancies
- **Bone metastasis with soft tissue mass**
  Thyroid carcinoma
  Renal tumors
- **Skeletal metastasis in children**
  Neuroblastoma
  Retinoblastoma
  Embryonal rhabdomyosarcoma
  Hapatoblastoma
  Ewings' tumor

Patterns of Bone Destruction (Lodwick's Classification)

Geographic (short zone of transition)	Moth-eaten (mixed lytic sclerotic areas)	Permeative (long zone of transition)
Histiocytosis X	Histiocytosis "X"	Aggressive bone tumor with rapid growth (Ewing's sarcoma)
Slow-growing benign tumor	Lymphoma	
Plasma cell myeloma	Ewing's sarcoma	
Metastasis	Multiple myeloma	
Granulomatous osteomyelitis	Osteomyelitis	
	Neuroblastoma	

Not only is breast cancer the most common primary tumor in women, but also its metastasis shows an unusual affinity for bone.
About 10 percent of metastasis from carcinoma breast produces osteoblastic lesions and in another 10 percent the lesions are mixed. Metastases from melanoma are usually lytic. Blood borne metastases are uncommon in carcinoma of uterus, cervix and ovary and are usually lytic, but may rarely be blastic (sclerotic) or mixed.

Metastatic spread of carcinoma to bone is a relatively late occurrence because the lung traps most tumor emboli. Bone metastasis is commonest in following carcinoma of following 5 organs → breast, bronchus, prostate, kidney and thyroid.

Primary Bone Tumors

Cartilaginous Benign Tumors
- Enchondroma
- Chondroblastoma
- Chondromyxoid fibroma.

Cartilaginous Malignant Tumors
Chondrosarcoma.

Osseous Malignant Tumor Malignant Tumors
- Bony island
- Ivory osteoma
- Osteoid osteoma.

Bone Lesions According to their Predominant/Primary Site of Occurrence/Origin

Epiphyseal	Metaphyseal	Diaphyseal
Chondroblastoma	Chondromyxoid fibroma	Fibrous dysplasia
Giant cell tumor	Osteochondroma	Eosinophilic granuloma
Subchondral cyst	Brodie's abscess	Metastasis
Aneurysmal bone cyst	Solitary bone cyst	Adamantinoma
Eosinophilic granuloma	Osteosarcoma	Leukemia, lymphoma
Chondrodysplasia punctata	Chondrosarcoma	Ewing sarcoma
Metastasis and myeloma after 40 years	Nonossifying fibroma	Nonossifying fibroma
Clear cell chondrosarcoma	Osteomyelitis	

Age (years)	Bone tumor
<5	Neuroblastoma
1–10	Ewing tumor (in diaphysis of long bones)
	Simple bone cyst
10–30	Chondroblastoma
	Chondromyxoid fibroma
	Osteoid osteoma
	Osteoblastoma
	ABC (5–20 years)
	Nonossifying fibroma
	Osteosarcoma (bimodal peak)
	Ewing tumor (in flat bones)
30–40	Primary lymphoma of bone
	GCT (20–45 years)
	Paraosteal sarcoma
	Fibrosarcoma
>40	Metastases
	Multiple myeloma
	Chondrosarcoma
	Osteosarcoma
	Chordoma (bimodal peak)
Any age	Chondroma
	Osteochondroma (peak in 2nd decade)

Pearls

- Can be regarded as normal variant → Fibrous cortical defect
- 'Celery-stick' appearance → Enchondromas
- 'Coat-hanger' appearance → Osteochondroma
- Codman tumor and 'Chicken-wire' calcification → Chondroblastoma
- Bony island → Enostosis
- Gardner syndrome → Osteoma
- Nidus and sclerotic rim; double density sign on RN scan → Osteoid osteoma (a hamartoma)
- Mineralized matrix → Osteoblastoma
- 'Driven snow' appearance → Pindborg tumor
- Fallen fragment/Hinged fragment sign → SBC (Unicameral bone cyst)
- 'Eggshell' covering of expansile cortex over surface of lesion → ABC
- 'Soap bubble' appearance → ABC
- 'Soap bubble' appearance → Chondromyxoid fibroma
- 'Soap bubble' appearance → Non-ossifying fibroma
- 'Soap bubble' appearance (and goes into corners) → GCT (Osteoclastoma)
- Soap bubble'/'Honeycomb' appearance → Adamantinoma/Ameloblastoma
- 'Floating tooth' sign → Eosinophilic granuloma, Adamantinoma

- Bone tumor of three Es (Epiphyseal, Eccentric, Expansile) → GCT (Osteoclastoma)
- 'Onion skin' appearance → Ewing sarcoma
- Resembling osteomyelitis → Ewing sarcoma
- Skip lesions → Osteosarcoma, Ewing sarcoma
- Bone tumor metastasizing to bone → Osteosarcoma, Ewing sarcoma
- 'Sunray'/'Sunburst' appearance → Osteosarcoma
- String sign (to differentiate from myositis ossificans) → Parosteal osteosarcoma
- 'Pop-corn'/nodular/mottled calcification → Chondrosarcoma
- Target calcification → Osseous lipoma
- Ground-glass appearance/Smoky matrix/Rind of orange → Fibrous dysplasia
- Shepherd's crook deformity → Fibrous dysplasia
- Leontiasis ossea (marked facial deformity) → Fibrous dysplasia
- Codman's triangle → Blood/pus/tumor (Osteosarcoma/Ewing tumor)

- Superscan on RN scanning → Breast/prostatic secondaries
- Winking owl sign → Metastasis involving pedicles of vertebra
- Corduroy/accordion vertebra/Vertical striations → Vertebral hemangioma
- Polka dot sign on CT → Vertebral hemangioma
- Geographical skull → Eosinophilic granuloma
- Physaliphorous cells → Chordoma
- Glycogen containing small round cells → Ewing tumor

Nonossifying Fibroma

- It may not be a neoplasm; may simply be a faulty ossification
- Seen in 8 to 20 years age group people (M>F)
- Asymptomatic
- Dimetaphyseal eccentric lesion
- Most often seen in distal tibia, distal femur, proximal tibia, proximal humerus, fibula may also be affected but ribs and ilium are rarely affected
- Solitary ovoid lucent lesion, located eccentrically within often-expanded cortex, scalloped margins and often multilocular on radiography
- Spontaneous regression without treatment is known.

Fibrous Dysplasia/FD (Jaffe-Lichtenstein Disease)

Its tumor-like lesion of the bone (nongenetic)

It can be monostotic or polyostotic.

The association of polyostotic fibrous dysplasia, patchy café-au-lait spots of skin pigmentation and sexual precocity, usually in girls, constitutes the McCune Albright syndrome.

Radiological features
- 'Ground-glass' or radiolucent area of trabecular alteration in the long bones with patchy sclerosis and expansion with cortical thinning and endosteal scalloping
- Smoky groundglass affected bony matrix is classical of FD
- Pathological fractures and deformities like 'shepherd's crook' deformity of femoral necks
- Asymmetrical thickening of skull vault with sclerosis at the base with multiple lucencies
- Obliteration with groundglass appearance of paranasal sinuses
- Leontiasis ossea (marked facial deformity).

Unicameral Bone Cyst, Simple/Solitary/Juvenile Bone Cyst

- *Age and Sex*: 3 to 19 years
- M:F = 3:1
- *Location*: Proximal humerus + femur (60–75%), fibula, calcaneum (at the base of its neck)
- After growth plate closure, 52 percent are in pelvis and calcaneum.
- *Site*: Metaphyseal (intramedullary expansile centric)
- *Prognosis*: Spontaneous regression mostly.

Radiologic features include
- Lytic geographic lesion, broad at metaphyseal end, narrow at diaphyseal end and longer than wide, "giving truncated cone appearance", with or without septa and endosteal scalloping.
- It's simply an expansile lesion without cortical disruption.
- *Fallen fragment sign* (10% cases), i.e. small-detached fragment floats in lytic defect is characteristic feature.
- *Hinged fragment sign* in which the fragments remains attached to the lytic area is another vital feature.

Osteoblastoma

- 30 to 40 percent in spine
- *Site*: Posterior element may involve body, if large.
- *Nature*: Expansile lesion with sclerotic/shell-like rim, foci of calcification.

Exostosis (Osteochondroma)

- Most common benign bone tumor
- Most occur at the growing ends of the bones
- Their growth ceases after skeletal maturity
- Most osteochondromas (cartilage cap tumor/exostosis) have cartilage caps no thicker than 5 mm, and a cap more than 20 mm in thickness is likely to be malignant
- Destruction of part of a well-formed calcified cap or ossified stem is also a radiological feature of osteochondroma favoring malignant transformation.

Multiple Exostoses (Diaphyseal Aclasis)

- Autosomal dominant inheritance
- Multiple flat/protuberant exostoses particularly at the ends of long bones, ribs, scapulae and iliac bones

- Cranial vault spared
- Long bone exostoses point away from the adjacent joint
- Failure of remodeling of bone ends resulting in deformities like short distal ulna (reverse Madelung deformity)
- Sarcomatous change suspected if rapid increase in size, or pain occurs.

Enchondromatosis/Multiple Enchondromas/Dyschondroplasia (Ollier's Disease)

- Nongenetic inheritance
- Asymmetrical shortening of affected bone/limb with joint deformity
- Radiolucency particularly in metaphyses with expansion of affected bone
- Areas of calcification within lesions
- Reverse Madelung deformity.

Enchondromatosis with Hemangiomas (Maffucci's Syndrome)

- Multiple enchondromas with cavernous hemangiomas in soft tissues
- Chondrosarcomatous metaplasia is recognized hazard (in 20% cases).

Osteoid Osteoma

Affects young people, 10 to 25 years of age.

Classical clinical presentation is pain during night time, which is relieved by aspirin.

Fifty percent percent are in femur or tibia, predilection for spine in 10 percent cases, usually in neural arch (sclerotic pedicle); however it can occur in almost any bone.

Usually cortical, but may be intramedullary or subperiosteal.

Radiological features
- Diaphyseal lesion.
- Cortically located lesions. Lucent **nidus** surrounded by reactive sclerosis. May have central fleck of target calcification in the center.
- Intramedullary lesions. Lucent nidus may be the only visible abnormality.
- *Spinal lesions:* Most often affects lamina. 60 percent are in lumbar spine. Mature sclerotic lesion may present as sclerotic 'Ivory pedicle' or 'ivory lamina'.
- Radionuclide bone scan may show "**double density sign**".
- Nidus of osteoidosteoma (which produces Pgs and Painproducing substances) is seen better with CT than with MRI.

Chondroblastoma (Codman's Tumor)

- Rare neoplasm
- Typically located in epiphysis of long bone
- Other epiphyseal origin tumors are:
  - Osteoblastoma
  - Subchondral cyst
- Generally benign
- 80 percent occur in 2nd decade
- Usually located eccentrically in epiphysis but may straddle the growth plate
- Classical 'Chicken-wire' calcification may be seen on HP
- X-ray spherical and well-defined lytic lesion with fine sclerotic margin
- Central punctate calcification is seen in only 10 percent cases
- Most common in femur followed by humerus and tibia.

Chondromyxoid Fibroma

- 10 to 30 years age
- Metaphyseal eccentric
- Proximal shaft of tibia most classical site
- It is eccentric without lobulations
- Lesion involving cortex and medulla with sclerotic border may show soap bubble appearance due to endosteal nodding.

Aneurysmal Bone Cyst

- Aneurysmal bone cyst (ABC) is regarded as non-neoplastic in nature and radiographically is characterized by an aggressively expanding and sometimes "blowout lesion" of bone.
- In addition to the conventional or primary ABC, an understanding of the significance of the following types of ABCs is required:
  - Secondary ABC
  - "Solid" ABC
  - Recurrent ABC
- Aneurysmal bone cysts are usually encountered in the first, second, and third decades of life, with 80 percent of patients being less than 20 years of age at time of diagnosis. There is a slight female preponderance.

- Although any bone of the skeleton may be affected, over 50 percent affect the large tubular bones of the body. Within a long bone, ABCs may be present exclusively in the metaphysis or show significant diaphyseal involvement as well.
- Distal of humerus is most common site.
- Although any vertebral level may be involved, ABCs are most frequently seen at the dorsal and lumbar levels. They arise in the posterior vertebral elements and may be confined to this region, but more commonly there is involvement of the body as well. Isolated involvement of the body is rare.
- *Radiographic features:* In long bones, the lesion tends to be predominantly metaphyseal and eccentric, with a predilection for maximum growth beyond the outer margins of the bone. The inner margin of the lesion is usually well-defined and the outer cortical surface is expanded or "ballooned". The appearance is that of an aggressive, rapidly growing, intraosseous abnormality. Although the appearance may simulate a sarcoma, the entities that usually tend to figure in the differential diagnosis (which is significantly influenced by patient age) are benign entities, such as chondromyxoid fibroma, simple bone cyst (especially in sites such as the proximal humerus) and, rarely, large non-ossifying fibroma. The expanding lesion may or may not have a soap-bubble pattern. Rarely, telangiectatic osteosarcoma of a long bone may mimic an ABC because of its metaphyseal location, purely osteolytic appearance, and balloon-like expansion.
- The radiograph is the most reliable imaging modality available for predicting the histological nature of a tumor or tumor-like lesion of bone, and an ABC is no exception to this rule.
- However, CT or MR imaging have important roles to play in depicting tumor extent when ABCs occur in vertebrae or flat bones.
- An interesting observation made initially on CT examinations and then on MR imaging of ABCs is the presence of fluid-fluid levels. This appearance is not exclusively seen in ABCs and has been described in a number of bone and soft-tissue abnormalities that include fibrous dysplasia, simple bone cyst, osteosarcoma, soft tissue hemangioma, synovial sarcoma, and even metastases.
- *Treatment:* The treatment of choice is complete curettage of the entire lesion, which may be followed by bone grafting.

Giant Cell Tumor

- These are benign epiphyseal bone tumors.
- Giant cell tumors (GCT) typically arise when the cartilaginous growth plate closes.
- They localize to the articular end of the bone.
- When this occurs, the histopathology is atypical; the cells contain large amounts of glycogen.

- GCT is uncommon before age 20 or after 50.
- Giant cell tumors have a preference for the knee.
- GCT is distinguished histologically by the vascularized network of plump stromal cells intermixed with multinucleated giant cells. It is the ubiquitous giant cell that creates the confusion in diagnosis. Many authors confuse a variety of lesions that contain giant cells with the true giant cell tumor (e.g. nonosteogenic fibroma, benign chondroblastoma, chondromyxoid fibroma, unicameral bone cyst, aneurysmal bone cyst, and hyperparathyroidism).
- The most common symptom is pain and swelling about the joint (usually the knee). The joints are tender, and motion is often limited.
- *Roentgenologic features:* The tumor is expansile and radiolucent and extends to the articular end of a long bone, most frequently the lower end of the femur and proximal end of the tibia.
- Giant cell tumor almost never occurs in the diaphysis or metaphysis of a long bone.
- Tumor invasion of the soft tissue occurs in 25 percent of cases.
- The gross appearance of a giant cell tumor is a fleshy, friable, reddish-brown lesion. Often, the lesion destroys the bone and extends into the soft tissue.
- *Treatment:* Excision (with bone grafting) is treatment of choice if one decides that resection is feasible, the boundaries of the tumor should be outlined.

Chondrosarcoma

- It is a malignant tumor originating in cartilage.
  Secondary chondrosarcoma arises in a pre-existing bony lesion like:
- Usually →
  - An enchondroma (**central type**)
  - An osteochondroma (**peripheral type**)
- Rarely in →
  - Chondromyxoid fibroma
  - Chondroblastoma
  - Synovial chondromatosis
  - Enchondromatosis
  - Maffucci's syndrome
  - Diaphyseal aclasis
- Most osteochondromas (**cartilage cap tumor/exostosis**) have cartilage caps no thicker than 5 mm, and a cap more than 20 mm in thickness is likely to be malignant. Destruction of part of a well-formed

calcified cap or ossified stem is also a radiological feature of osteochondroma favoring malignant transformation.
- **Age:** Peak incidence is at 50 years age.
- **Sex:** Slight male predominance (M:F is 1.5:1)
- **Common location:** Flat bones (pelvis, scapula), proximal femur and proximal humerus.
- *Radiological features*
    - Lytic lesion with endosteal resorption, periosteal reaction, periosteal new bone formation and bone expansion
    - Aggressive lytic lesion with narrow zone of transition and mottled calcification in a flat bone in elderly is highly suggestive of chondrosarcoma.
    - Multilobulated appearance with well-defined scalloping of endosteal surface and cortical destruction in more aggressive lesions
    - Soft tissue extracortical mass out of proportion to the size of the intraosseous lesion is characteristic
    - Being a chondroid tumor, presence of calcification (**dense/stippled/nodular/conglomerate popcorn-like/ring/arc-like calcification**) is characteristic feature.
    - P_X: The **prognosis** of chondrosarcoma is good when complete resection is achieved before metastatic spread.
    - The tumor shows poor response to radiotherapy and cytotoxic drugs.

Osteosarcoma

- Most common malignant primary tumor of bone in young adults and children
- 2nd most common primary malignant bone tumor after multiple myeloma
- It has **bimodal age distribution**: 10 to 25 years and >60 years with M:F = 3:2 to 2:1
- Constitutes 15 percent of all primary bone tumors confirmed at biopsy.
- Factors for secondary osteosarcoma:
    - Paget's disease
    - Diaphyseal aclasis
    - Enchondromatosis
    - Postradiation.

Location

Metaphysis is common site of origin (90–95%) with long bones affected in 70 to 80 percent cases; femur lower end (40–45%), tibia (16–20%) and 50 to 55 percent thus seen around knee; facial bones (8%), flat bones affected usually in age >50 years (ilium).

Radiographic Features

- Large osteosclerotic lesion (90%)
- Osteolytic lesion (fibroblastic)
- Aggressive periosteal reaction (sunburst/hair-on-end/onion-peel laminated periosteal reaction)
- Codman's triangle
- Moth-eaten bone destruction with cortical disruption
- Soft tissue mass with new bone formation (osseous/cartilaginous type)
- Physis does not act as barrier to tumor spread
- Spontaneous pneumothorax (due to subpleural metastasis)
- **String sign** → fine radiolucent line separating tumor mass from cortex seen in parosteal osteosarcoma.

CT Features

Metaphyseal bone lesion with:
- Soft tissue attenuation (nonmineralized part)
- Replacing fatty bone marrow
- Low attenuation (chondroblastic component/ hemorrhage/necrosis)
- Very high attenuation (mineralized matrix)
- Evaluate for extent of marrow and soft tissue involvement, epiphyseal invasion, joint and neovascular involvement and distant metastasis.

MR (Preferred Modality)

Tumor of intermediate signal intensity on T1W1 and high signal intensity on T2W1

Clearly defines marrow extent (best on T1W1), vascular involvement and soft tissue component (best on T2W1).

Radionuclide Bone Scan (NUC)

Intensity increased activity on blood flow, blood pool, delayed images (hypervascularity, new bone formation). Local extent, skip lesions, metastasis to bone and soft tissues detected. **Doughnut sign** (peripherally increased uptake with central photopenia on bone scan) is a classical feature. Soft tissue extension demonstrated especially on SPECT.

P_X: Treatment is radical surgery (e.g. amputation of limb) and high dose methotrexate chemotherapy.

Ewing's Sarcoma

- Ewing's sarcoma is the highly malignant primary bone neoplasm having specific cytogenetic analysis, i.e. t (11,12), is a PNET with 75 percent patients being under the age of 20 years and having male predilection.
- Histologically small oval/round tumor cells are seen arranged in sheets with occasional rosette-like pattern and most tumors are **PAS-positive** indicating presence of **glycogen** in the tumor cells.
- Mic-2 gene *(CD99)* mutation is characteristic.

Radiological Features

- Ill-defined osteolytic medullary lesion involving diaphysis
- Extension along the length of the marrow with permeative bone destruction
- Cortical saucerization
- Classical multilaminar periosteal reaction giving 'onion-peel' appearance
- Codman's triangles with elevated periosteum, although classically seen in osteosarcoma
- Soft tissue mass disproportionately large compared to the extent of osseous involvement, resembling osteomyelitis
- Bone sarcoma metastasizing to bone.

MRI is best modality for diagnosis and evaluation as–

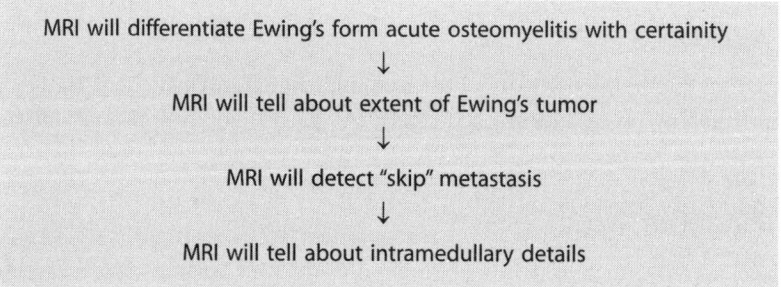

Chordoma

- It is a destructive bone tumor believed to arise from ectopic remnants of notochord/notochord cell rest.
- Its maximum incidence between 50 and 70 years.
- It is locally malignant with strong tendency to recur after excision.

- Predilection for sacral (50%) and cranial (40%) regions (the extreme ends of the axial skeleton).
- In sacrum at S_4 and S_5 and in cranium basisphenoid (clivus and dorsal aspect of sella).
- Above sacrum and below C_2, chordomas are rare.
- Radiologically appears as a oval or lobulated well-defined purely lytic mass in midline, which may contain calcification and a soft tissue component.
- Recurrence rate is high but it **metastasis occurs late**.
- Chordoma at the base of skull carries best prognosis.

Ameloblastoma

Most common malignant tumor of jaw

Middle-aged males are commonly affected

Occurs mainly in molar region of mandible

Radiologically the lesions are classically expansile, multilocular, and cystic with 'soap-bubble' or 'honeycomb' appearance and peripheral satellite defects, which are well demarcated.

Block excision of the involved part of bone should be carried out as following incomplete excision and re-exploration, recurrence is likely and the lesion may spread both locally and to the lungs.

Dentigerous/Follicular Cyst

It is found primarily in adolescents and young adults.

It is usually unilocular.

It is a cyst occurring in relation to the crown of unerupted tooth and although it becomes displaced, often for some distance, part of the crown is always in contact with the cyst.

The permanent mandibular 3rd molar and maxillary canines are especially affected.

Adamantinoma of Long Bone

- *Introduction*: Unusual neoplasm, almost always located in tibial shaft.
- *Clinical features*: Localized swelling and pain for several years.
- *Age*: Between 15 and 55 years.

Radiological Features

- An eccentric well-demarcated area of destruction usually involving the anterior portion of the tibial shaft.
- Slight expansion and cortical thinning, with a cystic or multiloculated appearance is usual.

- Periosteal reaction is not marked.
- Cortical destruction may be extensive.
- Margins of tumors vary from being sharply and clearly demarcated, with slight sclerotic areas, to a hazy zone of transition of several mm, comparable to that seen in giant cell tumors.

Histologically difficult to distinguish from metastatic adenocarcinoma, but component of the tumor may suggest an epithelial derivation.

Although the tumor continues to grow to a slow rate, it is featured by local recurrent and eventual lung metastasis.

> **Pindborg's tumor** is **calcifying odontogenic epithelioma**.
> It produces typical **"driven snow" appearance** on plain X-ray.

Best investigation for imaging of a bone tumor	⇒ MRI
Most sensitive investigation for bone metastases	⇒ Bone scan
Best investigation for bone metastases	⇒ MRI
Ideal agent for bone scan (scintigraphy)	⇒ ^{99m}Tc MDP
Double density sign on bone scintigraphy	⇒ Osteoid osteoma
"Doughnut sign" on bone scan	⇒ Osteosarcoma

JOINT DISEASES

- Few diseases and the most common joint involved/affected:
  - Gout→first metatarsophalangeal joint
  - Osteochondritis dissecans*→knee
  - Synovial enchondromatosis*→knee
  - Myositis ossificans*→around elbow
  - Premature osteoarthritis*→hip
- Osteomyelitis in diabetic foot*→metatarsal heads (first and fifth)

Radiological Features of Osteoarthritis/Degenerative Arthritis

- Joint space narrowing
- Subchondral sclerosis/eburnation
- Central and peripheral osteophytosis including tibial spiking in knees

- Subarticular cyst or Geode formation
- Loose bodies
- Joint deformities
- Heberden's nodes at DIP and Bouchard's nodes at PIP joints.

Osteoarthritis in Hands

The carpometacarpal joint of the thumb and the trapezioscaphoid joint are commonly affected in Osteoarthritis (OA), especially in females. These joints are seldom affected in RA. In OA, in contrast to RA, the distal interphalangeal (DIP) joints are most commonly affected. DIP joint prominences due to osteophytes are known as Heberden's nodes and those at PIP joints are called Bouchard's nodes.

Typical hand involvement in osteoarthritis includes DIP, PIP and 1st carpometacarpal joint and scaphotrapezial joints. DIP joint prominences due to osteophytes are known as Heberden's nodes and those at PIP joints are called Bouchard's nodes.

The architecture of the proximal end of the femur is determined by the magnitude of the forces acting upon the hip. A cone of compressive trabeculae extends from the load-bearing surface of the hip inferiorly to the medial cortex of the femoral neck. The tensile trabeculae arise from the lateral cortex and traverse the neck to the medial articular surface in a fanlike pattern. Between these is Ward's triangle, a zone of minimal pressure.

The type and the severity of OA is affected by the angle of Wiberg (an angle that defines the acetabular coverage of the femoral head). The less well developed the outer margin of the acetabulum, the smaller the angle of Wiberg, and the more likely it will be that the load-bearing segment will shift to the superior lateral part of the joint. OA joints frequently have an abnormal CE angle; migration of the femoral head is predominantly proximal or superolateral. In contrast, inflammatory joints have normal CE angles, and the femoral head tends to move in an axial or medial direction.

Rheumatoid arthritis	- Marginal bony erosions (bare area affected)
Scleroderma	- Most common site of bone erosion is distal phalanx and erosion + subluxation of thumb carpometacarpal joint is characteristic
Dermatomyositis/polymyositis	- Bone erosions very rare
SLE	- Nonerosive arthritis
Jaccoud's arthritis (classically develops following rheumatic fever)	- Late in the disease, "hook-erosions" may be seen
Multicentric reticulohistiocytosis	- Large "punched-out" erosions

Psoriatic	-	Erosions similar as in RA and seen at DIP, "mouse-ears" marginal erosion and cup-like erosions
Gout	-	Punched out erosions with sclerotic margins and overhanging bony edge
Reiter's disease	-	Calcaneal erosions (Lover's heel)

Juvenile Rheumatoid Arthritis (JRA)/Juvenile Chronic Polyarthritis/ Still's Disease

Patients are generally less than 16 years of age and have persistent arthritis of one or more joints for at least 6 weeks.

Rheumatoid factor is absent in about 90 percent cases.

Two forms:
1. Pauciarticular form (four or less joints involved)
2. Polyarticular (five or more joints involved).

Radiological Features

- Soft tissue swelling
- Synovitis with joint effusion
- Osteopenia
- Epiphyseal overgrowth (due to chronic synovitis and hyperemia)
- Cartilage loss, loss of joint space and bone erosions (late features)
- Ankylosis and deformities
- Early closure of epiphyseal plate may occur resulting in growth disturbances
- Atlanto-axial dislocation
- *In hands:* Florid periosteal reaction along the metacarpal and phalangeal shafts, loss of joint space, fine erosions and ankylosis.

The Plain X-ray Film Joint Changes of RA include

- Soft tissue changes
- Osteoporosis (Juxta-articular/juxtaepiphyseal)
- Joint space changes and alignment deformities

- Periostitis
- Bone erosions
- Secondary osteoarthritis.

Psoriatic Arthritis

Types
- True psoriatic arthritis (31%)
- Psoriatic arthritis resembling RA (38%)
- Concomitant RA with psoriatic arthritis (31%).

Radiological Features

Hands
- Asymmetrical involvement
- Ray distribution (all '3' joints of single ray involved; DIP, PIP, and MCP)
- *Sausage digits*
- Absence of osteoporosis
- Sparing of joint space (early)
- Erosions at DIP (*Gull wing* appearance)
- 'Cup-like' erosions
- Fluffy periosteal reaction
- Productive bone changes (periosteal reaction and proliferative new bone formation)
- 'Mouse ear' sign (joints flanked by fluffy new bone formation)
- 'Pensile in cup' or 'pestle in mortar' deformity
- 'Opera glass' or 'Main-en-lorgnette' deformity or 'telescoping'
- Tapering of proximal phalanges
- Acroosteolysis
- Ivory phalanx
- No ulnar deviation
- Fibular digital deviation
- Sharply demarcated adjacent bony surface (pathognomonic)
- Spontaneous joint fusion
- Destruction of IP joints of hands and feet with abnormal widening of joint space

- Neurotrophic changes at DIP joints with 'licked candy' appearance
- Arthritis mutilans.

Feet
- Similar changes as that of hand
- Feet affection less common and less severe than Reiter's syndrome
- Sausage toes
- Characteristic early changes at IP joints of great toe
- Calcaneal erosions
- Intertarsal ankylosis rarely
- Axial skeleton (SI joints and spine)
- Unilateral involvement common, when bilateral it is asymmetrical
- Sacroiliitis similar to AS, except that joint fusion does not occur and affection is asymmetrical
- Enthesitis
- Paravertebral ossifications/parasyndesmophytes (unilateral, asymmetrical).

Extra-articular involvement
- Silvery skin scales
- Thimble pitting of nails.

Ankylosing Spondylitis (Marie-Strumpell Disease or Bechterew Disease)

- Bamboo-spine (knobby spine, poker back or universal syndesmophytosis) is a characteristic feature of it.
- Syndesmophytes are gracile ossifications of the outer fibers of annulus fibrosus. They are marginal, delicate, vertically oriented, extending from edge or margin of one vertebral body to that of others.
- Syndesmophytes should be differentiated from the parasyndesmophytes or the paravertebral ossifications seen in psoriatic arthritis or Reiter's disease by which although vertically oriented are thicker, denser, non marginal extending from mid-body to mid-body, larger, coarse and may affect any part of spine to start with, without proper order.
- Other diagnostic radiological features of Ankylosing spondylitis are:
    - Bilateral symmetrical sacroiliitis (most specific)
    - Enthesitis (earliest pathological change)
    - Uncommon involvement of small joints of hand and feet.

Diffuse Idiopathic Skeletal Hypertrophy (DISH)/ Forestier's Disease/Senile Ankylosing Spondylitis

- Dense ossification is found in the cervical and especially the lower thoracic regions.
- Usually seen in elderly males.
- Bone is laid down often in continuity anteriorly and, in the thoracic region, on the right side, as the left-sided aortic pulsation prevents its deposition.
- The thick, flowing, florid, exuberant corticated plaques are extensive than that seen in degenerative changes producing the so-called 'dripping candle wax' appearance and may indent the esophagus.
- The SI joints may appear symmetrically fused on a plain film, without any erosion.
- Florid neo-ossification is also seen at exptraspinal sites, around the iliac crest, ischia, and above the acetabulum, and at the sites of ligamentous or tendinous insertions into bone.
- Similar changes are found in foot, especially on the calcaneus, where florid spur formation may be seen.
- Occasionally fusion between paired long bones may be seen
- Rarely, posterior ligamentous ossification (OPLL) encroaches on the theca and produces cord compression (often seen in Japanese patients).

Ossified Posterior Longitudinal Ligament

- Japanese disease.
- Best evaluated with CT (for ossification) and MRI (for evaluation of cord).
- Likely to progress to myelopathy with canal compromise of 60% and sagittal canal diameter of 8 mm.
- Cervical spine involvement is most common.
- Advanced cases of ossified posterior longitudinal ligament (OPLL) are easily recognized on routine radiography.
- MR is useful in assessing status of adjacent spinal cord.

Charcot's Joint

Repeated trauma to the joints in the absence of normal pain and proprioception will give rise to a severe destruction arthropathy known as Charcot's joint.

5 D's of Charcot's Joint

D - Disorganization
D - Density of bone increased

D - Debris within joint capsule
D - Destruction of bone
D - Deformity leprosy.

Causes of Charcot's Joint

- Diabetes (most common joint involved-tarsometatarsal joints)
- Neurosyphilis (knee joint)
- Syringomyelia (upper limb (shoulder) joint)
- Spina bifida (knee joint, foot joint)
- Congenital indifference to pain (ankle joint)
- Alcoholism (foot joint)
  - Leprosy (foot joints).

Developmental Dysplasia of the Hip (DDH)/Developmental Hip Dysplasia; DDH; Congenital Dysplasia of the Hip; Congenital Dislocation of the Hip; CDH

Causes, Incidence, and Risk Factors

- The hip is a ball and socket joint with the ball (called the femoral head) coming from the top part of the femur (thigh bone) and the socket (called the acetabulum) coming from the pelvis.
- The cause is unknown, but genetic factors may play a role.
- Problems resulting from very mild developmental dysplasia of the hip may not become apparent until the person is in their 30s or 40s.
- One or both hips may be involved.
- Risk factors include being the first child, being female, a breech delivery, and a family history of the disorder.
- It occurs in about 1 out of 1,000 births.
- DDH is 4 to 8 times more common in female infants than in male infants. This difference is believed to be the result of the increased levels of circulating estrogens and relaxin at the time of birth and an increased susceptibility to them.

Investigations
A hip radiograph is helpful in older infants and children.

But, ultrasound of the hip remains the most important imaging study and will demonstrate hip deformity.

Graf classification of infant hips based on the depth and shape of the acetabulum as seen on coronal ultrasonograms.

- *Type I:* Normal; characterized by a well-formed acetabular cup with the femoral head beneath the acetabular roof.
- *Type II:* Immature in infants less than three months of age and mildly dysplastic in infants older than three months; characterized by a shallow acetabulum with a rounded rim.
- *Type III:* Subluxated; characterized by a very shallow acetabulum with some displacement of the femoral head.
- *Type IV:* Dislocated; characterized by a flat acetabular cup and loss of contact with the femoral head.

Treatment

In early infancy, positioning with a device to keep the legs apart and turned outward (frog-leg position) will usually hold the femoral head in the socket. If there is difficulty in maintaining proper position, a cast may be applied and changed periodically to accommodate growth.

Surgery may be necessary if early measures to reduce the joint (put the joint back in place) are unsuccessful, or if the defect is first detected in an older child.

Crystal-Deposition Arthropathies and Periarthropathies

Disease	Composition of crystals	Site	Predilection (target area)	Radiologic hallmark
Gout	Sodium urates (negatively birefringent)	Articular and periarticular	First metatarsophalangeal articulation	Martei's overhanging edge sign
Pyrophosphate dihydrate crystal deposition disease (CPDD)	Calcium pyrophosphate dihydrate (CPDD) (positively birefringent)	Fibrocartilage and hyaline cartilage fiber-rich connective tissue synovial lining	Knee wrist	Chondro-calcinosis
Hydroxy apatite crystal deposition disease (HADD)	Calcium hydroxy apatite	Periarticular tendons and bursae	Shoulder	Mil shoulder

SOFT TISSUES
Causes of Soft-tissue Calcifications

Metastatic calcifications (disturbed calcium-phosphate metabolism)	Idiopathic calcifications (normal calcium-phosphate metabolism)	Dystrophic calcifications (normal calcium-phosphate metabolism)
Hyperparathyroidism Renal osteodystrophy Excess vitamin D Hypoparathyroidism Sarcoidosis Massive bone loss with plasmocytoma Leukemia, or extensive metastases	Collagenoses (e.g. systemic lupus erythematosus dermatomyositis CREST syndrome Tumorous calcinosis Calcinosis universalis (in children)	Burns Frostbites Severe soft-tissue injuries Compartment syndrome Tumors Osteonecrosis infarcts Tuberculosis

Soft Tissue Tumors

- MRI is investigation of choice for soft tissue tumors because:
    - MRI tells about extent of tumor
    - Relation with adjacent neurovascular bundle
    - Locating appropriate site of biopsy
- Rhabdomyosarcoma (30% cases) ⎫
- Fibrosarcoma (5% cases) ⎬ Lymphatic metastasis also seen
- Clear cell sarcoma
- Angiosarcoma
- Malignant fibrous histiocytoma
- Synovial cell sarcoma
- Askin tumor
- Elastofibroma (Benign).

Askin tumor (Primitive neuroectodermal tumors): Askin tumors are rare, malignant, small-cell tumors of neuroepithelial origin seen in children and adolescents. The Askin tumor is a sarcoma arising from the chest wall, often with rib involvement and a pleural effusion. Askin tumors are rare malignant neoplasms, seen predominantly in children and young adults. These tumors are heterogeneous on CT and T2-weighted MRI while on T1-weighted MRIs they have a density higher than that of skeletal muscle. Hemorrhage and necrosis are frequent findings.

Chapter 9

Endocrine Imaging

THYROID

Childhood Hypothyroidism (Cretinism) is Characterized by
- Delayed skeletal maturation
- Delayed dentition
- Delayed pneumatization of sinuses/mastoids
- Demineralization
- Dense vertebral margins with bullet shaped vertebrae
- Delayed closure/open wide fontanels/sutures
- Fragmented stippled epiphyses
- Hypoplastic phalanges of 5th finger
- Hypertelorism
- Wormian skull bones.

Adulthood Hypothyroidism
- Calvarial thickening/sclerosis
- Coxa vara with flattened femoral head
- Wedging of dorsolumbar vertebral bodies
- Premature atherosclerosis.

Tumors of Thyroid

- Primary (papillary carcinoma is most common)
- Secondary.

Metastatic tumor in thyroid

It comes from renal cancer. Other cancers, which are known to metastasize to thyroid, are melanoma and bronchogenic carcinoma.

ADRENALS

Imaging of Adrenals

Ultrasound

The adrenal glands are difficult to examine by ultrasound because of their small size and their location high in the abdomen, under the rib cage. Bowel gas from the stomach, duodenum, or colon often impairs visualization of the left adrenal gland, and a variety of patient positions and scan angles must often be tried before the adrenal glands can be examined adequately. The retroperitoneal fat, which provides optimal adrenal imaging by CT, impairs the ultrasound examination; thus, obese patients are poor candidates for ultrasound studies.

Computed Tomography

The single best imaging modality for examination of the adrenal glands is CT. In many cases, this is the only radiographic study required. The adrenal glands are well-visualized with contiguous 1 cm sections through the entire gland. Since the perirenal fat provides adjacent tissue of lower density, the adrenal glands are usually seen clearly, and intravenous contrast is not needed.

Radioisotope Scanning

The use of radionuclide labeled carriers that are incorporated in hormone synthesis is useful in identifying adrenal tumors. The major advantage of this technique is the ease of performing the examination and the ability to detect ectopic tumors, particularly pheochromocytomas. Disadvantages include limited availability of the materials and a relatively high dose of radiation to the patient.

The agent used to image adrenal cortical tumors has been 19-iodocholesterol labeled with iodine 131. However, NP-59-6 131I-odomethyl-19-norcholest-5 (10)-en-3-ol [NP-59] has an improved adrenal-to-tissue ratio and is now the preferred agent.

When a pheochromocytoma is suspected, metaiodobenzylguanidine (MIBG) labeled with iodine 131 is used. Iodine 123 has been used as the labeling isotope in patients with a normal 131I-MIBG scan but a strong clinical suspicion of pheochromocytoma. 131I MIBG remains the standard agent, with 123I MIBG reserved for problem cases.

Magnetic Resonance Imaging

As with CT, the adjacent perirenal fat provides sufficient contrast differences to image the adrenal glands, and differences in signal intensity, particularly on T2-weighted images, provide valuable information about the nature of adrenal masses.

Contrast material is not needed, but cardiac and respiratory gating have been used to improve image quality. For small adrenal lesions, surface coils provide better delineation.

Thus,
- The initial imaging of the adrenal glands is usually performed with CT due to its superior spatial resolution and the ability to perform routine thin slice imaging.
- Adrenal adenomas contain a large amount of lipid-laden cells, giving them a characteristic low density (fat density) appearance on CT scans.
- The radiologic findings of adrenal carcinoma show a large mass that usually envelops much of the area surrounding the involved adrenal gland. Most masses show degenerative and cystic changes, and 33 percent show calcification. CT and MRI findings thus reflect these pathologic changes that occur within these tumors. CECT shows vascularity in certain areas. With MRI, masses show low signal intensity on T1-weighted images and higher signal intensity on T2-weighted images when compared with liver. Signal intensity generally increases on opposed-phase chemical shift imaging. When CT or MRI is performed, tumors should also be staged.
- Adrenal gland hyperplasia secondary to pituitary or ectopic causes of Cushing's syndrome can have several imaging appearances. The most common pattern of it is diffuse bilateral enlargement without a focal mass. MRI has a secondary role in evaluation of patients with Cushing's syndrome because CT can better evaluate smaller adrenal masses. MRI signal intensity seen in adrenal hyperplasia closely follows that of the normal adrenal gland, rendering MRI less sensitive than CT in evaluating adrenal gland hyperplasia.
- In some cases of Cushing's syndrome secondary to hyperplasia, when evaluation of the pituitary gland does not reveal an adenoma, petrosal venous sampling may be valuable in determining the cause finally.

- 2/3rd of microadenomas of pituitary gland typically appear hypodense on dynamic, rapid sequence CECT scans, 1/3rd show "early" enhancement. Macroadenomas of pituitary gland have a variable appearance. Microadenomas are sometimes difficult to detect by MRI unless dynamic techniques are used. Macroadenomas typically parallel gray matter signal on all MR imaging sequences. Benign invasive adenomas cannot be distinguished from the rare pituitary carcinoma on imaging studies above.

Microadenomas are less than 10 mm and macroadenomas are of more than 10 mm size.

Cushing's Disease (Radiology)

Common findings
- Generalized osteopenia (fish vertebrae, wedge and compression fractures, insufficiency fractures in pelvis, mottled appearance of skull)
- Exuberant callus formation
- Osteonecrosis.

Uncommon findings
- Joints infections
- Neuropathic-like joints
- Delayed skeletal maturation
- Decreased osteophyte formation
- Tendon rupture
- Adrenal gland calcification
    - Idiopathic
    - Hemorrhage
    - Tuberculosis
    - Neuroblastoma
    - Ganglioneuroma
    - Phoechromocytoma
    - Histoplasmosis
    - Cysts
    - Addison's disease
    - Wolman's disease.

Adrenal Adenomas

Nonhyperfunctioning adrenal adenomas exceeding 1 cm are detected incidentally in about 1 to 3 percent of upper abdominal CT examinations. The number and size of these nodules increase with age and are most common in obese diabetics and elderly women. These 'silent' adenomas are thought to represent non-neoplastic overgrowth of adrenocortical cells of the zona fasciculata. They consist of cholesterol-laden clear cells, and usually contribute little to steroid production although there may be subtle biochemical changes. The appearance of nonhyperfunctioning and hyperfunctioning adenomas on cross-sectional imaging is similar.

On CT, adrenal adenomas show a much earlier and more rapid washout of contrast enhancement than do non-adenomas.

Lipid-poor adrenal adenomas show contrast enhancement washout nearly identical to that of the more common lipid-rich adenomas and significantly greater than that of nonadenomas. Although lipid-poor adenomas cannot be differentiated from nonadenomas on the basis of their CT attenuation value alone before or after contrast enhancement, they can be differentiated by their percentage enhancement washout and relative percentage enhancement washout with an acceptable sensitivity and high specificity.

Adrenal Carcinomas

Primary adrenocortical carcinomas are rare and highly malignant. Ninety percent produce steroids but only half cause symptoms related to excess hormone production. Functioning carcinomas most commonly result in Cushing's syndrome, but virilization or hyperaldosteronism may also occur. Most carcinomas are usually large (>6 cm in diameter) at the time of diagnosis and are more commonly seen on the left; about 10 percent are bilateral.

Adrenal Metastases

Adrenal metastases are most commonly form tumors of the lung, kidney, melanoma, breast, digestive tract and ovary (*in that order*). The adrenals are commonly involved in patients with lung and breast carcinoma on one or both sides by metastases.

Although with adrenal metastases, the primary is usually in lung and breast, melanoma, renal and gastrointestinal secondaries and secondary lymhomatous involvement are well known.

Pheochromocytoma

Intra-adrenal Pheochromocytoma

CECT has been the primary method of diagnosis for intra-adrenal pheochromocytoma. The accuracy of CT in detecting intra-adrenal pheochromocytomas is nearly 100 percent. It is 93 to 100 percent sensitive for adrenal ones. MRI is also excellent for evaluating intra-adrenal pheochromocytomas as these are generally larger than 5 cm size and the poorer spatial resolution of MRI is usually not a problem. Even a percentage of adrenal metastases have overlapping imaging findings. MIBG scanning can play a complementary role in evaluating intra-adrenal pheochromocytomas. It is 80 to 90 percent sensitive for adrenal one.

Extra-adrenal Pheochromocytoma

MIBG scintigraphy is extremely valuable in imaging of extra-adrenal and recurrent pheochromocytomas. MIBG is a precursor of catecholamines and therefore, is actively taken up in catecholamines producing tissues. After recurrent, metastatic or extra-adrenal lesions are sensitively discovered initially via whole body MIBG scanning, CT or MRI can then be performed for more accurate specific anatomic localization of lesion to be resected.

Neoplasms of Neuroendocrine Origin

- Pancreatic islet cell tumors
- Carcinoids
- Vipomas
- Apudomas
- Some pituitary adenomas
- Medullary thyroid cancers
- Pheochromocytomas
- Neuroblastomas
- Paragangliomas.

Radionuclide scans (somatostatin receptor scintigraphy and MIBG scan) have major role in localization of pancreatic islet cell tumors and their metastases and also investigation of gastrointestinal carcinoids, apudomas and related neuroendocrine tumors and their metastases.

Chapter 10

Head, Neck and Spine Imaging

GENERAL ASPECT AND SKULL RADIOGRAPH

Variations of Normal Sella

"J shaped sella"
In infants by the so called excavation caused by prominence of optic canal, roof results in J-shaped or omega sella.
Flattened sella with prominent sulcus chiasmaticus
- Normal varient
- Optic chiasm glioma
- Chronic hydrocephalus
- MPS
- Achondroplasia
- Neurofibromatosis (Sphenoid dysplasia).

Small pituitary fossa
- Normal varient
- Dystrophia myotonica
- Radiotherapy in childhood
- Hypopituitarism.

Cherry shaped sella → Hyopthyroidism

Radiographic Signs of Increased Intracranial Tension

In Infants and Children

- Large heads
- Thinning of skull vault
- Craniolacunae (if associated with meningocele)
- Excessive interdigitations of sutures
- Displacement of central part of anterior cranial fossa, i.e. cribriform plate downward
- Sutural diastasis (the first and most prominent sign)
- Sellar erosion is late sign in children
- Increased convolutional markings/'copper beaten' appearance (may be seen in normal children between 4 and 10 years age and craniosynostosis).

In Adults

- Erosion of posterior clinoid process (earliest sign)
- Interruption of the lamina dura at the base of the dorsum sellae (earliest sign)
- Slight porosis of anterior cortex followed by loss of lamina dura/cortex/compact bone
- Frank erosion of dorsum sellae (other causes may be hyperparathyroidism, nutritional, and local causes)
- Pineal displacement.

Differential Diagnosis of Calvarial Thickening

- Hypoparathyroidism
- Pseudohypoparathyroidism
- Pseudopseudohypoparathyroidism
- Chronic anemias
- Paget's disease
- Fibrous dysplasia
- Hyperphosphatasia
- Fluorosis
- Dilantin therapy.

Wormian Bones

These are intrasutural bony ossicles (>4 mm size) in lambdoid, posterior sagittal, temporosquamosal sutures of skull.

They can be seen in:
- Normal infants (up to 6 months of age)
- Idiopathic
- Down's syndrome
- Cleidocranial dysostosis
- Hypothyroidism
- Hypophosphatasia
- Healing phase of rickets
- Osteogenesis imperfecta
- Otopalatodigital syndrome
- Kinky hair syndrome
- Progeria
- Pachydermoperiostitis
- Primary acro-osteolysis (Hajdu-Cheney)
- Pyknodysostosis.

"Hair on end" or "Screw hair cut" skull
- Hemolytic anemia
- Thalassemia (a characteristic feature)
- Hereditary spherocytosis
- Sickle cell disease
- G-6-PD deficiency
- Iron deficiency anemia
- Neuroblastoma.

Craniosynostosis
- It is defined as premature closure of all cranial sutures.
- Primary craniosynostosis refers to closure of one or more sutures due to abnormalities of skull development.
- Secondary craniosynostosis results from failure of brain growth and expansion.

Platybasia

It refers to flattening of skull base.

It may be defined as an abnormal invagination or elevation of the floor of the posterior fossa. Instead of a normal downward and medial slope, the petrous pyramids are directed upward and medially.

Causes of platybasia/basilar invagination are:
- Achondroplasia
- Paget's disease
- Rickets
- Osteogenesis imperfecta (OGI), osteomalacia
- Cleidocranial dysostosis
- Hyperparathyroidism, Hurler syndrome
- Fibrous dysplasia.

Pathology of the Craniovertebral Junction

- Occipitoatlantoaxial anomalies
  - Down's syndrome
  - Achondroplasia
  - Congenital absence of the dens may also occur.
- Osseous dysplasias of the foramen magnum
  All causes of basilar impression including achondroplasia, Paget's disease, rickets, osteogenesis imperfecta (OGI), osteomalacia, cleidocranial dysostosis, hyperparathyroidism, fibrous dysplasia, mucopolysaccharidosis of the morquio type (in fact, this is the most common cause of death in this condition), Hurler syndrome, and craniometaphyseal dysplasia.
- Chiari malformations
- Syringohydromyelia
- Trauma
- Vascular conditions (The vertebral arteries, in traversing the craniovertebral junction area, may be affected in a number of ways which in turn may affect CVJ).
- Tumors (chordoma, ABC, dermoids, etc.) neoplasms at this site may be primary or may represent secondary involvement.
- Pseudotumor (chronic atlantoaxial subluxations)
- Spondyloarthropathies

- Rheumatoid arthritis (in rheumatoid arthritis, proliferative synovial tissue can cause destruction of the dens, lateral masses of the atlas, and the occipital condyles. The transverse and alar ligaments are also affected.)
  - JRA
  - Ankylosing spondylitis
  - Reiter's disease
  - Psoriatic arthropathy
- Infections (infectious lesions).

Physiological Intracranial Calcification

- Pineal gland (60% of adults, seen approximately 30 mm above highest posterior elevation of pyramids and pineal calcification more than 14 mm suggests pineal neoplasm)
- Habenular commissure (30%) and seen 4–6 mm anterior to pineal glands as posteriorly open C-shaped calcification
- Choroid plexus (10% most commonly in glomus within atrium of lateral ventricles)
- Arteriosclerosis (carotids, basilar and vertebral arteries)
- Basal ganglia
- Pituitary gland (rare)
- Dura mater
  - Falx cerebri (7%) and superior sagittal sinus
  - Tentorium
  - Dural plaques (frequently parasagittal)
  - Petroclinoid (12%) and interclinoid ligaments
  - Diaphragm sellae.

Basal Ganglia Calcification

- Physiological/idiopathic (primary) (typically bilateral and symmetric and commences in the region of head of caudate nucleus)
- Secondary to:
  - Hypoparathyroidism
  - Pseudohypoparathyroidism (Albright's syndrome)
  - Familial
  - Fahr's syndrome (Familial ferrocalcinosis)

- Cockayne's syndrome
- Lead and CO poisoning
- Methotrexate with radiation therapy (mineralizing microangiopathy of leukemia)
- Congenital toxoplasmosis (characteristically linear and associated with flaky subcortical calcifications).

Intracranial Calcification (Causes)

- **Physiologic:** Pineal, habenular, choroid plexus, dural, falx (cerebri, cerebelli) and tentorial, petroclinoid ligament, interclinoid ligament, basal ganglia, arteriosclerosis (ICA, basilar).
- **Infection:** TORCH. CMV (periventricular) and toxoplasmosis (diffuse), healed abscess, hydatid cyst, granulomas, cysticercosis the calcified stage (rice field/grain like calcification), paragonimiasis (soap bubble calcification), trichinosis.
- **Neoplasms:** Craniopharyngioma (40–80%), oligodendroglioma (50–70%), ependymoma (50%), chordoma (25–40%), meningioma (20%), pinealoma (10–20%), dermoid (20%), astrocytoma (15%), choroid plexus papilloma (10%), pituitary adenoma (3–5%), metastases (1–2 %, lung > breast > GIT). Medulloblastoma very rarely calcify.
- **Endocrinal:** Hyperparathyroidism, hypervitaminosis D, hypoparathyroidism, pseudohypoparathyroidism, CO or lead poisoning.
- **Arteriovenous:** Atherosclerosis, aneurysm and AV malformation, hemangioma, SDH, EDH and intracerebral hemorrhage, old chronic infarct.
- **Embryologic:** Neurocutaneous syndromes (Tuberous sclerosis—calcified subependymal nodules with subcortical calcification, neurofibromatosis, Sturge Weber syndrome—tramtrack calcification).
- **Miscellaneous:** Fahr's disease, mineralizing microangiopathy of leukemia, radiation necrosis, etc.

RADIOLOGICAL INVESTIGATIONS

Guidelines for CT, ultrasound and MRI in neuroimaging	
Condition	Recommended technique
Hemorrhage	
• Acute parenchymal	CT > MR
• Subacute/chronic	MRI
• Subarachnoid hemorrhage	CT, CTA, lumbar puncture → angiography
Aneurysm	Angiography > CTA, MRA
Ischemic infarction	
• Hemorrhagic infarction	CT

Contd...

Contd...

- Bland infarction — MRI > CT
- Carotid or vertebral dissection — MRI/MRA
- Vertebral basilar insufficiency — CTA, MRI/MRA
- Carotid stenosis — CTA > Doppler ultrasound, MRA

Suspected mass lesion
- Neoplasm, primary or metastatic — MRI + contrast
- Infection/abscess — MRI + contrast
- Immunosuppressed with focal findings — MRI + contrast

Vascular malformation — MRI +/− contrast

White matter disorders — MRI
    Demyelinating disease — MRI +/− contrast

Dementia — MRI

Trauma
- Acute trauma — CT (noncontrast)
- Shear injury/chronic hemorrhage — MRI

Headache/migraine — CT (noncontrast)/MRI

Seizure
- First time, no focal neurologic deficits — CT as screen
- Partial complex/refractory — MRI with coronal T2W imaging

Cranial neuropathy — MRI with contrast

Meningeal disease — MRI with contrast

Spine

Low back pain
- No neurologic deficits — MRI or CT after 4 weeks
- With focal deficits — MRI > CT

Spinal stenosis — MRI or CT

Cervical spondylosis — MRI or CT myelography

Infection — MRI + contrast, CT

Myelopathy — MRI + contrast > myelography

Arteriovenous malformation — MRI, myelography/angiography

Note: CT-Computed tomography; MRI-magnetic resonance imaging; MRA-MR angiography; CTA-CT angiography; T2W-T2-weighted.

Neurosonography

Advantage of USG over CT/MR for neurological imaging in infants

- Portable
- Cheap
- Multiplanar dynamic scanning

- Easy to perform
- Lack of ionizing radiations
- No need for sedation
- Especially best for screening for ICH, hydrocephalus and PVL.

The neurosonogram (5–7.5 MHz sector probe is preferable) is possible because of the following acoustic windows available in infants:

- Anterior fontanelle (till 12 to 14 months) → most vital window
- Foramen magnum (for posterior fossa evaluation)
- Squamous part of temporal bone.

Computed Tomography

Key Facts

- Generally 5–7 mm axial sections are taken which go parallel to the orbitomeatal line. For sella turcica we may take mainly coronal sections.
- "Beam hardening" artefacts significantly limit post-fossa imaging with CT.
- "Beam hardening" is not seen if MDCT (multidetector row CT) is used; however, MRI remains the best modality for neuroimaging.
- High ionizing radiation dose (2–3 mSv) is drawback
- CT is the single most sensitive tool for detecting:
  - Skull fractures
  - Acute hemorrhages (Acute SAH/EDH/SDH/ICH/IVH)
  - Pneumocephalus
  - Calcified lesions
    i. Oligodendroglioma
    ii. Craniopharyngioma
    iii. Retinoblastoma
    iv. Sturge-Weber syndrome
  - CSF rhinorrhea (CT-cisternography best).

Indications for Cranial and Spinal CT

- *CT is primary study of choice for*
  - Evaluation of an acute change in mental status
  - Evaluation of a focal neurologic findings
  - Acute trauma to the brain and spine

- Suspected acute subarachnoid hemorrhage
- Conductive hearing loss
- **CT is complementary to MRI**
  - In the evaluation of the skull base, orbit, and osseous structures of the spine.
  - In the spine, CT is useful in evaluating patients with osseous spinal stenosis and spondylosis, but MRI is often preferred in those with neurologic deficits.
  - CT can also be obtained following intrathecal contrast injection to evaluate the intracranial cisterns (CT cisternography) for cerebrospinal fluid (CSF) fistula, as well as the spinal subarachnoid space (CT myelography).

CT, however, can be quickly obtained and is widely available, making it a pragmatic choice for the **initial evaluation** of patients with acute changes in mental status, suspected acute storke hemorrhage, and intracranial or spinal trauma.

CT is more sensitive than MRI for visualizing acute bleed, calcific lesions, and fine osseous detail.

Hypodense Brain Lesions on CT

- Infarct
- Nonhemorrhagic contusion
- Brain tumors
- Brain edema
- Metabolic encephalopathy
- Hypertensive encephalopathy
- Pseudotumor cerebri
- Encephalitis.

Hyperdense Brain Lesions

- Intracranial calcification
- Infection (TORCH)
- Neoplasms
- Endocrinal (Hypoparathyroidism)
- Embryologic (Neurocutaneous syndromes)
- Arteriovenous lesions (aneurysms, AVM, hemangioma, SDH, SAH, EDH, ICH)
- Lipoma
- Lipoid proteineosis
- Lissencephaly.

Ring-enhancing Lesions in Brain on CT Scan

- Cerebral abscess (73%)
- Epidural/subdural empyema
- Tuberculoma (regular or irregular ring with or without central/target enhancement is characteristic; however, MRI may be able to differentiate it from neurocysticercosis)
- Neurocysticercosis (especially in colloidal and granular-nodular stage)
- Toxoplasmosis (especially in HIV)
- Metastasis (33%)
- Glioblastoma multiforme (48%)
- Resolving infarct/hematoma
- Radiation necrosis
- Lymphoma
- Demyelinating disease (e.g. 'open-ring' sign in tumefactive demyelination)
- Other brain tumors which may show are glioma (high grade), meningioma, leukemia, craniopharyngioma, acoustic neuroma, abnormal pituitary–uncommon causes.

Gyriform Enhancement on CT Scan Brain

- *Focal*
  AV malformation
  Infarct (reperfusion)
  Cerebritis
  Glioma.
- *Widespread*
  Meningitis
  Carcinomatosis
  Lymphoma
  Sarcoidosis.

Cerebral Angiography

- With currently available catheter and guidewire technology, the *"transfemoral route"* is now almost exclusively used for catheterization of cerebral vessels and puncture of axillary artery or direct carotid punctures are only rarely performed.
- Most diagnostic cerebral angiography can be performed under la.
- Most frequently used catheters are 4F or 5F with a tapered I-shaped tip or a mani catheter.

- In old or hypertensive patients best is to use reverse curve catheter (side winder catheter).
- Once catheter has been positioned in an appropriate vessel (ica, cca, eca or vertebral artery), a double flush technique–withdrawing blood into one syringe and saline flushing from another is used, to minimize risks of embolism.
- LOCM is recommended for cerebral angiography.

(pneumonic: "cf-fc", i.e. Cerebral–femoral artery, fluorescein–cubital vein)

Magnetic Resonance Imaging

MRI

- While clinical MRI currently makes use of the ubiquitous hydrogen proton, research into sodium and carbon imaging appears promising.
- *Basic principle*
    - Magnetic resonance is a complex interaction between:
        i. Hydrogen protons in biologic tissues,
        ii. Static strong magnetic field (the magnet)
        iii. RF coil: Energy in the form of radiofrequency (Rf) waves of a specific frequency introduced by coils placed next to the body part of interest.
- The MRI image consists of a map of the distribution of hydrogen protons, with signal intensity imparted by both density of hydrogen protons as well as differences in the relaxation times of hydrogen protons on different molecules.
- Many different MR pulse sequences exist, and each can be obtained in various planes. The selection of a proper protocol is vital.

T1 and T2 relaxation times
- The rate of return to equilibrium of perturbed protons is called the *relaxation rate*.
- The relaxation rate varies among normal and pathologic tissues.
- The relaxation rate of hydrogen proton in a tissue is influenced by local interactions with surrounding molecules and atomic neighbors.
- Two relaxation rates T1 and T2, influence the signal intensity of the image.
- So-called T1-weighted (T1W) images are produced by keeping the TR and TE relatively short.
- The T1 relaxation time is the time, measured in milliseconds, for 63 percent of the hydrogen protons to return to their normal equilibrium state, while the T2 relaxation is the time for 63 percent of the protons to become dephased owing to interactions among nearby protons.

- The intensity of the signal within various tissues and image contrast can be modulated by altering acquisition parameters, such as the interval between Rf pulses (TR) and the time between the Rf pulse and the signal reception (TE).

Some Common Intensities on T1- and T2-weighted MRI Sequences

Image	TR (interval between Rf pulses)	TE (interval between Rf pulse and signal reception)	Signal intensity			
			CSF	Fat	Brain	Edema
T1W	Short	Short	Low	High	Low	Low
T2W	Long	Long	High	Low	High	High
FLAIR	–	–	Low	Low	High	Low

- Fat and subacute hemorrhage have relatively shorter T1 relaxation rates and thus higher signal intensity than brain on T1W images.
- Structures containing more water, such as CSF and edema, have long T1 and T2 relaxation rates, resulting in relatively lower signal intensity on T1W images and a higher signal intensity on T2W images.
- Gray matter contains 10 to 15 percent more water than white matter, which accounts for much of the intrinsic contrast between the two on MRI.

MRI sequence	More sensitive for
T2W images are more sensitive than T1W images for:	• Edema • Demyelination • Infarction • Chronic hemorrhage
T1W imaging is more sensitive for:	• Subacute hemorrhage • Fat-containing structures
FLAIR images are more sensitive than standard spin echo images for:	• Any water-containing lesions or edema • Chronic SAH • DAI
Gradient echo imaging is most sensitive to magnetic susceptibility generated by:	• Blood, calcium, and air • Indicated in patients with traumatic brain injury to assess for subtle confusions and shear microhemorrhages

Note: Fluid-attenuated inversion recovery (FLAIR) is a useful pulse sequence that produces T2W images in which the normally high signal intensity of CSF is suppressed.

Technical Advantages

- MR images can be generated in any phase without changing the patient's position (Multiplanar Capability).
- Each sequence, however, must be obtained separately and takes 1–5 min on average to complete.
- Three-dimensional volumetric imaging is also possible with **MRI**, resulting in a volume of data that can be reformatted in any orientation on a workstation to highlight certain disease processes.

Field strength of the magnet is directly related to signal to noise ratio.

- While 1.5 Tesla magnets have become the standard **high-field MRI units**, 3T–8T magnets are now available and have distinct advantages for many *special applications* or MRI especially in the brain and musculoskeletal systems.

Type of MRI study	Utility
Perfusion and diffusion imaging	– Are EPI techniques that are useful in early detection of ischemic injury of the brain and may be useful together to demonstrate infarcted tissue as well as ischemic but potentially viable tissue at risk of infarction (e.g. the ischemic penumbra) – Diffusion-weighted imaging (DWI) assesses microscopic motion of water; restriction of motion appears as relative high signal intensity on diffusion-weighted images – DWI is the most sensitive technique for detection of acute cerebral infarction of <7 days' duration and is also sensitive to encephalitis and abscess formation, all of which have reduced diffusion and result in high signal on diffusion-weighted images
Perfusion MRI	– Involves the acquisition of EPI images during a rapid intravenous bolus of gadolinium contrast material – Relative perfusion abnormalities can be identified on images of the relative cerebral blood volume, mean transit time, and cerebral blood flow – Delay in mean transit time and reduction in cerebral blood volume and cerebral blood flow are typical of infarction. In the setting of reduced blood flow; a prolonged mean transit time of contrast but normal or elevated cerebral blood volume may indicate tissue supplied by collateral flow that is at risk of infarction. pMRI imaging can also be used in the assessment of brain tumors to differentiate intra-axial primary tumors from extra-axial tumors or metastasis.

Contd...

Contd...

Diffusion tract imaging (DTI)	– Derived from diffusion MRI techniques. Preferential microscopic motion of water along white matter tracts is detected by diffusion MR, which can also indicate the direction of white matter fiber tracts. This new technique has great potential in the assessment of brain maturation as well as disease entities that undermine the integrity of the white matter architecture
fMRI of the brain	– An EPI technique that localizes regions of activity in the brain following task activation. Neuronal activity elicits a slight increase in the delivery of oxygenated blood flow to a specific region of activated brain. This results in an alternation in the balance of oxyhemoglobin and deoxyhemoglobin, which yields a 2–3 percent increase in signal intensity within veins and local capillaries. Further studies will determine whether these techniques are cost-effective or clinically useful but currently preoperative somatosensory and auditory cortex localization is possible. This technique has proved useful to neuroscientists interested in interrogating the localization of certain brain functions.

Hyperintense (bright) on T1 MRI	*Hyperintense (bright) on T2 MRI*
• Early subacute hemorrhage • Fat • Gelatine sponge • Gadolinium • Highly protein rich lesions, e.g. mucinous material • Infections of fungal origin • Posterior pituitary gland (due to hormonal secretion) • Melanin	• Water • CSF • Cyst • Edema • Tumors (but all) • Demyelination

Positron Emission Tomography

- Positron emission tomography (PET) relies on the detection of positrons emitted during the decay of a radionuclide that has been injected into a patient.
- The most frequently used moiety is 2-[^{18}F] fluro 2-deoxy-D-glucose (FDG), which is an analog of glucose and is taken up by cells competitively with 2-deoxyglucose.
- Multiple images of glucose uptake activity are formed after 45 to 60 min.
- Images reveal differences in regional glucose activity among normal and pathologic brain structures.

- A lower activity of FDG in the parietal lobes has been associated with Alzheimer's disease. FDG PET is used primarily for the detection of extracranial metastatic disease.
- Combination PET–CT scanners, in which both CT and PET are obtained at one sitting, are replacing PET scans alone for most clinical indications.
- Fuctional images superimposed on high-resolution CT scans result in more precise anatomic diagnoses.

CONGENITAL MALFORMATIONS OF BRAIN

Hydrocephalus

- Congenital hydrocephalus in infants and young children may be classified as communicating or nonobstructive and noncommunicating or obstructive types.
- In communicating hydrocephalus there is free communication between the ventricles and basal cisterns, with obstruction to the flow of CSF in the subarachnoid space or basal cisterns causing all ventricles to enlarge and prominent basal cisterns.
- In noncommunicating hydrocephalus flow is obstructed within ventricular system, usually at aqueduct of Sylvius, 3rd or 4th ventricle.
- The ventricles above the level of obstruction are dilated and below it are normal.
- Aqueductal stenosis is the **most common cause of congenital hydrocephalus** causing dilatation of 3rd and 4th ventricle.

Ultrasonography is best investigation for detection of hydrocephalus in infancy.

Vein of Galen Malformation

VGM is frequently referred to as vein of Galen aneurysm, but this is a misnomer because it is not true aneurysm. It usually represents dilatation of vein of Galen caused by a vascular malformation that is fed by large arteries of the anterior and posterior cerebral artery circulation.

Sonographically, a galenic malformation appears as an anechoic, cystic mass between the lateral ventricles. It lies posterior to the foramen of Monro, superior to the third ventricle and primarily in midline. Identification of large feeding vessels differentiates this lesion from other cystic masses. Hydrocephalus may or may not be present and calcification may occur, especially if there is thrombus in the malformation. Differential diagnosis includes *arachnoid cysts, cysts associated with corpus callosal agenesis, and porencephaly*. However, once VGM is suspected, the diagnosis can be readily confirmed with Doppler ultrasound.

Arnold Chiari I Malformation

Chiari I Malformation (Cerebellar Ectopia and Seen in Adulthood)

Definition: Descent of otherwise normal cerebellar hemispheres below the foramen magnum, usually involving tonsils.

Features: Peg like, pointed tonsils displaced into upper cervical canal:
- 0 to 10 years → 6 mm at least
- 10 to 30 years → 5 mm
- 30 to 40 years → 4 mm

Associated anomalies: Syringomyelia (30–60%), hydrocephalus (20–25%), basilar invaginations (25–50%), Klippel-Feil syndrome (5–10%) and atlanto-occipital assimilation (1–5%).

Chiari II Malformation (Childhood)

Definition: Descent of dysplastic cerebellar hemisphere below the foramen magnum, usually involving inferior vermis, which is everted instead being inverted, causing 4th ventricle to reduce to a coronal cleft and medulla oblongata to elongate and kink.

Features

Skull and dura	Brain	Ventricles	Spine and cord
Calvarial defects (Lacunar skull Luckenschadel)	Inferior displaced vermis	Hydrocephalus (90%)	Myelomeningocele (100%)
Small posterior fossa	Medullary spurs/kink	Batwing frontal horns	Syringohydromyelia
	Beaked tectum	Elongated tube-like 4th vent.	Diastematomyelia
Heart-shaped incisura	Interdigitating gyri	Fenestrated falx	Incomplete/absent C_1 arch
Hypoplastic tentorium	Towering cerebellum	Large mass intermedia	
Gaping foramen magnum	Polymicrogyria	Colpocephaly	
Concave clivus and petrous ridge	Heterotopias	Callosal agenesis	

Chiari type III and IV are extremely rare.

Dandy-Walker Malformation: Features

Skull and Dura

- Large posterior fossa (increased volume)
- High tentorial insertion (Lambdoid torcular inversion)
- High transverse sinus.

Ventricles and CSF Spaces

- Fourth ventricle floor present
- Ventricle open dorsally to large posterior fossa cyst
- Hydrocephalus in 80 percent cases.

Cerebellum, Vermis, Brainstem

- Vermian cerebellar hemispheric hypoplasia
- Vermian remnant anterosuperiorly everted above cyst
- Cerebellar hemispheres winged anterolaterally in front of cyst, heterotopias and cerebellar dysplasia may also occur
- Brain stem may be hypoplastic, compressed.

Associated CNS Anomalies

- Corpus callosal agenesis (20–25%)
- Heterotopias, gyral anomalies, schizencephaly
- Cephaloceles.

Disorders of Sulcation and Cellular (Neuroblast) Migration are:
- Lissencephaly (smooth brain)
- Nonlissencephalic cortical dysplasia (agyria-pachygyria complex)
- Heterotopias
- Schizencephaly (split-brain)
- Unilateral megalencephaly

Disorders of Diverticulation and Cleavage are:
- Holoprosencephaly
- Septo-optic dysplasia
- Arhinencephaly

Lissencephaly

Lissencephaly refers to brain with absent or poor sulcation. It can be complete (synonymous with agyria) or incomplete (synonymous with nonlissencephalic cortical dysphasia or agyria-pachygyria complex). It is the most severe form of neuronal migration anomalies (autosomal recessive). Type I lissencephaly shows cortex with diminished white matter; broad, flat gyri; smooth gray-white matter interface; with absent or shallow sulci and gyri with **'figure of eight' appearance** of cerebrum on axial images due to shallow widened vertically oriented Sylvain fissures.

Nonlissencephalic Cortical Dysplasia

The agyria-pachygyria complex has recently been reclassified into a more general category nonlissencephalic cortical dysplasia, which is characterized by irregular "bumpy" gyral pattern (Polymicrogyria) and relative paucity of underlying white matter or areas of both agyria and pachygyria. Pachygyria means focal areas of thickened, flattened cortex.

Heterotopias

Gray matter heterotopias are collections of otherwise normal neurons in abnormal locations secondary to arrest of neuronal migration. Heterotopias can be laminar (band-like) or nodular, focal or diffuse.

Schizencephaly

It is a gray matter lined CSF filled cleft that extends from the ependymal surface of brain through the white matter to the pia. It is of two types:
1. Type I or closed lip type—cleft walls are in apposition.
2. Type II or open lip type—cleft walls are separated.

Unilateral Megalencephaly

The hamartomatous overgrowth of part or all of one cerebral hemisphere with localized neuronal migrational anomalies. The hemisphere is enlarged as compared to opposite normal side. Ipsilateral ventricle is often enlarged.

Holoprosencephaly

It is classically divided into three types by the degree of brain cleavage.
1. Alobar holoprosencephaly (most severe): Brain is an uncleaved/undifferentiated holosphere with a central primitive monoventricle and fused thalami seen on imaging as a completely unsegmented rim of brain that surrounds a large central CSF filled cavity.
2. Semilobar holoprosencephaly (moderately severe).
3. Lobar holoprosencephaly (mildest form): Nearly complete brain cleavage.

Arhinencephaly

Absent olfactory bulbs and tracts.

NEUROCUTANEOUS SYNDROMES (PHAKOMATOSES)

The phakomatoses (Greek "phakos" = mole or freckle) are a unique group of congenital neuroectodermal disorders that share the characteristics of central nervous system (CNS) and skin tumors. Neurofibromatosis, tuberous sclerosis, von Hippel-Lindau disease, and Sturge-Weber syndrome are the major members of this group. Less common neurocutaneous syndromes include *basal cell nevus syndrome, Osler-Weber-Rendu disease, ataxia-telangiectasia, Klippel-Trenaunay syndrome, and the blue-rubber-bleb-nevus syndrome*. These diseases share several features, including special involvement of organs of ectodermal origin (retina, skin, nervous system), the tendency to form benign neoplasms ("hamartomas," "phakomas"), the gradual progression of lesions throughout childhood and adolescence, and the predisposition to malignant transformation.

Neurofibromatosis

Two distinct forms known:
1. NF-1 (von Recklinghausen disease) → accounts for 90 percent of all cases
2. NF-2 (Central neurofibromatosis; MISME complex).

Clinical Features

- Café-au-lait spots
- Axillary freckling
- Subcutaneous/plexiform neurofibromas
- Overgrowth or hypertrophy

- Subaortic valve stenosis and other cardiac anomalies
- Coarctation of abdominal aorta
- Renal and cerebral artery aneurysms
- Optic gliomas
- Neurofibrosarcoma
- Lisch (iris) nodules
- MEN
- Exophthalmos.

Radiological Features

- Macrocephaly and cranial asymmetry
- Bone defects in orbits (**Bare orbit/empty orbit sign**) or lambdoid suture
- Orbital enlargement
- Intracerebral neoplasms
- Kyphoscoliosis
- Dural ectasia and posterior vertebral scalloping
- Enlargement of intervertebral foramen and **dumb-bell** tumors
- Anterior meningoceles
- Notching of ribs (ribbon ribs)
- Pulmonary interstitial fibrosis
- Limb asymmetry (hyper or hypoplasia)
- Soft tissue hypertrophy
- Subperiosteal cortical cystic lesions
- Multiple metaphyseal cortical defect
- Pseudoarthrosis of tibia
- Hypophosphatemic osteomalacia
- Multiple or plexiform neurofibroma in GIT.

Sturge-Weber Syndrome (Encephalotrigeminal Syndrome/ Meningofacial Angiomatosis)

- Congenital facial port wine stain (nevus flammeus) along distribution of trigeminal nerve
- Leptomeningeal venous angiomas
- 'Tram track or Railroad track' gyriform cortical calcifications (>2 years age)

- Hemiatrophy of brain (ipsilateral)
- Ipsilateral choroid plexus angiomatosis
- Sphenoid dysplasia (elevated sphenoid wing)
- Thickened calvarium
- Choroidal capillary venous angiomas.

Tuberous Sclerosis (Bourneville's Disease/EPILOIA)

Incidence: 1:10,000–50,000
Inheritance: Autosomal dominant (Low penetrance)
　　　　　　　Chromosomes 9 and 11
Clinical features: Classic **triad of** seizures, low IQ and adenoma sebacium

CNS Lesion

- Cortical tubers
- Benign white matter lesions
- Subependymal nodules (95%)
- Subependymal nodules may bulge into the ventricular system, resembling *candle drippings* or giving *candle guttering* appearance on CT brain.
- Typically located in lateral ventricles along striothalamic groove, often calcified (increases with age)
- Subependymal giant cell astrocytoma **(SGCA)** typically located at foramen of Monro.
- *Miscellaneous lesions:* Retinal Phakomas
　　　　　　　　　　　　Aneurysms
　　　　　　　　　　　　Nonatheromatous vascular stenosis
　　　　　　　　　　　　Mild nonspecific ventricular enlargements

Non-CNS Lesions

- Shagreen patch
- Adenoma sebaceum
- Subungual fibromas
- Ash leaf macules
- Café-au-lait spots
- Bilateral multiple renal angiomyolipomas
- Multiple bilateral cortical cysts

- Interstitial lung disease indistinguishable from lymphangioleiomyomatosis
- Cardiac rhabdomyoma
- 'Flame shaped' sclerotic bone islands especially affecting pelvis.

von Hippel-Lindau Disease (Cerebelloretinal Hemangioblastomatosis)

As with tuberous sclerosis and neurofibromatosis, a wide array of organ system involvements may occur, but clinical manifestations are generally limited to four lesions: spinal and cerebellar hemangioblastoma, retinal angioma, pheochromocytoma, and renal cell carcinoma. The skin is seldom involved. An autosomal dominant pattern of inheritance is accepted, but a number of sporadic cases have been reported.

Symptoms related to retinal angiomatosis, the von Hippel part of the disease, are the presenting feature in 16 percent of patients. Approximately 40 percent of patients may have no retinal disease at all. The angiomas are multiple and bilateral in approximately 35 percent of patients and tend to cause progressive loss of vision due to retinal detachment, glaucoma, uveitis, or retinal inflammation with exudate and hemorrhage. Photocoagulation is the preferred treatment for smaller angiomas.

Hemangioblastomas occur in 40 percent of patients and account for the greatest morbidity and mortality associated with the syndrome. The neurologic complications most commonly become apparent during late adolescence or early adulthood and are dominated by progressive cerebellar ataxia, papilledema, and headache. Tonsillar herniation and obstructive hydrocephalus may develop if the lesion blocks the aqueduct or foramina of the fourth ventricle. Rarely, a vascular bruit may be audible over the head. The majority of hemangioblastomas occur in the cerebellum, although medullary or spinal lesions may be seen about 5 percent of the time. Involvement of the cerebral hemispheres is exceedingly rare. About 90 percent of cerebellar hemangioblastomas are lateral in position. The lesions may be multiple in 15 percent of cases. There is usually little surrounding edema, and calcification is extremely uncommon.

Spinal cord hemangioblastomas are usually located on the posterior aspect of the cord, and symptoms depend on which nerve roots are involved. Up to 70 percent of spinal lesions are associated with syringomoyelia.

MRI is rapidly replacing CT as the study of choice in the evaluation of CNS hemangioblastoma. It more accurately defines the lesion's extent and characteristics, associated syringomyelia, and the mass effect on adjacent neural structures, including tonsillar herniation. Gd-DTPA optimizes visualization of the small mural nodule.

Renal cell carcinoma is reported to occur in approximately 40 percent of patients and is the presenting symptom of the syndrome in 10 percent of this group. The neoplasm is bilateral in 65 percent, and multiple lesions are seen 85 percent of the time. The average age at diagnosis is 41 years, as opposed to the average age of 58 for diagnosis of renal cell carcinoma in the general population. Because of this high-risk, annual screening CT is recommended, beginning at age 20. Benign renal cysts may be seen in approximately 60 percent of cases; small cysts may be difficult to distinguish from solid tumors due to partial averaging.

Pheochromocytoma occurs in 15 percent of patients affected with von Hippel-Lindau disease and is bilateral in 40 percent. Other coexisting abnormalities include pancreatic cysts (72%), hepatic cysts (17%), splenic cysts (7%), and epididymal cysts (7%).

Polycythemia, possibly related to the production of erythropoietin, may occur in association with hemangioblastoma (15%) or renal cell carcinoma (10%), and often remits following tumor excision. Hemoglobin levels, often exceeding 16 g/dL, are not uncommon.

Ataxia-Telangiectasia (Louis-Bar Syndrome)

As its name suggests, ataxia-telangiectasia is a neurocutaneous disorder characterized by progressive cerebellar ataxia associated with telangiectasias of the bulbar conjunctiva and skin. This autosomal recessive condition has recently attracted considerable interest because of its association with limited immunocompetence. Decreased or absent IgA, secondary to decreased synthesis, has been found in nearly all patients. One may also find decreased circulating antibodies, lymphopenia, and failure of delayed hyper-sensitivity reactions. There is usually a rudimentary thymus at best, with a paucity of Hassall's corpuscles, associated with a generalized decrease in overall lymphoid tissue mass.

Clinically, the child appears normal at birth. The first signs appear in infancy and progress steadily, manifested by cerebellar ataxia, apraxia of ocular movement, and choreoathetosis. The child learns to walk and talk but is severely dysarthric and chairfast by the second decade. The cutaneous and conjunctival telangiectasias generally follow the onset of ataxia by several years. Mental deterioration may occur in the later stages of the disease. The disease is relentlessly progressive, and death usually occurs by the second or third decade of life from recurrent sino-pulmonary infections or a reticuloendothelial neoplasm, most frequently large-cell lymphoma. Of all the immunodeficiency disorders associated with an increased frequency of lymphoma, ataxia telangiectasia is the only one with constitutional chromosome abnormalities. Lymphoid cells in this disease have a high frequency of chromosomal breaks at the loci on chromosome 14 that are associated with the genes for proteins crucial to T-cell and B-cell function. These breaks could result in an increased likelihood of oncogene translocation and activation, with resulting T-cell or B-cell neoplasia.

Pathologic changes within the CNS consist of cerebellar cortical atrophy with extensive loss of Purkinje and granule cells. Spinocerebellar tract and posterior column degeneration, affecting the gracile more than cuneate fasciculi, may be seen in many cases of longer duration. In a few cases, vascular abnormalities similar to those seen in skin and mucous membranes have been found scattered throughout the white matter of the brain and spinal cord. There may be a loss of pigmented cells in the substantia nigra and locus ceruleus, and cytoplasmic inclusions (Lewy bodies) in remaining cells. The anterior lobe of the pituitary may contain scattered large cells with bizarre nuclei. Changes in the peripheral nervous system are less well documented. Demyelination, small ganglion cells, and a paucity of satellite cells with bizarre, atypical nuclei have been observed within the dorsal root ganglia. Neurogenic muscular atrophy with a loss of anterior horn cells at all levels of the spinal cord has been reported.

Radiographic manifestations are generally limited to identification of the recurrent bronchopulmonary infections, intercurrent neoplasia, and thymic dysgenesis on CT and chest radiographs. As such, imaging has a minimal role in the diagnosis of this syndrome. Although not yet reported, it is conceivable that the spinocerebellar degeneration will be visualized on high-resolution MRI.

IMAGING IN DEMENTIA

Disease	Imaging
Alzheimer's disease	Entorhinal cortex and hippocampal atrophy
Frontotemporal dementia	Frontal and/or temporal atrophy; spares posterior parietal lobe
Dementia with Lewy bodies	Posterior parietal atrophy; hippocampi larger than in AD
Creutzfeldt-Jakob disease	Cortical ribboning and basal ganglia or thalamus hyperintensity on diffusion/flare MRI
Vascular	Cortical and/or subcortical infarctions, confluent white matter disease

STROKE AND VASCULAR DISORDERS

Brain Stroke

Diffusion MR (DWMRI)

DWMRI is an MR sequence that detects reduction of microscopic motion of water, is the most sensitive technique for detecting acute ischemic stroke and is also useful in the detection of encephalitis, abscesses, and prion diseases.

Hyperacute Stroke

Abnormalities seen on diffusion weighted MR are irreversible and represent core of infarct, whereas the area of perfusion/diffusion mismatch surrounding the core as seen on combined perfusion and diffusion imaging indicates potentially salvageable tissue (ischemic penumbra).

Acute Stroke

- CT scanning is the initial modality of choice for imaging in patients with acute stroke especially to rule out hemorrhage. CT signs like *hyperdense MCA sign*, obscuration of lentiform nucleus, insular ribbon loss sign and loss of CM differentiation are not always seen in ischemia.
- Structural changes develop after 6 hours and reaches peak between 24 and 48 hours after the onset of ischemia when irreversible changes mostly occur and thrombolysis not used.

However, the most sensitive investigation for cytotoxic edema due to ischemia and the most sensitive MR technique for detection of early parenchymal changes following an ischemic insult is MR diffusion imaging with 'light bulb' sign positive. DWMRI can detect ischemia as early as at half hour after stroke.

Subacute Stroke

The effects of structural breakdown and disruption of the BBB dominate in subacute phase of infarct.

MR diffusion can distinguish between old and acute or subacute infarcts and can help to pinpoint the vascular territory of most of the lesions.

Chronic/Old Stroke

Late changes on CT and MRI are well-delineated areas of encephalomalacia with focal trophy. The radiodensity on CT and signal intensity on MRI of the affected area approaches that of CSF. MRI is much more sensitive in showing evidence of previous hemorrhagic stroke since hemosiderin is taken up by macrophages and can persist for years.

Lacunar Infarcts

- The term lacunar is used to describe small infarcts—by convention, infarcts measuring less than 1.5 cm in greatest dimension.
- Such infarcts are a manifestation of small vessel disease, and are particularly common in hypertension.
- Basal ganglia, thalamus, pons, internal capsules, and cerebral white matter are common sites for these lesions.

- Lipohyalinosis causing occlusion of small penetrating branch arterioles is the basic underlying pathology.

Diffusion weighted MRI (DWMRI) provide the best method for determining whether a lacunar infarct is old or recent.

Hypertensive Hemorrhage

Location of hypertensive hemorrhage

Putamen/external capsule	60 to 65 percent
Thalamus	15 to 25 percent
Pons	5 to 10 percent
Cerebellum	2 to 5 percent
Subcortical white matter	1 to 2 percent

In contrast to hypertensive hemorrhage, hemorrhages in amyloidosis are characteristically multiple, spare the basal ganglia and brainstem and are located at CM junction. The most common nonglial hemorrhagic primary intracranial tumor is pituitary adenoma. The most common glial hemorrhagic primary intracranial tumors are anaplastic astrocytoma and glioblastoma multiforme.

Germinal Matrix Hemorrhage (Most Common Site of IC Hemorrhage in Neonates)

- It is the most common form of intracranial hemorrhage occurring in the highly vascular gelatinous subependymal tissue adjacent to lateral ventricles in which the cells that compose the brain are generated and it usually involutes by 32 to 34 weeks of gestation.
- Germinal matrix is located above caudate nucleus in the floor of lateral ventricle (caudothalamic groove)
- Grades of periventricular or germinal matrix or subependymal hemorrhage (**Papile classification**):
  Grade I. Confined to germinal matrix on one/both sides
  Grade II. Intraventricular extension
  Grade III. Intraventricular extension with ventricular enlargement
  - Mild
  - Moderate
  - Severe
  Grade IV. Extension into brain parenchyma

Subarachnoid Hemorrhage

Causes
Spontaneous: Ruptured aneurysm (72%)
AVM (10%)
Hypertensive hemorrhage
Tumors
Embolic hemorrhagic infarction
Blood dyscrasias
Anticoagulants
Eclampsia
Intracranial infections
Spinal vascular malformations
Cryptogenic (6%)

Trauma
Clinical features: 'Worst headache of life'/ 'thunderclap' headache.

Investigation
- NCCT is 60 to 90 percent accuracy, higher within first 4–5 days of the onset (pseudodelta sign and cortical vein sign)
- MRI is relatively insensitive in acute SAH (first 48 hours of onset)
- FLAIR-MRI is best for chronic SAH
- Although CT scan is the most important primary investigation in SAH, angiography will be required if surgery is to be undertaken.
- Following confirmation of SAH by CT or LP, a **'four-vessel' angiogram** is performed for further evaluation, which includes injection of contrast into either ICA (CCA if there is atheromatous disease at carotid bifurcation) and of at least one vertebral artery, but if reflux of contrast to display contralateral PICA does not occur, the contralateral vertebral artery is also catheterized.

The rationale is base on the fact that ruptured aneurysm is the most common cause of spontaneous SAH and that up to 20 percent of aneurysms are multiple.

> FLAIR (fluid attenuation and inversion recovery) MRI sequence is more sensitive than CT in detecting chronic hemorrhage (a small amount of blood). After 2 or 3 days when methemoglobin is formed, high signal can be seen on T1WI, and this persists even when the blood is no longer visible on CT.

Cerebral Aneurysms

There are three basic types of intracranial aneurysms:
1. Saccular/Berry aneurysms
   - Developmental/degenerative
   - Traumatic
   - Mycotic
   - Oncotic
   - Flow related
   - Vasculopathic
   - Drug related.
2. Fusiform aneurysms
3. Dissecting aneurysms.

Berry Aneurysms

- These are true aneurysms, i.e. they are dilatations of a vascular lumen due to weakness of all vessel wall layers. The sac is composed only of intima and adventitia. The internal elastic membrane is reduced or absent.
- 90 percent are located in circle of Willis arising on anterior circulation, with anterior communicating artery being most common, followed by posterior communicating artery and then MCA bifurcation.
- Usual age of presentation is 40 to 60 years age.
- They usually present with subarachnoid hemorrhage (most common presentation).
- Giant aneurysms (> 2.5 cm diameter) are likely to produce mass effect like oculomotor palsy due to aneurysm in cavernous sinus or arising from origin of posterior communicating artery.
- Ruptured aneurysms often have an irregular shape and may show a 'nipple' or 'tit' indicating the site of rupture.
- Vasospasm is leading cause of disability and death from aneurysm rupture.

Sudden onset headache, vomiting and neck stiffness in a hypertensive male without focal neurological deficit points towards clinical diagnosis of ruptured intracerebral aneurysm, causing subarachnoid hemorrhage. On CT scan some bleeding patterns have been associated with particular aneurysm locations.

Hemorrhage located predominantly within the	Probable site of aneurysm
Blood in interhemispheric tissue	Anterior communicating artery aneurysms
Blood in sylvian fissure	Middle cerebral artery aneurysm
Fourth ventricle hemorrhage	Posterior fossa aneurysms
Frontal horn blood	Anterior communicating artery lesions

The most common cause of spontaneous brain parenchymal hemorrhage is ruptured **charcot-bouchard microaneurysm.**

Arteriovenous Malformations (AVMs)

- Intra-arterial angiography is the method of choice for confirmation of cerebral AVMs and dural fistulas.
- For cavernomas, capillary telengiectasias and developmental venous anomalies MR is investigation of choice, while for cerebral AVMs and dural fistulae MRI is screening or initial test of choice.
- Intra-arterial angiography should comprise an injection of all possible feeding vessels of an AVM, which frequently amounts to a four-vessel study.
- **Particularly important DSA features are** the venous drainage pattern, premature filling of veins and slow flow compartments.
- The main disadvantage of noninvasive vascular imaging (CTA or MRA) is their lack of temporal resolution compared to intra-arterial angiography, which provides physiological information about the transit time of contrast and speed of shunting through the AVM.
- "Multiple serpiginous flow voids", which are tightly packed strongly favor diagnosis of AVM.

Hypertensive Encephalopathy (Posterior Reversible Encephalopathy Syndrome)

It occurs predominantly in the posterior cerebral artery distribution. It has been postulated that the posterior cerebral artery and its branches are less successful at autoregulation than other cerebral vessels, accounting for the increased passage of fluid across its endothelium into the parietal and occipital lobes. This may be seen in eclampsia or other hypertensive conditions. White matter changes resulting from hypertensive encephalopathy usually are confluent and reversible. *Pregnanacy related encephalopathy syndrome* (PRES) is the newer term coined for HE due pregnancy induced hypertension.

INTRACRANIAL INFECTIONS

Leptomeningitis and Meningoencephalitis

Haemophilus influenzae is the most common pathogen in purulent meningitis during the first year of life, whereas *Staphylococcus* pneumonia and infection with *Escherichia coli* and *Staphylococcus aureus* are more common in childhood and in individuals 30 years or older.

Meninges are not seen on CT, they are seen on MRI, hence MRI is best.

Ventriculitis and ependymitis are well demonstrated with CT and MR because of enhancement of the lining of the ventricular walls. In bacterial leptomeningoencephalitis, thickening and enhancement of the leptomeninges, subdural collections, and focal areas of parenchymal edema or cerebritis may be seen. The formation of intraventricular septa in ventriculitis is a relatively frequent complication and can be the cause of shunt failure. When the inflammatory process is localized to the base of the brain, the cranial nerves usually are involved. Extension to vascular structures may produce arteritis, leading to thrombosis with subsequent infarcts.

Subdural serous collections are a frequent complication of *H. influenzae* meningitis in children. Subdural empyemas may occur if those collections become infected.

Meningitis may be difficult to detect with CT or MR in the early stages. Obliteration of the subarachnoid spaces and enhancement of the basal cisterns and interhemispheric and sylvian fissures because of hyperemia and inflammatory exudates may be seen. Compression of the lateral ventricles also may be observed with localized cerebritis from brain edema. CT and MR may detect vascular thrombosis and infarcts as a complication of meningitis. In some cases, radionuclide or CT cisternography may be useful in detecting CSF fistulae at the base of the skull that could be the source of recurrent meningitis. HRCT temporal bone may sometimes reveal rare predisposing factor for recurrent meningitis like pseudo-Mondinis malformation.

Cerebritis and Cerebral Abscess

Cerebral abscesses may occur as the result of direct extension of an infectious process, as the result of embolic phenomena, or in an area of pre-existing cerebritis. Direct extension typically is from infection of the paranasal sinuses, the middle ear, or the mastoid air cells (**Temporal lobe abscess**). Skull fractures also can contribute to the development of cerebral abscess. Septic emboli typically originate in the setting of bacterial endocarditis, pneumonia, or congenital cardiac disease (**Frontal lobe abscess**).

Most abscesses occur near the corticomedullary junction. This is thought to be secondary to the large vascular supply in this region. They most commonly are found in the distribution of the middle cerebral artery, with frontal and temporal lobe involvement most frequent.

During the second week, the abscess is clearly seen as a well-defined lesion by CT and MR. Demonstration of a well-formed capsule or mature abscess is important, since it is an indication for drainage or surgical resection. MR is superior to CT in the detection and characterization of abscess formation, particularly in the early stages of its evolution.

Subdural and Epidural Empyemas

H. influenzae is common underlying cause.

Subdural and epidural empyemas are manifested as semilunar-shaped extra-axial fluid collections that are of low-attenuation fluid on CT and hyperintense on T2-weighted MR images. The density or intensity of the collection on CT or MR varies according to the age of the empyema and usually are isodense or isointense to the adjacent brain in the late stages. The capsule of the empyema generally enhances with contrast because of granulation tissue or inflammatory hyperemia of the adjacent cerebral cortex and microthrombosis of the cortical veins.

The sequelae of meningitis can be manifested by communicating hydrocephalus, periventricular and meningeal calcifications, fibrosis, focal areas of encephalomalacia producing porencephaly, and diffuse or focal ventricular dilatation caused by cortical atrophy.

Cryptococcosis

- Cryptococcosis, also known as torulosis, is caused by the *Cryptococcus neoformans* and is widely disseminated worldwide.
- The fungus is inhaled with primary involvement of the lungs.
- Cryptococcois of the CNS is demonstrated on CT and MR as meningitis with enhancement of the leptomeninges. Additional findings include abscesses, intraparenchymal cryptococcomas, and hydrocephalus.
- Cryptococcus meningoencephalitis is the most common mycosis found in the CNS and can be fatal within months after first diagnosis.
- On CT or MR, parenchymal inflammatory reaction can be seen adjacent to enhancing granulomatous lesions, which can vary in size.

Commonly, small cryptococcomas or gelatinous pseudocysts can be seen in the basal ganglia with extension along the Virchow-Robin perivascular spaces.

Tubercular Meningitis

It is characterized by a thick, gray gelatinous exudate that predominantly involves the basilar cisterns. NECT scan shows "ex plaque" dural thickening and 'popcorn' like dural calcification especially around the basilar cisterns. CECT may show abnormal meningeal enhancement. However, atrophy and cerebral infarction may be a striking feature.

Thus, following are hallmarks of tubercular meningitis
- Cerebral atrophy.
- Dural thickening and calcification in area around basal cistern.
- Enhancing basal exudates with predominantly involving basilar cisterns (diagnostic).
- The generalized arteritis involving basilar vessels, particularly the supraclinoid internal carotid arteries and middle cerebral arteries segmental branches and patient may develop infarcts.
- Noncommunicating hydrocephalus due to blockage of foramen of Magendie and Luschka by the exudate.
- Ring enhancing lesions of tuberculomas if any.
- Calcified tuberculomas.

Toxoplasmosis

A ring enhancing lesion with an eccentric nodular area of enhancement; called eccentric target sign is typical of toxoplasmosis.

Herpes Simplex Encephalitis (HSE)

- HSV 2 in neonates, HSV 1 in children, adults (usually activation) of latent infection in Gasserian ganglion.
- Most common viral encephalitis.
- Fulminant, necrotizing, hemorrhagic viral infection.
- Predilection for limbic system (**temporal lobes, cingulate gyri, subfrontal region**) in older children, adults

- *CT*:
  - Often normal early in the disease.
  - Low-density lesions in temporal lobes with mild mass effect are common initially.
  - Hemorrhage is **highly suggestive** of HSE and is seen later in the disease course.
- It shows strikingly increased density of cortical gray matter and diffuse low attenuation in white matter
- CECT shows the ill-defined patchy or gyriform enhancement in neonatal HSE.
- *MR*: Gyral edema
  - Hemorrhage in late stages.
  - Temporal lobe hyperintense on T_2 WI ± enhancement in early stage.

Neurocysticercosis

Brain is most commonly affected, especially the gray white matter interface. In neurocysticercosis on imaging studies, findings vary with stage, from nonenhancing cyst (CSF density) with mural nodule (vesicular stage) to cyst wall enhancement in form of ring like enhancement (colloidal vesicular stage) to an isodense cyst with a hyperdense calcified scolex with surrounding perilesional edema and enhancement of contrast still persisting (granular nodular stage) to a small calcified nodule without mass effect or enhancement in the last stage (nodular calcified stage).

Stages of neurocysticercosis are
- Vesicular
- Colloidal
- Nodular
- Granulonodular

} MRI is best for these stages

- Calcified CT is best.

Hematogenous spread to ocular tissues, particularly extraocular muscles of eye, may occur in cysticercosis presenting with above said features on CT scan.

Japanese Encephalitis

Several patients with severe Japanese encephalitis have presented with bilateral thalamic lesions that have often been hemorrhage.

DISEASES OF DEMYELINATION (ACQUIRED)

Distinctive features of various leukodystrophies (Congenital diseases of dysmyelination)							
Leukodystrophy	Enzyme deficiency	Inheritance	Location	Subcortical involvement*	Corticospinal tract involvement	Enhancement	Other features†
Lysosomal storage disease							
Metachromatic leukodystrophy	Arysulfatase A	Autosomal recessive	–	(Y)	Y	N	Tigroid pattern
Krabbe disease	Galactocerebroside aspartoacylase	Autosomal recessive		(Y)	Y	Y	High CT attenuation
Mucopolysaccharidosis							
Peroxisomal disorders							
ALD	Acyl-CoA synthetase	X-linked recessive	Parieto-occipital	(Y)	Y	Y	
Zellweger syndrome		Autosomal recessive					Gyral abnormality
Mitochondrial dysfunction							
Leigh disease						Y	
MELAS syndrome	–	–	Parieto-occipital	Y	–		Migrating infarct
Kearn-Sayre syndrome							
Canavan disease	–			Y			Macrocephaly
Unknown cause							
PMD	–	X-linked recessive		Y	Y	N	Tigroid pattern
Alexander			Frontal	Y		Y	Macrocephaly

*(Y) indicates delayed subcortical white matter involvement
† MR imaging features (except in Krabbe disease)

Amyotrophic Lateral Sclerosis

It is characterized by progressive muscle weakness, limb and truncal atrophy and bulbar signs and symptoms. Mean age at diagnosis at 57 years. Disease progression is relentless; half the patients are dead within 3 years and 90 percent have died by 6 years following symptom onset.

Non-tau inclusions and degeneration in spinal motor neurons and pyramidal tracts (corticospinal tracts) usually produce no specific sign on MRI except for occasional signal changes on T2WI. T2WI disclose high signal areas along the large myelinated pyramidal tract fibers in the posterior limb of the internal capsule and cerebral peduncles in about 25 percent cases.

Multiple Sclerosis

Common neurological disorder characterized by disseminated plaques of demyelination and gliosis throughout the neuraxis.

The classical sites involved in multiple sclerosis (lesions on MRI) are:
- Periventricular deep white matter (perpendicular to the callososeptal interface–Dawson fingers on MRI)
- Optic pathways
- Brain stem
- Spinal cord
- Cerebellar white matter and peduncles.

MRI is far more sensitive than CT in the demonstration of MS plaques, and accuracy of nearly 100 percent can be obtained. The most characteristic feature is periventricular nodular hyperintense lesions on T2WI, most numerous posteriorly and plaques are also well shown at GW matter interfaces. Contrast enhancement after giving gadolinium occurs in acute phase.

MR Imaging in Wilson's Disease

- Basal ganglia lesions are most often bilateral and symmetrical.
- The putamina shows striking increase in T2 signal intensity. This is present to a lesser degree in other deep gray matter structures.
- Thalamic lesions are often present but typically spare the dorsomedial nuclei.
- White matter tracts including the dentatothalamic, corticospinal, and pontocerebellar tracts are commonly involved.
- The claustrum may show high T2 signal intensity.
- The midbrain is bright on T2-weighted images with relative sparing of its deep nuclei giving rise to the so-called Panda sign.

PRION Disease

"Cortical Ribboning" with increased intensity in basal ganglia (~90% patients) is finding on MRI–T2 scan.

MESIAL TEMPORAL LOBE EPILEPSY SYNDROME

- Mesial temporal lobe epilepsy (MTLE) is the most common syndrome associated wtih complex partial seizures and is an example of a symptomatic, partial epilepsy with distinctive clinical, electroencephalographic, and pathologic features.
- High-resolution MRI can detect the characteristic hippocampal sclerosis that appears to be essential in the pathophysiology of MTLE for many patients.
- Recognition of this syndrome is especially important because it tends to be refractory to treatment with anticonvulsants but responds extremely well to surgical intervention.

Characteristics of the mesial temporal lobe epilepsy syndrome

Laboratory studies
- Unilateral or bilateral anterior temporal spikes on EEG.
- Hypometabolism on interictal PET
- Hypoperfusion on interictal SPECT
- Material-specific memory deficits on intracranial amobarbital (Wada) test.

MRI findings
- Small hippocampus with increased signal on T2-weighted sequences
- Small temporal lobe
- Enlarged temporal horn
- Atrophy of ipsilateral fornix and mammillary bodies

Pathologic findings
Highly selective loss of specific cell populations within hippocampus in most cases

Treatment
Refractory to treatment with anticonvulsants but responds extremely well to surgical intervention (temoral lobectomy)

PML

- The diagnosis of PML is frequently suggested by MRI.
- MRI reveals multifocal asymmetric, coalescing white matter lesions located periventriculary, in the centrum semiovale, in the parietal-occipital region, and in the cerebellum.
- These lesions have increased signal on T2 and FLAIR images and decreased signal on T1-weighted images.

- PML lesions are classically nonenhancing (90%) but may rarely show ring enhancement, especially in more immunocompetent patients. PML lesions are not typically associated with edema or mass effect.
- CT scans, which are less sensitive than MRI for the diagnosis of PML, often show hypodense nonenhancing white matter lesions.

BRAIN TUMORS

WHO classification of the brain tumors:
- Astrocytic tumors (**the most common glial tumors**)
    - Astrocytoma (WHO grade II)
      Variants: protoplasmic, gemistocytic, fibrillary, mixed
    - Anaplastic (malignant) astrocytoma (WHO grade III)
    - Glioblastoma multiforme (WHO grade IV)
    - Pilocytic astrocytoma [noninvasive, WHO grade I]
    - Subependymal giant cell astrocytoma [noninvasive, WHO grade I] (**classically seen in tuberous sclerosis**)
    - Pleomorphic xanthoastrocytoma [noninvasive, WHO grade I]
- Oligodendroglial tumors (**the most common brain tumor in adults to calcify**)
    - Oligodendroglioma (WHO grade II)
    - Anaplastic (malignant) oligodendroglioma (WHO grade III)
- Ependymal cell tumors
    - Ependymoma (WHO grade II)
      Variants: cellular, papillary, epithelial, clear cell, mixed
    - Anaplastic ependymoma (WHO grade III)
    - Myxopapillary ependymoma
    - Subependymoma (WHO grade I)
- Mixed gliomas
    - Mixed oligoastrocytoma (WHO grade II)
    - Anaplastic oligoastrocytoma (WHO grade III)
    - Others (e.g. ependymo-astrocytomas)
- Neuroepithelial tumors of uncertain origin
    - Polar spongioblastoma (WHO grade IV)
    - Astroblastoma (WHO grade IV)
    - Gliomatosis cerebri (WHO grade IV)

- Tumors of the choroid plexus
  - Choroid plexus papilloma (**most common brain tumor in infants**)
  - Choroid plexus carcinoma
  - Choroid plexus lipoma (**'bracket calcification' is pathognomonic feature**)
- Neuronal and mixed neuronal-glial tumors
  - Gangliocytoma
  - Dysplastic gangliocytoma of cerebellum (Lhermitte-Duclos)
  - Ganglioglioma
  - Anaplastic (malignant) ganglioglioma
  - Desmoplastic infantile ganglioglioma
  - Central neurocytoma
  - Dysembryoplastic neuroepithelial tumor
  - Olfactory neuroblastoma (esthesioneuroblastoma)
- Pineal parenchyma tumors
  - Pineocytoma
  - Pineoblastoma
  - Mixed pineocytoma/pineoblastoma
- Tumors with neuroblastic or glioblastic elements (embryonal tumors)
  - Medulloepithelioma
  - Primitive neuroectodermal tumors (PNET)
    i. Medulloblastoma (**most common posterior fossa tumor in childhood**)
    ii. Cerebral primitive neuroectodermal tumor
  - Neuroblastoma
    i. Variant: ganglioneuroblastoma
  - Retinoblastoma (**most common orbital tumor in childhood, presence of calcification is pathognomonic**)
  - Ependymoblastoma
- Tumors of the sellar region
  - Pituitary adenoma
  - Pituitary carcinoma
  - Craniopharyngioma (**most common brain tumor in childhood and most common brain tumor in childhood to calcify**)

- Hematopoietic tumors
  - Primary malignant lymphomas
  - Plasmacytoma
  - Granulocytic sarcoma
  - Others
- Germ cell tumors
- Tumors of the meninges
  - Meningioma **(the most common extra-axial tumor)**
    Variants: Meningothelial, fibrous (fibroblastic), transitional (mixed), psammomatous, angiomatous, microcystic, secretory, clear cell, chordoid, lymphoplasmacyte-rich, and metaplastic subtypes.
  - Atypical meningioma
  - Anaplastic (malignant) meningioma
- Non-meningothelial tumors of the meninges
  - Benign mesenchymal
  - Malignant mesenchymal
  - Primary melanocytic lesions
  - Hemopoietic neoplasms
  - Tumors of uncertain histogenesis (hemangioblastoma) – **most common primary posterior fossa tumor in adults**.
- Tumors of cranial and spinal nerves
  - Schwannoma (neurinoma, neurilemmoma)
    Cellular, plexiform, and melanotic subtypes
  - Neurofibroma
    i. Circumscribed (solitary) neurofibroma
    ii. Plexiform neurofibroma
  - Malignant peripheral nerve sheath tumor (Malignant schwannoma)
- Local extensions from regional tumors
  - Paraganglioma (chemodectoma)
  - Chordoma
  - Chondroma
  - Chondrosarcoma
  - Carcinoma
- Metastatic tumors **(most commonly from carcinoma breast in female and bronchogenic carcinoma in males)**

- Unclassified tumors
- Cysts and tumor-like lesions
  - Rathke cleft cyst
  - Epidermoid
  - Dermoid
  - Colloid cyst of the third ventricle
  - Enterogenous cyst
  - Neuroglial cyst
  - Granular cell tumor (choristoma, pituicytoma)
  - Hypothalamic neuronal hamartoma
  - Nasal glial heterotopia
  - Plasma cell granuloma

Tumors of brain are usually better demonstrated on **MRI** than on CT due to **greater inherent soft tissue contrast.**
- An additional advantage of MRI is its ability to provide **direct multiplanar imaging, which helps to define the relationship of the tumor to adjacent structures,** and thus helps in planning of surgery and facilitates the distinction between intra-axial and extra-axial tumors.
- MRI is vastly superior to CT in evaluating posterior fossa tumors as CT is frequently hampered by **beam-hardening artifact** from the base of skull.
- *CNS tumors* can be primary and secondaries.

Intracranial Metastases

- These are overall more common than primary brain tumors.
- About 25 percent of patients with cancer die with intracranial metastases.
- Lung cancer is most commonly the primary malignancy.
- Chest CT scans and brain MRI as the initial diagnostic studies can identify a biopsy site in most patients.
- Hemorrhage into the metastasis.
  - Melanoma, germ cell tumors, and renal cell cancers have a particularly high incidence of intracranial bleeding.

The tumor mass and surrounding edema may cause obstruction of the circulation of cerebrospinal fluid, with resulting hydrocephalus
- CT scan and MRI are equally effective in the diagnosis of brain metastases.

- CT scan with contrast should be used as a screening procedure.
- If a single lesion or no metastases are visualized by contrast-enhanced CT, MRI of the brain should be performed.
- Gadolinium-enhanced MRI is more sensitive than CT at revealing meningeal involvement and small lesions, particularly in the brainstem or cerebellum.

Neoplasms, which Calcify Commonly

- Craniopharyngioma (40–80%)
- Oligodendroglioma (50–70%)
- Ependymoma (50%)
- Chordoma (25–40%)
- Meningioma (20–25%) → 'brain stone'
- Pinealoma (10–20%)
- Dermoid (20%)
- Astrocytoma (15%)
- Choroid plexus papilloma (10%)
- Pituitary adenoma (3–5%)
- Metastases (1–2 percent, lung > breast > git)

Medulloblastoma calcifies very rarely.

Medulloblastoma

- It is the most malignant infratentorial PNET
- **Incidence:** It is the most common (1/3rd) neoplasm of posterior fossa in childhood (followed by cerebellar pilocytic astrocytoma). It accounts for 15 to 25 percent of primary CNS tumors in children. Rare in adults (<1% primary CNS tumors).
- **Age:** 75 percent cases < 15 years of age, with slight male predominance.
- Medulloblastoma tends to metastasize early, widely and massively throughout the CSF (**drop metastases**—the subarachnoid metastatic spread). Disseminated CSF metastases coat the brain like continuous frosting on a cake giving **"sugar-icing or zuckerguss" appearance**.

Brain tumors seen as a cystic lesion with enhancing mural nodule on CT/MR:
- Hemangioblastoma
- Ganglioglioma

- Pilocyctic astrocytoma
- Glioblastoma multiforme
- Pleomorphic xanthoastrocytoma.

Hemorrhage into a brain tumor is seen with:
- Metastatic tumors associated with intracerebral hemorrhage are:
  - *Choriocarcinoma*
  - *Malignant melanoma*
  - *Renal cell carcinoma*
  - *Bronchogenic carcinoma*
- Glioblastoma multiforme (in adults)
- Medulloblastoma (in children)
- *Imaging:*
  - *CT*: Typically pear or heart shaped midline vermian mass that displaces fourth ventricle anteriorly. They are often homogeneously hyperdense (70%) on NECT and show moderately strong, relatively homogeneous enhancement on CECT (97%). Atypical CT features include cystic/necrotic areas (10–16%), calcification (13%), hemorrhage (3%) and supratentorial extension.
  - *MRI*: Typical medulloblastoma fills the fourth ventricle often extending inferiorly through the foramen of Magendie into cisterna magna and are heterogeneously hypointense to gray matter. On T1W1 and on T2W1 it varies from hypo- to hyperintense.

CSF Seedlings of Intracranial/Brain Tumors (known as Drop Metastases)
- Brain tumors causing spread via CSF are
  - Medulloblastoma and other primitive neuroectodermal tumors
  - Anaplastic glioma
  - Ependymoma
  - Germinoma
  - Pineoblastoma, pineocytoma
- Less common causes include
  - Choroid plexus carcinoma
  - Teratoma
  - Angioblastic meningioma
  - Craniopharyngioma

Craniopharyngioma

- Bimodal age of distribution (6–10 years and second peak in fifth decade)
- Half of the childhood suprasellar tumors are craniopharyngiomas
- Calcification is present in over 80 percent of childhood cases, but is often absent in the less common adult cases
- Histologically two types occur →
  - Adamantinomatous (childhood variety, predominantly cystic, calcified)
  - Squamous-papillary (Adulthood; predominantly solid).

Oligodendroglioma

Uncommon glioma constituting 2 to 5 percent of all primary brain tumors
   Peak age to get affected being 35 to 45 years.
   Frontal lobes are most commonly involved.

Imaging features
- Oligodendroglioma is the most common intracranial tumor to calcify.
- 'Nodular or clumped' calcification is seen in 70 to 90 percent of all cases.
- Heterogeneous partially calcified mixed density hemispheric mass that often extends peripherally to cortex.
- Overlying skull may show pressure erosion.
- Cystic degeneration is common.
- Necrosis or gross hemorrhage rare.
- Mild/moderate nonhomogeneous enhancement is common.

- Comprise about 15 percent of gliomas in adults.
- More benign course.
- More responsive to cytotoxic treatment than astrocytomas.
- Occur chiefly in supratentorial locations; frontal lobe being most common site.
- Fifty percent contains areas of calcification; in fact, oligodendroglioma is the most common tumor in adults to calcify, which is best seen with CT scan.
- Are surgically well treatable.

Meningioma (Extra-axial Brain Tumor)

It is derived from "arachnoid cap cells"
   Peak incidence 45 years (30–75 yrs)
   M:F = 1:2 to 1:4
   Associated with neurofibromatosis type 2 and basal cell nevus syndrome

Histological types
- Fibroblastic
- Transitional
- Meningothelial/syncitial
- Angioblastic (malignant)

It can also be classified as:
- Globular (most common)
- Enplaque
- Multicentric.

Location

About 90 percent are supratentorial
- Convexities of lateral hemispheres (most common site/type of meningioma)
- Parasagittal
- Sphenoid ridge and middle cranial fossa
- Frontobasal at olfactory groove

   Infratentorial rare (cerebellar convexity, tentorium cerebelli, CP angle, clivus)
   Spine (12%) (Intradural but extramedullary).

Imaging Features

X-ray skull
- Hyperostosis at site close to or within bone
- Calcification (psammomatous)
- Enlarged meningeal grooves and marked vascular markings
- Enlarged foramen spinosum
- Blistering of paranasal sinuses with or without sclerosis (**pneumosinus dilatans**)

CT Scan
- Extra-axial SOL (hyperdense/isodense)
- Cortical buckling
- Calcification (circular/medial pattern)
- Hyperostosis of adjacent bone
- Intense uniform enhancement on CECT.

MRI
- Hypo- to isointense on T1W1 and iso to hyperintense on T2WI
- Dural tail sign (curvilinear area of enhancement).

Angiography
- "Mother-in-law" sign (contrast media shows up early and stays late into venous phase)
- "Sunburst/Spoke-wheel" pattern of tumor vascularity with hypervascular cloud like stain.

Spinal Meningioma

Meningioma is vascular spinal cord tumor, and is characteristically seen as an extramedullary, intradural, homogeneously enhancing lesion especially common in middle aged females.

The majority of primary extramedullary and intradural tumors of spinal cord are comprised of meningiomas and neurofibromas.

These lesions are well circumscribed and can be difficult to distinguish from each other morphologically. Enhancement in both tumors is frequently intense and homogeneous. On long TR, long TE images the signal of neurofibromas may increase greater than that of meningioma. The greater amount of fibrous connective tissue and calcifications within the substance of meningiomas may account for this finding.

Meningiomas are also more common in the thoracic region and more commonly occur in middle-aged women. They are generally entirely intradural in location and usually have a broad base of origin along the dura. Enhancement along the dural margins at the site of tumor attachment may be a result of en plaque extension.

Neurofibromas may be entirely intradural or extradural but may also have components in both compartments. The extension of a neurofibroma through the neural foramen with components in the intraspinal and lateral foraminal regions accounts for the typical 'dumbbell' appearance.

Bone erosion, although present with meningiomas, occurs more commonly with neurofibromas.

Vestibular Schwannoma (Acoustic Neuroma)

- Most are benign neoplasms arising from Schwan cell (schwannomas) of the nerve sheaths.
- Vestibular schwannoma arises eccentrically from the sheath and compresses the parent nerve rather than invading it.
- It is the most common CP angle tumor, followed by meningioma and epidermoid cyst.
- All cranial nerves except I and II, which are in fact white matter tracts of the cerebrum, have nerve sheaths, but schwannomas usually grow on the sensory nerves, most frequently from the superior vestibular division of vestibulocochlear nerve (acoustic neuroma) and with decreasing frequency, from trigeminal, glossopharyngeal and lower cranial nerves.
- Pure motor cranial nerves rarely form schwannomas.
- The acoustic neuroma produces symptoms initially by compressing the nerves in the narrow confines of the internal auditory canal.
- As the tumor enlarges it produces a funnel-shaped enlargement or erosion of the temporal bone and protrudes through the internal acoustic meatus to compress cranial nerves VIII, V, VII, and other brain stem and cerebellar structures (**Ice-cream cone sign on MRI**).
- The **earliest sign of an acoustic neuroma** is the spontaneous appearance of episodic dizziness with problems in speech discrimination.

  - Acoustic neuroma is the most common CP angle tumor.
  - Gd-enhanced MRI is investigation of choice.
  - It shows brilliant enhancement on CEMRI.
  - Arises most often from superior division of vestibular nerve.

- Additionally, another early sign of acoustic neuroma is a depressed or absent corneal reflex.
- Late signs of acoustic neuromas include facial nerve palsy, sensory loss to the entire ipsilateral side of the face, gait unsteadiness, taste disturbance, and a diminished corneal reflex.
- Nystagmus due to acoustic neuroma is coarse and slow upon gaze directed to the side of the lesion and is rapid and fine when gaze is directed away from the side of the lesion. The affected labyrinth fails to respond to caloric testing.
- It is important to consider the presence of cerebellopontine angle tumors in all patients with persistent unilateral tinnitus and hearing loss and mild vestibular symptoms which persist between attacks.
- Multiple cranial nerve schwannomas are found in neurofibromatosis type 2 and bilateral vestibular schwannomas are pathognomonic (sine qua non) of NF-2. Recently, NF-2 is called as **MISME complex** (Multiple inherited schwannomas, meningiomas and ependymomas). Cranial nerve tumors almost invariably show marked contrast enhancement.

- Acoustic (vestibular) schwannomas (neuromas) account for 80 percent of cerebellopontine lesions
- Plain skull radiograph or conventional tomography shows widened porus acusticus and internal auditory meatus (IAM).
- MRI is much more sensitive than CT in detection of small lesions. MRI is now the method of choice for the investigation of suspected vestibular schwannomas than can be diagnosed or excluded on high-resolution, thin section, T2 weighted fast spin-echo images of CP angles, capable of resolving the 7th and 8th nerves in detail. If the findings are equivocal, gadolinium-enhanced MRI is best.

Pituitary Tumor

Pituitary tumor	Percent
Prolactinomas	35
Somatotrophic (Acromegaly and gigantism)	25
Corticotrophinoma (Cushing and Nelson syndrome)	05
Miscellaneous and mixed	15
Nonsecretory	20

PITUITARY IMAGING

- Sagittal and coronal T1-weighted MRI imaging, before and after administration of gadolinium.
- Apart from pituitary gland, also there is clear delineation of:
  - Hypothalamus
  - Infundibular stalk
  - Surrounding suprasellar cisterns
  - Cavernous sinuses
  - Sphenoid sinus
  - Optic chiasm.
- Pituitary gland height ranges from 6 mm in children to 8 mm in adults, during pregnancy and puberty, the height may reach 10 to 12 mm (**Eister's rule**).
- The upper aspect of the adult pituitary is flat or slightly concave, but in adolescent and pregnant individuals, this surface may be convex (physiologic pituitary enlargement).
- The stalk should be midline and vertical.
- Posterior pituitary (high phospholipid content) gives a "pituitary bright spot".

- Anterior pituitary is slightly heterogeneous on MRI, and signal intensity resembles that of brain matter on T1-weighted imaging.
  Adenoma density is usually lower than that of surrounding normal tissue on T1-weighted imaging.
- CT scan is indicated to define the extent of bony erosion or the presence of calcification.

In children, the most common extracranial malignancy that involves the skull base is rhabdomyosarcoma. It is the most common soft tissue sarcoma in children and the head and neck is the most common site of their affection. Imaging of rhabdomyosarcoma in children varies with the location of the lesion. In head and neck region, CT and MRI are used to detect the origin, extent and staging, including the assessment of bony and intracranial invasion. In addition, on MRI the appearance of lesion reflects its morphology.

Leukoencephalopathy is mineralizing microangiopathy of leukemia seen in patients of leukemia treated with methotrexate and radiotherapy in the form of craniospinal irradiation.

Lipoma of Corpus Callosum

Bracket calcification is uncommon but characteristic finding of corpus callosal (CC) lipoma. There is often marginal calcification where they merge with adjacent cortical tissue, which can be of a characteristic 'brackets' type that occasionally permits diagnosis from a simple PA X-ray film of skull. Azygos or single ACA (fused pericallosal arteries) and partial or complete CC agenesis may be associated sometimes.

HEAD TRAUMA

In head trauma the imaging study of choice is CT scan.

Usually contrast study is not needed for head injury *per se*.

Skull radiographs have extremely limited value as compared to CT except in evaluation of skull fractures that to depressed skull fracture/fracture base of skull.

Indications for CT include:
- Loss of consciousness
- Altered mental status
- Focal neurologic signs
- Clinically suspected basilar
- Depressed skull fracture
- Penetrating wound (e.g. bullet)
- Suspected acute SAH/EDH/SDH/parenchymal hematoma.

Indications for MR include:
- Post-concussive symptomatology
- Suspected *diffuse axonal injury*, critical contusion or primary brainstem injury
- Vascular damage (e.g. pseudoaneurysm formation due to basilar skull fracture)
- Diagnosis of small sub/epidural hematoma.

Skull Fractures

These, in newborn are most commonly linear and simple but may occasionally be depressed without a fracture line, a so-called 'ping-pong' or pond fracture.

Growing skull fractures (leptomeningeal cysts) usually occur after severe head injuries early in life. The dura mater underlying a linear fracture is torn.

CT is best investigation to detect skull fractures.

'Blow-out' fracture usually involves the orbital floor with 'trap-door deformity' on skull AP view and CT is best technique to study orbital fractures.

	EDH	*SDH*
Incidence	1–4 percent overall	10–20 percent overall
Etiology	Associated # in 85-95 percent cases. Lacerated middle meningeal artery/dural sinus in 70–85 percent cases and venous "OOZE" or MMA tear without # in 15 percent cases only	Stretching, tearing of bridging cortical veins
Location	Between skull and dura. Cross dural attachments but not sutures. 95 percent supratentorial, 5 percent bilateral	Between dura and arachnoid. Cross sutures but not dural attachment. 95 percent supratentorial, 15 percent bilateral
Imaging	CT: Biconvex displaced gray white interface. 2/3 hyperdense, 1/3 mixed	CT: a. Acute SDH: Crescentic. 60 percent hyperdense, 40 percent mixed b. Subacute SDH: May be nearly isodense with cortex neomembrane, underlying vessels may enhance. c. Chronic SDH: Hypodense with enhancing membrane. May be loculated. Rehemorrhage can cause mixed density. 1–2 percent of very old SDH calcify.

Transtentorial Herniation

Ascending → displacement of cerebellum cephalad through tentorial incisura
Features:
- Superior vermian cistern effaced
- 4th ventricle is compressed and anteriorly displaced
- Quadrigeminal plate cistern is deformed
- Anterior displacement of midbrain
- Aqueductal compression and obstructive hydrocephalus

Descending →
- *Anterior*: Uncal herniation (most common)
- *Posterior*: Herniation of parahippocampal gyrus
- *Total*: Herniation of entire hippocampus

Features:
- Brain is shifted away from herniating temporal lobe
- Ipsilateral CP angle cistern dilatation
- Obliteration of all basal cisterns with increasing herniation
- Displacement of midbrain
- PCA may be compressed against the tentorial incisura, resulting in occipital lobe infarction
- Kinking of perforating vessels that arise from circle of Willis result in basal ganglia and midbrain infarction
- Periaqueductal necrosis
- Secondary midbrain or duret hemorrhage (in corpus callosum and dorsal midbrain)
- Kernohan's notch
- Compressive craniaolopathies.

Central transtentorial herniation of brain is common in children with progressive hydrocephalus.

Diffuse Axonal Injury

It is a frequent result of traumatic deceleration injuries and a frequent cause of persistent vegetative state in patients.

Diffuse axonal injury (DAI) is the most significant cause of morbidity in patients with traumatic brain injuries, which most commonly are the result of high-speed motor vehicle accidents.

Typically, the process is diffuse and bilateral, involving the lobar white matter at the gray white matter interface. The corpus callosum frequently is involved, as is the dorsolateral rostral brainstem. *The most commonly involved area is* the frontal and temporal white matter, followed by the posterior body and splenium of the corpus callosum, the caudate nuclei, thalamus, tegmentum, and internal capsule. Internal capsule lesions are associated more frequently with hemorrhage than are the other lesions and are secondary to the proximity of the lenticulostriate vessels.

CT Diagnostic Criteria of Diffuse Axonal Injury

- Single or multiple small intraparenchymal hemorrhages in the cerebral hemispheres (<2 cm in diameter)
- Diffuse cerebral edema with compression of basal cisterns
- Intraventricular hemorrhage
- Hemorrhage in the corpus callosum
- Small focal areas of hemorrhage adjacent to the third ventricle (<2 cm in diameter)
- Brain stem hemorrhage.

Stages of involvement described by Adams et al according to the anatomic location of the lesions:
- Stage I: Involves the parasagittal regions of the frontal lobes, periventricular temporal lobes, and, less likely, the parietal and occipital lobes, internal and external capsules, and cerebellum.
- Stage II: Involvement of the corpus callosum, in addition to the white matter areas in stage I. The involvement of the corpus callosum carries a poorer prognosis.
- Stage III: Involves the areas associated with stage II, with the addition of brainstem involvement.

MRI with T2-weighted, and FLAIR images is more sensitive in depicting tissue changes than is CT. It is the preferred examination (particularly with gradient-echo sequences), although CT examination may demonstrate findings suggestive of DAI and is more practical and available in today's medical milieu.

Traumatic Facial Nerve Palsy/Facial Nerve Trauma

The seventh, i.e. facial nerve contains motor, sensory, and parasympathetic fibers. Among its functions are the vital control of facial expression, taste to the anterior two thirds of the tongue, and salivary and lacrimal gland secretion

The facial nerve can be divided into 6 segments. From proximal to distal, they include the intracranial, meatal, labyrinthine, tympanic, mastoid (i.e. vertical), and extratemporal segments.

Two of these segments are outside the temporal bone. In the proximal portion, the intracranial segment extends from the brainstem to the internal auditory canal (IAC). In the distal portion, the extratemporal segment extends from the stylomastoid foramen to the muscles of the face.

Of particular relevance in temporal-bone trauma are the intratemporal segments. The meatal segment extends from the porus of the IAC to the meatal foramen. The meatal foramen represents the narrowest (0.68 mm) portion of the facial canal. The nerve runs superior to the transverse crest and anterior to the vertical crest (Bill bar) of bone at the distal IAC before entering the facial canal. The shortest segment, the labyrinthine segment (3-5 mm), extends from the meatal foramen to the geniculate ganglion. Its initial lateral course is followed by an anterior curve between the basal turn of the cochlea and the vestibule. The end of the labyrinthine segment is marked by the formation of the geniculate ganglion. In this region, the greater superficial petrosal nerve carrying fibers to the lacrimal gland leaves anteriorly from the ganglion by means of the hiatus of the facial canal. The greater superficial petrosal nerve travels anteriorly carrying parasympathetic fibers, for instance, to the lacrimal gland.

The Schirmer test for tear secretion is purportedly useful to assess the function of this branch. Adequate tear secretion implies a site of lesion distal to the geniculate ganglion.

The tympanic segment courses in a posterior direction following a 40-80° turn of the first genu at the geniculate ganglion. The facial nerve then enters the medial tympanic cavity, running in the facial canal and curving around the oval window niche. At this point, the nerve runs superior to the oval window niche where the bone of the facial canal can be thin and where it may be dehiscent in as many as 55 percent of individuals. The distal tympanic segment lies just anterior and inferior to the lateral semicircular canal, where the nerve curves through its second genu and begins its vertical descent. Most intratemporal traumatic injuries occur in the perigeniculate region and labyrinthine segment.

The mastoid (i.e. vertical) segment of the facial canal is the longest of all segments (10–14 mm). It extends from the pyramidal process to the stylomastoid foramen. The stapedius muscle lies medial to the facial nerve and receives its motor branch in this segment. Tympanometry with stapedial-reflex measurement is performed to assess the function of the facial nerve at this level.

Lastly, the chorda tympani nerve, which carries efferent fibers to the submandibular and submaxillary glands and special afferent (taste) fibers from the tongue branches from the facial nerve in this segment.

The facial nerve is the most susceptible to injury of all the cranial nerves. More than 40 causes of facial paralysis are known. Trauma is a distant second to idiopathic or Bell palsy as a cause of facial nerve paralysis. Approximately 5 percent of people who have trauma have temporal bone fractures. These fractures are classified with respect to the axis of the petrous ridge and include longitudinal, transverse, and mixed (or oblique) types. Longitudinal fractures are most common (70-80%), followed by transverse (10-20%) and mixed (10%) fractures. Facial paralysis most commonly occurs after transverse fractures of the temporal bone (50%). However, paralysis also occurs after longitudinal fractures (25%).

The facial nerve is a complex nerve with motor, sensory, and parasympathetic contributions. Motor fibers originate in the facial nucleus and innervate the posterior belly of the digastric muscle, stylohyoid muscle, stapedius muscle, and muscles of facial expression. The facial nerve carries cutaneous sensory fibers from the EAC, tympanic membrane, and areas of the external ear and postauricular region are carried to the fasciculus solitarius. The geniculate ganglion represents the nucleus of the sensory root of the facial nerve. Parasympathetic fibers originating in the superior salivatory nucleus and entering the facial nerve as the nervus intermedius innervate the lacrimal, submandibular, and sublingual glands, as well as glands of the nose, sinuses, and palate. Also included in this portion of the facial nerve are special.

Classic longitudinal fractures extend from the temporal squamosa along the roof of the EAC and petrous apex to the foramen lacerum. The fracture injures the tympanic membrane, facial canal, and middle ear, resulting in ossicular disruption and conductive hearing loss. Because the otic capsule is made of dense bone, the fracture line often courses around this structure.

In contrast, transverse fractures extend from the jugular foramen in an anterolateral direction across the petrous pyramid ending at the foramen spinosum or foramen lacerum. In its course, the fracture line may traverse the otic capsule, resulting in sensorineural hearing loss. *High-resolution CT scan of the temporal bone* can reveal findings diagnostic of temporal bone fracture.

Patients with traumatic facial paralysis often are *treated empirically with* a short course of oral steroids. In contrast to idiopathic facial paralysis or Bell palsy, no studies confirm or dispute the utility of steroid treatment after traumatic facial paralysis. The potential risks of using corticosteroids in a patient with multiple trauma and possible risk of infectious complications must be weighed against the unknown probability for benefit in decreasing the risk of permanent facial paralysis. A typical course of high-dose prednisone is 1 mg/kg for up to 10 days followed by a tapering regimen.

	Benign intracranial hypertension	Benign intracranial hypotension
Synonym	Pseudotumor cerebri	Spontaneous CSF leak
Etiology	Drug (vitamin A, Quinolones, etc.), steroid therapy and diseases like lateral sinus thrombosis. Addison's, Hypoparathyroidism, SLE implicated	Idiopathic/Low CSF volume headache
C/f	Sudden or gradual headache with vision disturbance Enlargement of blind spot	Postitional head pain: It begins when the patient sits or stands upright and resolves upon reclining. The pain, which is occipitofrontal, is usually a dull ache but may be throbbing.
Investigations	Isotope brain scan, CT, MRI normal	– MRI with gadolinium is the initial study of choice.

Contd...

Contd...		– A striking pattern of diffuse meningeal enhancement is so typical that in the appropriate clinical context the diagnosis is established. – The source of CSF leakage may be identified by spinal MRI, by CT myelogram, or with ^{111}In-DTPA CSF studies – In the absence of a directly identified site of leakage early emptying of ^{111}In-DTPA tracer into the bladder or slow progress of tracer across the brain suggests a CSF leak
Rx	– Patient improves spontaneously after a few months – Acetazolamide – Oral glycerol – Dexamethasone may be required – Cerebral decompression is rarely necessary	*Mild cases:* – Increase in fluids, especially caffeine, and rest – Intravenous caffeine is safe and can be curative *Moderate-to-severe cases:* – Abdominal binder – Autologous Epidural blood patch (blood patch is also effective for post-LP headache)

ENT RADIOLOGY

Anatomy of Nose

Lateral Nasal Wall

- Superior turbinate meatus: Post-ethmoidal air cells drain into it and sphenoid sinus drains via sphenoethmoidal recess. However, superior turbinate being small may not be always identified.
- Middle turbinate meatus: Most important area, forms OMC where anterior ethmoid air cells, maxillary and frontal sinuses drain into it.
- Inferior turbinate meatus: Largest turbinate. Nasolacrimal duct drains into its anterior part.
- Frontal recess: Frontal sinuses communicate the medial meatus of ipsilateral half of nasal cavity by means of a passage called frontonasal canal/frontal recess. Anterior to frontal recess and anterior end of middle turbinate is the bony prominence of frontal process of maxilla known as **Agger nasi**; cells in it drain into ethmoid infundibulum.

- **Osteomeatal unit/complex (OMC):**
    - OMC is the normal aerated channel which provides airflow and mucociliary clearance for sinuses.
    - It is the key area for pathogenesis of chronic sinus diseases.
    - It is the cross road for drainage of most paranasal sinuses.
    - It is the center of interest due to functional endoscopic sinus surgery (FESS).
    - The concept that obstruction of OMC results in ethmoid, frontal and maxillary sinusitis is fundamental to FESS.
    - Well-identified on coronal CT with patient prone and head hyperextended.
    - Anterior ethmoidal air cells, maxillary and frontal sinuses drain into it.

Components of OMC include:
- Middle meatus
- Maxillary sinus ostium and infundibulum
- Anterior and middle ethmoidal air cells ostia and ethmoidal infundibulum
- Frontal recess/frontonasal duct
- Bulla ethmoidalis
- Hiatus semilunaris
- Uncinate process
- Sphenoethmoid recess and superior meatus (included by some authors).
    - In several areas of OMC, two mucosal layers come into contact with one another thus increasing the likelihood of local impairment of mucociliary clearance. Secretions may then be retained at the site, creating potential for infection even without osteal closure.
- **Uncinate process** is thin, curved lamina of bone from the lateral side of ethmoidal labyrinthine that forms a portion of lateral nasal wall. It projects downwards and backwards and ranges from 1 to 4 mm in height and 14 to 22 mm in length. Superior edge of uncinate process is free and forms medial boundary of hiatus semilunaris.
- **Ethmoidal infundibulum** is a trough shaped air space that is below bulla and above and lateral to uncinate process. It receives drain from anterior and middle ethmoid air cells and frontal and maxillary sinuses.

   The infundibulum may be narrowed if there is concha bullosa (pneumatized middle turbinate) and Haller cell (ethmoid air cells at orbital floor).

- **Hiatus semilunaris** is curvilinear opening of lateral wall of that is above uncinate process and below the bulla ethmoidalis. This opening separates uncinate process from ethmoidal bulla and serves as connection between infundibulum and middle meatus.

- Middle ethmoidal air cell produces a round swelling called **bulla ethmoidalis** on lateral wall of middle meatus.

    Onodi cells are most posterior ethmoidal cells that surround optic canal, related to optic nerve.
- Thus, the normal variants like abnormal course of free edge of uncinate process, a concha bullosa, large Haller's cell or Onodi cells may be a cause for obstruction, causing chronic sinonasal disease and should be well commented in CT PNS report for ease in FESS.

Water's view (occipitomental view)

Demonstrates: Maxillary sinuses (mainly), frontal sinuses, maxillae, inferior orbital rim, zygomatic arches, zygoma, nasal septum, anterior nasal spine and orbit floors.

Technique: Patient sits erect facing (PA) the erect Bucky; chin is raised so that orbitomeatal line is at 45° to film plane and patient touching the X-ray film plate with his nose and chin.

Caldwell's view (occipitofrontal view)

Demonstrates: Frontal and ethmoid sinus mainly. Orbit, superior orbital fissure, sphenoid wings and petrous ridges are also seen.

Technique: Patient touches a vertical X-ray film plate with nose and forehead (by cervical flexion) with 15° caudal tube tilt. Orbitomeatal line is perpendicular to the cassette. X-rays pass horizontally.

Base of skull or submentovertical view or full axial or Hirtz's view

Demonstrates: Foramen magnum, foramen ovale and spinosum, mandible, sphenoid and ethmoid sinuses, petrous ridge, hard palate, occipital bone and mastoid process.

Technique: Patients sit erect with dorsal aspect against Bucky, neck is hyperextended until the orbitomeatal line is parallel to the film plane and horizontal central rays are directed in the midline to a point midway between the mandibular angles (kV used: 90).

Towne's view or half axial view (occipitofrontal 40°)

Demonstrates: Dorsum sellae, posterior clinoid process, foramen magnum, occiput, parietal bones, lambdoid sutures, structures in petrous bone (bony labyrinth, IA canal).

Stockholm 'C' (Stenver's) view

Demonstrates: Internal auditory meatus (enface) and the petrous temporal bone (medial part). Both right and left petrous bones must be examined for comparison.

IAM and canal lie 1–2 cm above the ipsilateral temporomandibular joint. Normally both IAM orifices are equal in size and this enables destruction or distortion of bony margins to be detected early.

Chapter 10 ❖ Head, Neck and Spine Imaging

Technique: Patient's is prone, head turned to bring the median sagittal plane parallel to and interpupillary line, vertical/perpendicular to the tabletop. Patient is comfortable by raising shoulder remote from the side being examined. A gap of 10 cm between patient couch and table is kept to ensure early rotation of Bucky tray.

Central rays are directed 10° cephalad and 25° from vertical, enters the head through occipital bone, 6 cm behind and 1 cm below external auditory meatus, remote from cassette. It is now perpendicular to long axis of petrous bone.

Schuller's view
Demonstrates: Mastoid bone and middle ear.

Lateral view
Nasal bone fracture (Jarjavay's fracture).

Radiographic view	Demonstration of
Water's view (occipitomental view)	Maxillary sinuses/antra (mainly), sphenoid sinuses, ethmoidal sinuses.
Caldwell view (occipitofrontal view)	Frontal and ethmoidal sinuses (mainly), nasal cavity and orbits
Towne's view (half axial view)	Dorsum sellae, posterior clinoid process, foramen magnum, occiput, parietal bones, lambdoid sutures, structures in petrous bone (bony labyrinthine, IA canal)
Stenver's (Stockholm C) view	Medial part of petrous bone and its tip with internal auditory meatus (IAM) enface
Schuller's view	Mastoid
Submentovertical (Hirtz's or basal skull or full axial) view	Structures of the base of skull (foramina and canals), foramen magnum, petrous bone, middle ear structures, mastoid air cells
Ruggiero projection and oblique four-point landing projection	Optic canal
Fronto-occipital (petrous) view	Both internal auditory canals
Chausse's view	Jugular foramen
Jug handle view	Zygomatic arches
Lateral view	All paranasal sinuses with two sides superimposed
Rhese view	Posterior ethmoidal air cells, optic foramen
Pineal view	Internal auditory canals
Stryker's view	Shoulder
Skyline view	Patella
Ferguson's view	Sacroiliac joints
Cahoon view	Styloid process
Skull lateral	Sphenoid sinus

Foramen/canal/fissure	Best projection
Superior orbital fissure	Occipitofrontal view
Optic canal	Optic canal view
IAM	Perorbital
Pterygoid (vidian) canal	Occipitofrontal view
Carotid canal	Submentovertical view
Foramen ovale	Submentovertical view
Foramen spinosum	Submentovertical view
Jugular foramen	Submentovertical view
Foramen magnum	Lateral; submentovertical view
Anterior condylar or hypoglossal canal	Reversed Stenver's view
Optic foramen	Rhese view

CT PNS (Multislice Machine and Coronal Sections)

The use of computed tomography (CT) or sinus radiography is not recommended for routine cases, particularly early in the course of illness (i.e. at <7 days), gives the high prevalence of similar abnormalities among cases of acute viral rhinosinusitis. In the evaluation of persistent, recurrent, or chronic sinusitis, CT of the sinuses is the radiographic study of choice (contrast not required). But for neoplasms of nose and sinuses.

Adenoid (Lymphoid) Tissue Hypertrophy

The amount of adenoid tissue within the nasopharynx varies greatly among patients. The adenoid mass is most commonly found in the mid-portion of the nasopharynx and, depending on its thickness, projects over a variable distance into the nasopharyngeal air space (*Air crescent sign* on lateral nasopharyngeal radiograph). The margins of the mass are sharply delimited and often lobular in configuration. The lateral pharyngeal recess (fossa of Rosenmuller) may be obliterated by the adenoid tissue. The adenoid mass does not extend into the deep-tissue planes of the nasopharynx and thus can be differentiated by CT from malignancies and inflammatory lesions

Thornwaldt Cyst

It results from the failure of regression of notochordal tissue in the posterior nasopharyngeal area and communication with the nasopharyngeal lumen provides a pathway for ingrowth of respiratory epithelium, forming a potential space in the midline of the nasopharynx. With inflammation, the space may become filled with fluid to form a cyst, which is lined by respiratory epithelium and contains little or no lymphoid tissue. The cyst may be asymptomatic but in some cases gives rise to persistent posterior nasopharyngeal drainage, dull occipital headache, and an unpleasant taste. Such cysts have been seen in all age groups, with the peak incidence among persons aged 15 to 30 years. There is no sex preponderance. They are seen as a smooth, midline, sacular mass or pouch of 1 cm to 2 cm in diameter in the posterior superior angle of the nasopharynx.

Juvenile Nasopharyngeal Angiofibroma

- It is a tumor of adolescent boys.
- It typically presents as nasal mass with recurrent epistaxis.
- Life-threatening hemorrhage has occurred from biopsy and therefore radiological features are relied upon to establish diagnosis.
- It is the most common benign nasopharyngeal tumor, which can grow enormously and invade local vital structures.
- *Age:* Teenagers (peak 15 year); almost exclusively in males.
  It is highly vascular mass supplied primarily by internal maxillary artery.
- *Extensions:*
  - Posterolateral wall of nasal cavity; via pterygopalatine fossa into retroantral region, orbit; Middle cranial fossa and laterally into infratemporal fossa
- *Radiological features:*
  - Widening of pterygopalatine fossa (90%) with anterior bowing of posterior antral wall, invasion of sphenoid sinus through floor of sinus (66%), widening of inferior orbital fissure (orbital spread) and superior orbital fissure (middle cranial fossa spread).
  - Angiography is not required to establish the diagnosis, but has valuable role in preoperative therapeutic embolization to reduce blood loss.
  - **CECT is investigation** of choice for diagnosis and evaluation of the mass.
  - It shows bright intense contrast enhancement immediately and long erosion and invasion can be best visualized.
  - A reliable imaging sign is erosion of medial pterygoid plate and enlargement of sphenopalatine foramen.
  - HRCT allows accurate diagnosis since these tumors start in pterygopalatine fissure, which enlarge before they extend. MRI is reliable for defining tumor extension, which may involve the posterior nasopharynx, middle cranial fossa and infratemporal fossa.

- MRI shows intermediate signal intensity on T1W1 with discrete punctate areas on hypointensity.
- Biopsy is contraindicated.

Combination of CT and CEMRI may be required for accurate diagnosis imaging which reveals an enhancing mass, which arises from the posterolateral nasal wall adjacent to sphenopalatine foramen.

Nasopharyngeal Carcinomas

- Most nasopharyngeal malignancies are either keratinizing or nonkeratinizing squamous-cell carcinomas (80%).
- Nasopharyngeal carcinomas *arise most frequently* posterosuperiorly in the region of the lateral recess (*fossa of Rosenmuller*).
- Early blunting of the pharyngeal recess may be the first sign of a nasopharyngeal tumor. However, asymmetry may occur normally, and this should be kept in mind when such a recess is evaluated.
- Serous otitis media as a consequence of eustachian tube obstruction can be detected on CT as opacification of the middle-ear cavity and mastoid air cells. This is best demonstrated with the bone window setting.
- Exophytic tumors project into the nasopharyngeal air space over a variable distance. Large tumors may extend to the choanal area or extend inferiorly to the oropharynx with inferior and anterior displacement of the soft palate. A crater within the exophytic tumor reflects ulceration, which may be visible in the contour of the mass. Deep infiltration is characterized by obliteration of fascial planes and muscles. Tumor in the parapharyngeal space is reflected by loss of the normal fatty density that surrounds the deglutitional muscles.

Primarily infiltrating carcinomas cause only slight asymmetry in the contour of the nasopharyngeal air space in axial and coronal images.

Intracranial extension, a common finding in advanced lesions, occurs primarily through the *foramen lacerum*. Skull invasion is characterized by lytic bone destruction, and occasionally a sclerotic reaction may be elicited by the tumor cells. The most common areas with bone destruction are, in order of decreasing frequency, clivus, foramen lacerum, and surrounding middle cranial fossa, floor of the sphenoid sinus, and foramen jugulare. *Bone destruction is best evaluated by CT using the bone window technique.* Coronal scans in addition to axial sections are mandatory in the assessment of the skull base.

Nodal spread may be bilateral in midline tumors. The following incidents of lymph node metastases have been reported: *jugulodigastric nodes* (70%), upper cervical nodes (66%), jugulo-omohyoid nodes (34%), spinal accessory nodes (28%), and inferior cervical nodes (20%). Any lymph nodes found on CT to be greater than 1.5 cm in diameter should be suspected of being metastatic.

OPHTHALMIC RADIOLOGY

Optic Nerve Enlargement

While radiography offers limited usefulness in assessing orbital and periorbital abnormalities, tomographic imaging such as ultrasound, CT and MRI produce images in thin slices-eliminating tissue superimposition - and are more accurate for soft tissue lesion detection and characterization.

Tubular Type

- Neoplastic
  Optic nerve glioma
  Optic nerve sheath meningioma
  Metastasis
  Lymphoma
  Leukemia.
- Non-neoplastic
  Perineural hematoma
  Papilledema
  Optic perineuritis
  Compressive neuropathy
  Patulous subarachnoid space.

Fusiform Type

Optic nerve glioma
Optic nerve sheath meningioma.

Escrescent Type

Meningioma from middle fossa
Meningioma from periorbita
Optic nerve sheath meningioma
Optic nerve glioma
Vascular anomaly.

Enlargement of One or More Extraocular Muscles

Neoplastic
- Orbital apex tumor
- Rhabdomyosarcoma
- Lymphoma
- Metastasis.

Non-neoplastic
- Graves' disease
- Myositis pseudotumor
- Contiguous inflammation
- Arteriovenous fistula (congestion)

This has many causes, most commonly, Graves' disease (50%). The second most common cause is myositic pseudotumor (8%).

Inflammatory Orbital Pseudotumor

The idiopathic form is probably related to an abnormal immune response; acute and chronic forms of inflammatory orbital pseudotumor often respond to steroid therapy. It is classified according to the orbital anatomy involved: (1) acute orbital myositis, (2) chronic orbital myositis, (3) dacryoadenitis, (4) perineural inflammation, and (5) lymphoid hyperplasia. As these groupings suggest, orbital pseudotumor presents in many ways, most frequently as an enlargement of one of the extraocular muscles (myositis) or as an orbital tumor mimicking lymphoma.

An extremely pathognomonic feature of pseudotumor of orbit is its dramatic response to steroid therapy.

Vascular Intraorbital Tumors

Various tumors of vascular origin present in the orbit are capillary hemangioma, cavernous hemangioma, hemangiopericytoma, lymphangioma, and vascular malformation. Of these, the cavernous hemangioma is the most common benign tumor of the orbit in adults and is usually located in the intraconal space.
- Lymphangioma and capillary hemangiomas are not capsulated.
- Hemangiopericytoma although not strictly a meningioma, is a meningeal tumor with an especially aggressive behavior.

- Capillary angioma is a tumor of early childhood. It forms a soft, bluish mass, which may involve any part of the orbit, including the eyelid. US shows it as a well-defined anterior soft lesion with small irregular echoes. CDFI shows pathognomonic features with high flow within immature vessels in a hypervascularized mass. Since these tumors regress either spontaneously or after steroids, CT is only indicated tumors with retrobulbar extension.
- *Cavernous hemangioma:* The most common primary retrobulbar tumor, is a slow-growing, well-defined, rounded or oval mass consisting of large vascular spaces surrounded by a firm capsule. Usually it flies within the muscle cone, displacing the optic nerve, and is well-depicted by US, CT and MRI. Phleboliths are not uncommon.
  - CT reveals a well-defined homogeneous rounded tumor, enhancing moderately after injection of intravenous contrast medium. The MRI signal is rather characteristic, equal to muscle signal on T1-weighted images and marked hypersignal relative to fat on T2-weighted images. Strong but heterogeneous contrast enhancement is the rule.
  - The diagnosis may be confirmed by US, since these lesions have a specific 'honeycomb' US pattern of alternating weak and strong echoes, corresponding to their structures. Their reflectivity is high and the attenuation is moderate.

Optic Nerve Gliomas

These are usually benign pilocytic astrocytomas occurring in children.

About 30 percent to 40 percent of these tumors are intraorbital at the time of diagnosis; the remainder will be partially intracranial. The optic canal is enlarged by this tumor in most cases. The optic nerve may appear diffusely enlarged, with a fusiform shape, or irregularly thickened. The tumors are usually inseparable from the nerve. The contrast enhancement is less than in meningioma. Approximately 10 to 30 percent of optic gliomas occur in patients with neurofibromatosis.

CT appearance of the intraorbital optic nerve glioma shows fusiform enlargement of the nerve with tapering at both ends (in the axial view) in the early phase. As it enlarges, it appears as a large, centrally positioned intraconal mass that enhances slightly with contrast.

Retinoblastoma

- Most common intraocular tumor of childhood
- Malignant primary neoplasm of retina that arises from neuroectodermal cells of retina (pigment layer)
- About 94 percent of cases are sporadic.

- May be a congenital lesion that is present but not usually apparent at birth; average age of diagnosis is 13 months.
- Principal symptom = Unilateral blindness
- Primary sign = Leukocoria
- It is bilateral in about 30 percent cases
- When bilateral, follows AD with complete penetrance pattern
- Chromosome 13 mutation (100% in B/L and 15% in U/L)
- *Histopathology:* Flexner Wintersteiner rosettes
- It is a PNET
- The most common second malignancy in survivors of retinoblastoma is osteosarcoma.

Morphologic forms
- Endophytic
- Exophytic
- Diffuse form

Type based on location
- Unilateral (70%)
- Bilateral (30%)
- Trilateral (<1%) → Bilateral RB plus pineal or suprasellar tumor
- Tetra/Quadrilateral (<0.1%) → Bilateral RB plus pineal and suprasellar mass.

CT Scan

Best to detect calcification in the tumor (a pathognomonic sign). However, calcification in the tumor can also be detected on *ultrasound scan*.

Calcification intraocular mass centered posteriorly in globe with moderate or intense CT with punctate or finely speckled calcification (<90%) with or without extraocular extension.

MRI

Best for seeing extraocular extension.

Treatment
- Small sized tumor → RT (Plaque or ext. beam) with/without vitreous seeding
- Large RB +– local extension enucleation +– External beam RT.
- Unilateral tumor without invasion has excellent progress.

Reese-Ellsworth classification is useful in predicting visual prognosis following radiotherapy.

NECK IMAGING

The understanding of various neck spaces is important for CT and MRI imaging of the neck.

Suprahyoid Neck Spaces

- Pharyngeal mucosal space -PMS
- Parapharyngeal space -PPS
- Masticator space -MS
- Parotid space -PS
- Carotid space -CS
- Retropharyngeal space -RPS
- Danger space -DS
- Perivertebral space -PVS

Infrahyoid Neck Spaces

- These spaces continue largely unchanged from above the hyoid:
    - Carotid space
    - Retropharyngeal space
    - Danger space
    - Perivertebral space
- Two new major spaces:
  1. Visceral space
  2. Posterior cervical space

Cystic Lymphangiectasis/Lymphangioma/Cystic Hygroma

It is a congenital malformation of lymphatic system producing posterolateral neck swelling.

It is known to be associated with Turner's syndrome.

Diagnosis is confirmed by ultrasound, which shows a multilocular cystic mass in neck, extending into mediastinum/axilla/pleural space or by CT/MRI, which show a thin-walled cyst containing septae and fluid attenuation.

Branchial Cyst

Branchial cysts are embryological cysts derived from the cervical pouch.

First branchial cleft cyst results in cyst near external auditory canal or parotid gland.

Second branchial cleft cyst is most common (95% of all branchial cleft anomalies) and present as mass in anterior triangle of neck close to the angle of mandible. **Type II** second branchial cysts are most common among the four types of second branchial cleft cysts and are classically located at anteromedial border of sternocleidomastoid muscle, lateral to carotid space and at posterior margin of submandibular gland in close proximity to internal and external carotid artery.

Third branchial cleft cyst present as posterior cervical space mass.

Parasympathetic Paragangliomas (Chemodectomas, Glomus Tumor)

These arise from the paraganglia that exist in various locations in the body, the most common head and neck sites of these tumors being the carotid body/bifurcation (**carotid body tumor/chemodectoma/ potato tumor**), jugular foramen (glomus jugulare) and middle ear (Glomus tympanicum) and vagus nerve (glomus vagale).

- **Glomus jugulare** is situated in the jugular bulb adventitia immediately below the middle ear.
- **Glomus tympanicum** are the paragangliomas that are localized to cochlear promontory in the middle ear cavity.
- **Glomus jugulotympanicum** tumors extend from jugular foramen into the middle ear cavity.
- The "salt and pepper" appearance is typical for paraganglioma on MR scan study.
- **Pheochromocytoma of adrenal medulla is the most common paraganglioma.**
- Other extra-adrenal sites are spine, mediastinum and para-aortic.

Salivary Gland Tumors

Salivary gland tumors occur in the parotid gland (80%), in the submandibular gland (10%), in the minor salivary glands (9%), and in the sublingual glands (1%). The incidence of malignancy in salivary gland tumors is 25 percent in the parotid gland, 47 percent in the submandibular gland, 65 percent in the minor salivary glands, and 90 percent in the sublingual glands.

Of all parotid gland tumors, 70 percent are benign mixed tumors, the favorite location for which is in the posterior inferior portion of the superficial portion of the parotid gland. Only 11 percent to 12 percent of all parotid tumors occur in the deep portion of the gland.

Of salivary gland tumors, 95 percent are of epithelial origin. The World Health Organization classifies epithelial tumors as adenomas, mucoepidermoid tumors, acinic cell tumors, and carcinomas; nonepithelial tumors are hemangiomas, lymphangiomas, neuromas, lymphomas, and sarcomas. Metastases to the salivary glands also occur.

CT is more sensitive than conventional sialography and thus is the method of choice to demonstrate masses within or outside the salivary glands.

Three patterns of tumor appearance have been described on CT:
1. The encapsulated round pattern, most likely to be benign
2. Lobular pattern of encapsulation, tending to be more aggressive
3. The infiltrating, poorly defined mass, representing the most aggressive or malignant configuration.

Pathological Classification

- Seventy five percent of tumors occur in parotid gland, 15 percent are malignant
- Ten percent of tumors occur in submandibular gland, 30 percent are malignant
- Fifteen percent of tumors occur in minor salivary glands, 50 percent are malignant.

Benign

- Pleomorphic adenoma (mixed parotid tumor)
- Adenolymphoma (Warthin's tumors)
- Hemangioma in children
- Lymphangioma in children
- Intermediate
- Mucoepidermoid tumors
- Acinic cell carcinoma
- Oncocytoma.

Malignant

- Adenoid cystic carcinoma
- Adenocarcinoma
- Squamous cell carcinoma.

Pleomorphic adenomas (Mixed tumors) are the most common tumors of the parotid gland and account for 80 to 90 percent of tumors in the parotid).

> Most common benign tumor of salivary glands → Pleomorphic adenoma
> Most common tumor of major salivary glands → Pleomorphic adenoma
> Most common tumor of minor salivary glands → Malignant tumors
> Most common site of pleomorphic adenoma in parotid is → Superficial lobe, more common in females.
> Malignant transformation takes place in 2 to 70 percent of cases.

Pleomorphic Adenoma

- Initially described as a 'mixed' tumor
- Accounts for 75 percent of parotid and 50 percent submandibular tumors
- Believed to have both epithelial and mesothelial elements
- Now appears to arise from ductal myoepithelial cells
- Male:female ratio approximately equal
- May undergo malignant change but risk is small
- Requires excision with 5 to 10 mm margin as local implantation of cells can lead to recurrence.

Warthin's Tumor (Papillary Cystadenoma) (Also known as Adenolymphoma)

- It is the second most common benign tumor of the salivary gland
- Usually occurs in elderly patients
- Male:female ratio is approximately 4:1
- Accounts for 15 percent of parotid tumors
- Ten percent of tumors are bilateral
- Rare in other salivary glands, occurs almost exclusively in the parotid gland
- Produces a hot spot in Tc^{99} Pertechnetate scan, so a clear-cut diagnosis can be made preoperatively without biopsy
- Warthin's tumor never undergoes malignant change.
- Treatment of benign neoplasm is surgical excision of the affected gland or, in the case of parotid, excision of the superficial lobe with facial nerve dissection and preservation. The minimum surgical procedure for neoplasm of the parotid in superficial lobe is superficial parotidectomy.

Malignant Salivary Tumors

- Adenoid cystic, adenocarcinomas and squamous cell tumors are rare
- All are usually high grade tumors

- Prognosis is often poor regardless of treatment
- Adenoid cystic tumors have tendency for perineural spread into the brain
- Also develop distant metastases to the lung
- Cannon-ball metastases may be present for years without symptoms
- Overall 5-year survival is approximately 50 percent.

Sialosis (Asymptomatic Parotid Enlargement)

Sialosis is the term given to a condition characterized by non-neoplastic, noninflammatory chronic or recurrent enlargement of the salivary glands. It most commonly involves the parotid glands and is associated with many conditions, including malnutrition, alcoholic cirrhosis, diseases of the endocrine glands including diabetes, with the administration of certain drugs, and with excessive starch ingestion. Sialosis is probably the commonest disturbance of the parotid glands in adults. *Salivary gland scintigraphy* can be very helpful in distinguishing between sialosis and involvement of the salivary glands by Sjögren's syndrome.

SPINE RADIOLOGY

Imaging modalities

Plain Radiography

The standard frontal and lateral films are useful in detecting bony abnormality, alignment and fractures. Obviously they do not demonstrate the soft tissues of the spine (e.g. disk, cord or ligaments) and are therefore of limited use.

Computed Tomography

Usually the patient lies in the computed tomography (CT) scanner. The scout view is obtained and then selected levels are scanned axially. If the slices are thin enough, good quality sagittal reformation can be performed. In trauma, CT is useful in detecting fractures and bony fragments. It is of limited sensitivity for imaging the soft tissues and is therefore sometimes performed after myelography (CT myelogram). However, in most centres magnetic resonance imaging (MRI) is preferred for imaging the soft tissues. Occasionally intravenous contrast is given. In the postoperative patient this is usually to distinguish scarring from the normally enhancing dura and epidural tissue.

Magnetic Resonance Imaging

In many circumstances MRI is now the modality of choice for spinal imaging. Usually Ti- and T2-weighted images are obtained in the axial and sagittal planes. The soft tissue contrast and particularly cerebrospinal fluid/spinal cord distinction is good. This enables excellent visualization of disk, ligaments, spinal cord and nerve roots. The long scan times mean that motion artefacts can degrade the images considerably. However, quicker sequences are being developed to overcome this. MRI cannot be performed in the presence of certain contraindications' or in patients who are claustrophobic or too heavy for the scanner. In these circumstances, either myelography or CT are performed.

Myelography

Myelography has largely been superceded by MRI. It is an invasive procedure that necessitates a lumbar puncture (or even occasionally a lateral cervical puncture) and installation of nonionic water-soluble contrast media into the subarachnoid space. There is strict adherence to a maximum dose of contrast media. Cord compression, impingement and nerve root compression can be demonstrated. Side-effects include headache, fits and other contrast reactions. Infections and implantation dermoids are rare.

Angiography

Spinal angiography is only rarely performed. If an arteriovenous malformation is suspected from the MRI or myelogram then angiography can be used to confirm the diagnosis and possibly to perform therapeutic embolization. The spinal cord has a variable vascular anatomy. The spinal arteries usually arise from the intercostal and lumbar arteries. They can be selectively catheterized from a standard femoral approach. There is definite morbidity including ischemia of the cord.

Discography

This is an uncommon investigation of back pain rather than cord or nerve root symptoms. A spinal needle is introduced from the posterolateral approach (avoiding the spinal cord) into the annulus of the disk (usually lumbar) under fluoroscopic control. Contrast is introduced to demonstrate any herniation. The sensation at the time of injection is compared to the original symptoms in an attempt to localize the cause of the symptoms. This technique is also the preliminary to chemical nucleolysis when chymopapain is injected into the annulus.

Vertebral Lesions

D/D of Intervertebral Disk Calcification

- Acromegaly
- Alkaptonuria
- Amyloidosis
- Ankylosing spondylitis
- Chronic infection
- CPPD
- Degenerative disk disease
- DISH
- Gout (rare)
- Hemochromatosis
- Homocystinuria
- Hyperparathyroidism
- Spinal fusion
- Wilson's disease.

Normal Variant

Curvatures/Curves of Spine

A healthy adult spine has four curves when viewed from the side, located in the neck (cervical spine), midback (thoracic), low back (lumbar) and base of the spine (sacrum).

Upon entering the world, a newborn has only two curves in the spine: the midback and the base of the spine. These two curves are called the primary or *kyphotic* curves. They have an apex or "hump" at the back of the body. The curves in the neck and low back develop later and are termed secondary or *lordotic* curves. The curve in the cervical spine develops as the child begins to lift his head and the neck muscles are strengthened. The curve in the lumbar spine results as the child starts to crawl. **The lordotic curves have an apex at the front of the body.** These four curves — two primary and two secondary; are extremely important in the spine (both adult and child), for this is how the body handles the stress of gravity. If these curves do not exist, the body's center of balance is shifted, causing undue stress on the spinal column and spinal cord.

Scoliotic curves less than 30° at skeletal maturity tend not to progress regardless of curve pattern. Important prognostic factors in thoracic curves are the **Cobb angle**, apical vertebral rotation, and the Mehta angle. In lumbar curves, factors of prognostic value are the degree of apical vertebral rotation, the Cobb angle, the direction of the curve, and the relationship of the fifth lumbar vertebra to the iliac intercrest line.

Cupid's bow vertebra—two parasagittal posterior concavities on inferior aspect of vertebral body.

Congenital Anomalies of the Vertebral Bodies

- Asomia—absent vertebral body
- Hemivertebra (*Ventral sclerotome* defect)
- Butterfly vertebra—failure of fusion of lateral halves (complete cleft in the vertebral body)
- Block vertebra—congenital vertebral fusion
- Bar vertebra.

'H' Shaped Vertebra

Basically cortical infarction of blood supply results in 'H' shaped vertebral bodies in which the central portion is compressed from subchondral infarcts, seen characteristically in **Sickle cell disease** and other anemias and Gaucher disease.

Striated (Vertical Striations)/Corduroy/Accordion/Honey Comb Vertebra

Vertebral hemangioma.

(*Note:* 'Polka-dot' sign → small punctate sclerosis in the vertebral body on CT scan is diagnostic of vertebral hemangioma)

Vertebra Plana/Wafer Thin Vertebra/Dollar Vertebra (Pneumonic → FETISH)

- **F**racture (trauma, osteogenesis imperfecta)
- **E**osinophilic granuloma
- **T**umor (metastasis, myeloma, leukemia)
- **I**nfection
- **S**teroids (avascular necrosis)
- **H**emangioma.

Ivory Vertebra

- Lymphoma
- Osteoblastic secondaries

- Sickle cell disease
- Trauma
- TB spine
- Fluorosis
- Renal osteodystrophy
- Osteopetrosis
- Myelosclerosis
- Multiple myeloma
- Chordoma
- Chronic sclerosing osteomyelitis of Garre
- Hemangioma
- Osteosarcoma
- Paget's disease.

"Picture Frame" Vertebra

Paget's disease.

"Square-shaped" Vertebra

Ankylosing spondylitis (occurs due to Romano's lesion, i.e. vertebral body ostitis and anterior longitudinal ligament calcification).

Limbus Vertebra

PID (Intraosseous herniation of disk material at the junction of vertebral body rim of central part and end plate).

"Sandwich"/"Hamburger" Vertebrae (Sclerotic End plates Alternate with Radiolucent Mid Bodies)

- Osteopetrosis
- Myelofibrosis.

"Bullet Shaped" Vertebra

- Hypothyroidism

- Achondroplasia
- Morquio syndrome.

"Fish Mouth"/Biconcave Vertebra

- Osteomalacia
- Osteoporosis
- Paget's disease
- Hyperparathyroidism
- Gaucher disease.

"Beak-shaped" Vertebra

Mucopolysaccharidosis.

"Wedge-shaped" Vertebra

Osteoporosis
Trauma.

"Pancake" Vertebra

Overall flattening of vertebra seen in osteoporosis.

Ghost (Bone within Bone) Vertebra

Follows stressful event during vertebral growth phase in childhood
- Stress line of unknown cause
- Leukemia
- Heavy metal poisoning
- Hypothyroidism
- Hypoparathyroidism
- Scurvy
- Rickets
- TB.

"Winking-owl" Eye Sign

Metastasis in spine (pedicles).

Anterior Scalloping of Vertebra

- Multiple myeloma
- Aortic aneurysm
- Lymphadenopathy
- TB.

Posterior Scalloping of Vertebra

- Dermoid/lipoma
- Meningioma/ependymoma
- Neurofibromatosis
- Marfan syndrome
- Ankylosing spondylitis
- Acromegaly
- Syringohydromyelia
- Hydrocephalus
- Achondroplasia
- Mucopolysaccharidoses
- Ehlers-Danlos syndrome.

Causes of anterior scalloping of vertebra
- Aortic aneurysm
- Lymphadenopathy
- Tuberculosis
- Multiple myeloma.

Causes of posterior scalloping of vertebra
- Communicating hydrocephalus
- Ependymoma
- Dermoid lipoma
- Ankylosing spondylitis
- Posterior meningocele

- Achondroplasia
- Neurofibromatosis
- Marfan syndrome
  - Ehlers-Danlos syndrome
  - Mucopolysaccharidoses.

Cervical Spine Trauma/Injury

Fractures limited to the vertebral body or posterior elements are considered *stable*; those involving both the vertebral body and posterior elements are considered *unstable*.

Hyperflexion Injury (Most Common Mechanism of Injury)

- Odontoid fracture
- Simple wedge fracture (stable)
- Teardrop fracture (unstable)
- Bilateral facet lock (unstable)
- Spinous process fracture (**Clay Shoveler's fracture** C6, C7/T1) (stable)
- Anterior subluxation.

Hypertension Injury

- Extension teardrop fracture
- Neural arch fracture of C1
- Subluxation
- **Hangman's fracture** (unstable, traumatic spondylolisthesis of C2 over C3).

Flexion Rotation Injury

- Unilateral facet lock (**Bowtie sign** on lateral view and **naked facet sign** on CT).

Vertical Compression

- Jefferson's fracture (comminuted burst fracture C1)
- (Pseudo-Jefferson → Lateral offset of lateral masses of C_1 without fracture of C1)
- **Minimum study for cervical trauma includes:**
  AP open mouth projection

AP lower cervical spine
Right and left oblique
Lateral view.

- **Additional projections required may be**
Swimmer's lateral view to demonstrate C7—T2 more clearly
Flexion and extension lateral cervical projections to evaluate atlanto-axial stability and intersegmental motion. Pillar view to demonstrate articular pillars, facet joints.
Devis series (seven views)
With the history of trauma and suspected fracture/dislocation, least movement of cervical spine or no movement of cervical spine should be done, hence, cross table lateral instead of upright lateral is preferable.

> With the history of trauma and cervical fracture/dislocation least movement of cervical spine or no movement of cervical spine should be done hence cross table lateral is ideal view, as the neck is not moved and stabilization is not hampered. Most initial treatment is hard cervical collar and bed rest. But in a patient with cervical spine (C5-C6) fracture dislocation, it being unstable cervical spine injury will require instrument fixation.

Failure to visualize the seventh cervical vertebra and the CT/T1 junction is the most common error made in the radiographic assessment of cervical spine injury.

Fractures of atlas are quite common and at times are radiographically obscure. Therefore, C2 should be scrutinized for evidence of injury in every case.

Fractures of odontoid are quite common, the diagnosis of which is often difficult because the fractures are minimally displaced and therefore obscure.

Fractures of First Cervical Vertebra, i.e. Atlas

Relatively uncommon
Two types known
- Most common type is an isolated fracture (nondisplaced and bilateral) of the posterior or neural arch of the atlas (hyperextension injury), which is mechanically stable and neurologically benign.
- **Jefferson fracture** is an common injury characterized by disruption of the anterior and posterior arches of the atlas, which results from force delivered to the top of the skull when the force is transmitted through the occipital condyles to the superior articular surfaces of atlas resulting in fracture disruption. However, neuronal loss (quadriplegia) is unlikely to occur.

- CT is best means of visualizing the fracture sites.
- Fusion of vertebrae may be required for treatment.

Fractures of Second Cervical Vertebra, i.e. Axis

Quite common
May be radiographically obscure

Types
- Hangman's fracture dislocation of neural or posterior arch of C2 produced by hyperextension force in judicial hanging. Often associated with dislocation of C2 on C3, hence it is also known as traumatic spondylolysis of axis
- Fracture of odontoid/dens fractures
- Extension tear drop fracture of anteroinferior corner of the body of C2 avulsed by the intact anterior longitudinal ligament
- Rotational subluxation or physiological dislocation of atlantoaxial relationship.

Tubercular Spondylitis or Pott's Spine

It is infection and destruction of the vertebral body and intervertebral disk by *Mycobacterium tuberculosis* (named after a surgeon in London, **Percival Pott, 1714–1788**, who also worked out the association of scrotal cancer with coal tar in chimney sweepers).

Incidence: It accounts for about 25 to 60 percent of skeletal TB.

Age and sex: Children and adults; M > F

Location: Upper lumbar and lower thoracic spine (L_1 most common); typically more than one vertebra affected. In 80 percent cases vertebral body is affected, with predilection for anterior part adjacent to end plates.

Spread
- Hematogenous via Batson's paravertebral venous plexus
- Contiguous into the disk by penetrating subchondral and cartilaginous end plates.
- Subligamentous spread beneath the anterior and posterior longitudinal ligaments to the adjacent vertebrae.
  Pulmonary lesions are not seen in about 50 percent of these patients.

Radiological Features

Spine radiograph
- Demineralization (**the first sign**)
- Mild contour irregularity of anterior and lateral aspect of vertebral body due to erosion from subligamentous extension of tubercular abscess (**gouge effect**)
- Loss of the intervertebral disk space (however, maintained longer than in pyogenic arthritis)
- Collapse of vertebral body, angular kyphotic deformity (**gibbus**)
- **"Vertebra within vertebra"** appearance (growth recovery lines)
- **Ivory vertebra** (due to reossification as healing response to osteonecrosis)
- Anterolateral scalloping of vertebral bodies
- Large fusiform paraspinal bulge due to cold abscess in paravertebral gutters/psoas, commonly bilateral. The abscess may extend into groin and thigh
- Amorphous/teardrop-shaped **calcification in paraspinal region** (nontuberculous abscess rarely calcifies)

MRI is the **investigation of choice** for diagnosis of the disease and evaluation of its complications.

Complications of Pott's Spine

- Kyphoscoliosis
- Bony ankylosis
- Osteonecrosis
- Spinal cord compression from abscess, granulation tissue, bone fragments and arachnoiditis
- Extensive spread of abscess
- Amyloidosis.

Tubercular spondylitis is known as Pott's disease. The others in the spectrum of skeletal tuberculosis include:
- Infection in appendicular skeleton
- Caries sicca (shoulder joint TB)
- Spina ventosa (tubercular dactylitis)
- Pott's puffy tumor (solitary tubercular focus with button sequestrum and cold abscess in scalp and calvarium)
- Weaver's bottom (tuberculous subgluteal bursitis).

Chapter 11

Obstetrics and Gynecological Radiology

ULTRASONOGRAPHY IN PREGNANCY

By transvaginal ultrasonography (TVS) the earliest sign of pregnancy in the form of gestational sac seen at 5th menstrual week, corresponds to predicted β-hCG levels of 1000 mIU/mL.

Mean gestational sac diameter by TVS (mm)	Predicted age (weeks)	Predicted hCG range (mIU/mL)
2 (Earliest seen)	5.0	629–2188
6	5.5	1226–4256
10	6.0	2483–8075
14	6.5	4894–15726
18	7.0	9343–31621
22	7.5	17560–64570

- For USG in pregnancy frequency of USG probe used is 3.5 to 5 MHz.
- The earliest embryonic structure, however, is yolk sac that is detectable by USG, which can be seen using TVS during 5th menstrual week itself.
- The earliest unequivocal sign of pregnancy using sonographic evaluation is demonstration of the "gestational sac".
- The gestation in the uterine cavity starts with formation of choriodecidual layer after blastocyst implantation into the endometrium surrounded by echogenic gestational sac measuring 0.1 mm

known as **intradecidual sign** where endometrial thickening occurs first, followed by visualization of following on the ultrasound study:
- Gestational sac w/o embryo or yolk sac = 5 weeks
- Gestational sac + yolk sac w/o embryo= 5.5 weeks
- Heart beat embryo < 5 mm = 6 weeks
• Recording the presence or absence of fetal life can generally be accomplished by real-time ultrasound by 6th week (TAS) or 5th week (TVS) counting from first day of last menstrual period.
• The routine use of Doppler in pregnancy remains controversial, with concern about the increased power intensities when compared with imaging levels and with the widespread use of TVS.

Transvaginal sonographic landmarks	
Menstrual age	Landmark
4 weeks	Choriodecidual thickening; chorionic sac
5 weeks	Chorionic sac (5–15 mm); yolk sac/embryo complex
6 weeks	Embryonic heart motion seen
7 weeks	Embryo/fetal movement; prominent rhombencephalon
8 weeks	Physiologic bowel herniation; arms and legs seen

TRANSVAGINAL USG

Transvaginal USG (TVS) is more informative in first trimester. In TVS, images are of enhanced quality (5–7.5 MHz transducer). Full bladder is not required. Fetal heart sounds are audible as early as 10th week. It is superior to transabdominal USG in placenta previa. Use of transvaginal probe can detect the following events by one week earlier than transabdominal.

14d–Fertilization
18d–Conceptus enters uterus (morula)
20d–Blastocyst
23rd–Implantation and primary yolk sac

Detection of fetal structures by ultrasound		
Fetal structure	TVS	TAS
Gestational sac	4½ weeks (2–3 mm)	5 weeks (5 mm)
Double decidual sign	—	5 weeks
Yolk sac	5 weeks	6–7 weeks
Fetal heart beat	5½ weeks	6½ weeks
Embryo	6 weeks	6–7 weeks
Head	8 weeks	9 weeks
Ventricles	8½ weeks	11 weeks
Fetus	—	10 weeks (30–35 mm)
Face	—	10 weeks
4-chamber heart	—	16 weeks
Spine	7–8 weeks	12 weeks

Ideal Time for US

First trimester—8–9 weeks
Second trimester—18–20 weeks

Best for gestation age—1st trimester US
1st trimester: CRL
2nd trimester: BPD
3rd trimester: FL, HC

- Double decidual sac sign — 2 concentric echogenic rings surrounding at least a part of gestational sac (decidua parietalis + decidua capsularis).
- Pseudogestational sac — ectopic pregnancy — single echogenic layer of decidua surrounding endometrial cavity fluid collection.

Parameters for Estimation of Fetal Age by Ultrasound

Gestational sac size
- Parameter used for dating between 6 and 12 weeks menstrual age. Identified as early as 5 weeks on transabdominal scan.
- *Accuracy*: 7 days.

- CRL (crown-rump length)
  - Used up to 12 weeks MA
  - Identified by 7 weeks MA on transabdominal scan
  - Accuracy: 5–7 days
- Biparietal diameter (BPD)
  - Excellent parameter for estimating GA in 2nd trimester > 12 weeks MA.
  - Less reliable for dating in 3rd trimester because of increasing biologic variability.
- Abdominal circumference (AC)
  - Measured at level of vascular junction of umbilical vein with left portal vein ("hockey-stick" appearance)
  - Better predictor of fetal weight than BPD.
- Femur length (FL)
  - The length of diaphysis of fetal femur is often used for gestational age prediction and given accurate estimate of gestational age in third trimester.

Variability Associated with Fetal Age: Estimates Derived from Anatomic Parameters

Parameter	Age variability (weeks)			
	6–14	12–18	24–30	36–42
CRL	±0.4	–	–	–
BPD	–	±1.2	±2.2	±3.2
FL	–	±1.6	±2.8	±4.0
HC	–	±1.2	±2.1	±2.7
AC	–	±1.7	±2.2	±3.0
BPD, HC, AC, FL	–	±1.1	±1.8	±2.3

Umbilical Cord

The umbilical cord normally contains three vessels—two arteries and a vein, which are protected by Wharton's jelly. It is important to document the number of vessels in the cord. *Single umbilical artery* occurs in up to one percent of cases. Ten to twenty percent of these cases have malformations including:
- Trisomies 13 and 18
- Anomalies of the urinary tract, central nervous system and heart
- Omphalocele

- Sirenomelia, and
- VATER association.

Human Placenta

- It is discoid, deciduate and **hemochorial.**
- It develops from—fetal (4/5th)—chorionic frondosum and maternal (1/5th) decidua basalis.
- Its development begins at 6th week of gestation and is completed by 12th week.

Placental demonstration, localization, and distinguishing it from surrounding portions of chorion and the underlying myometrium is generally possible form 12 weeks gestation onward.

PATHOLOGICAL CONSIDERATION IN OBSTETRICS USG

Complications of Early Pregnancy

- Blighted ovum
  - Gestation sac with no yolk sac or fetal pole
  - TVS: Sac diameter > 20 mm with no yolk sac
- Missed abortion
  - Fetus smaller than expected for sac size
  - Fetus formless
  - Embryo >6 mm with no evidence of cardiac pulsations
- Incomplete abortion
- Inevitable abortion
  - Gestational sac and fetus detach from implantation site and lie in lower uterine segment
  - Cx dilated
- Ectopic pregnancy
- Hydatidiform mole
  - Normal sac growth rate—1.1 mm/d
  - Normal hCG doubling time—48 hours.

Polyhydramnios

Definition: Polyhydramnios means amniotic fluid volume more than 1,500 to 2,000 cu cm at term.

USG features:
- Single largest pocket devoid of fetal parts/cord > 8 cm in vertical direction
- Amniotic fluid index (AFI) 20–24 cm.

Intrauterine Growth Retardation

Although no single criterion permits confident diagnosis of intrauterine growth retardation (IUGR) (here history of smoking relates), there are three key parameters that can be used in combination to establish the diagnosis with greater certainty:
1. Estimated fetal weight (using AC, corrected BPD and femur length)
2. Amniotic fluid volume
3. Maternal blood pressure status.

However, it is generally accepted that the size of fetal trunk correlates most strongly with the overall size of fetus and that an abdominal weight can be calculated from the measured abdominal circumference. Using estimated fetal weight to identify babies below 10th percentile gives positive predictive value of 55 percent at 38 weeks.

Doppler ultrasonography can be used to assess uteroplacental and fetal blood flow. This can be accomplished by using either continuous-wave or pulsed (duplex) Doppler.

With continuous-wave Doppler, a waveform arising from the umbilical arteries is identified. This waveform can be quantified by calculating the systolic-diastolic ratio and comparing it with established values. In some cases of intrauterine growth retardation (IUGR) due to uteroplacental insufficiency, the systolic-diastolic ratio will be elevated.

Even though the predictive value of continuous-wave Doppler for IUGR is relatively low, reversed diastolic flow has important implications because these fetuses are usually severely hypoxic.

Recent studies have also used color Doppler sonography to obtain a waveform from the middle of the cerebral artery of the fetus. In head-spared IUGR, diastolic flow to the brain is increased, an indication that the head is spared from the diminished flow to the body.

Intrauterine Fetal Death (IUD)

- Specific signs of fetal death is absent cardiac/somatic motion
- Nonspecific signs of fetal death (not seen before 48 hours after death):
  - Spalding sign—overlapping fetal skull bones
  - 'Halo' sign of head—due to scalp edema
  - Dolichocephaly

- Same/decreased BPD measurement compared with prior exam
- Gas in fetal vascular system
- Skin edema and fetal maceration
- Increased echoes in amniotic fluid.
• Vanishing twin—disappearance of one twin *in utero* due to complete resorption/anembryonic pregnancy
• Fetus papyraceous—compression and mummification of one fetus with risk also to the surviving fetus.

Immune Hydrops Fetalis (Erythroblastosis Fetalis): Features

- Anasarca (skin edema)
- Fetal ascites
- Pleural effusion
- Pericardial effusion
- Hepatosplenomegaly
- Placentomegaly (>6 cm)
- Increased umbilical vein diameter
- Increased flow in MCA.

Placental enlargement is not a feature of nonimmune hydrops fetalis.

Cystic Hygroma

It is a congenital malformation of the lymphatic system resulting in a uni- or multi-loculated fluid-filled mass. It is most often located in the posterior neck and is frequently associated with Turner's syndrome (XO karyotype). The lymphatic abnormality may be localized or may occur in conjunction with more generalized lymphedema. Sonographically, a thin-walled cystic lesion is seen, often with fine septations. In the generalized form, skin thickening, pleural effusions, and ascites may be seen.

Posterior Urethral Valve

Varying degree of chronic urethral obstruction due to fusion and prominence of plicae colliculi, normal concentric folds of urethra.

Posterior urethral valve is the most common obstructive uropathy seen in male child and can be reliably diagnosed by ANC ultrasound.

Bilateral hydronephrosis of varying degree, distended bladder and posterior urethra in a male fetus is highly suggestive of PU valve on ANC ultrasound.

Ultrasound Marker is Associated with Greatest Increased Risk for Trisomy 21 in Fetus

Nuchal fold thickening (edema) of ≥6 mm is the most sensitive and specific single marker of mid-trimester detection of Down syndrome.

Ultrasound markers of trisomy	
Major markers	*Minor markers*
Nuchal fold edema	Brachycephaly
Major cardiac anomaly	Clinodactyly
Choroid plexus cysts	Duodenal atresia
Short femur and/or humerus	Flat facies
Pyelectasis ≥4 mm	Hypoplasia of 5th digit
Hyperechoic bowel	Sandal gap toes
Echogenic intracardiac focus	Ventriculomegaly
	Wide iliac angle

Hydrocephalus

Obstetric ultrasound study is one of the best methods for antenatal diagnosis of hydrocephalus as it is noninvasive and hazard-free not only to fetus but also to mother.

However, assessment prior to GA of 20 weeks may be difficult, as ventricles constitute a large portion of cranial vault.

Signs suggestive of fetal hydrocephalus on obstetric USG study are
- Atrial size >10 mm
- Dangling "choroid plexus" sign
- Banana sign
- Lemon sign
- BPD > 95th percentile
- ± Polyhydramnios.

Neural Tube Defects

Incidence 1:500 = 600 live births

Recurrence risk = 3 to 4 percent

It includes:
- Spina bifida
- Anencephaly
- Acrania
- Encephalocele
- Porencephaly
- Hydranencephaly
- Iniencephaly
- Microcephaly
- Corpus callosal agenesis
- Lissencephaly
- Arachnoid cyst
- Choroid plexus cyst
- Vein of Galen aneurysm.

Following are the appropriate methods according to the duration of pregnancy for antenatal diagnosis of certain chromosomal and neuronal anomalies:
- 8–10 weeks = Chorionic venous sampling (CVS)
- 12–11 weeks = Amniocentesis
- 16 weeks to term = Percutaneous umbilical blood sampling (PUBS).

Anencephaly

It is the most common congenital defect of CNS resulting due to failure of closure of the rostral end of the neural tube by 5 to 6 weeks. Incidence is 1 in 1000 births and recurrence rate 3 to 5 percent.

The main sonographic feature of anencephaly is symmetric absence of the skull vault, and the cerebral hemispheres but relative preservation of brainstem and portion of midbrain. Although on ultrasonographically the diagnosis can be suspected by 12 to 13 weeks of gestation, it is more reliable by around 15 to 16 weeks, when the ossification in normal calvarial bones is more obvious.

Ectopic Pregnancy

It means implantation outside the endometrial cavity presenting with classical clinical triad:
(a) Pelvic pain, (b) Abnormal PV bleeding, and (c) Palpable adnexal mass.

Location:
- Tubal (95%)
  - Ampullary (75–80%)
  - Isthmic (10–15%)
  - Fimbrial (5%)
  - Cornual/interstitial (2–4%)
- Other (5%)
  - Abdominal
  - Ovarian
  - Interligamentary
  - Cervical

USG features:

Uterus
- Absence of intrauterine pregnancy
- Thickening of endometrium (hyperechoic)
- Sloughing of endometrium (decidual cast)
- Decidual cyst seen at junction of endometrium and myometrium
- Pseudogestational sac (single parietal decidual layer surrounding an anechoic fluid collection in uterine cavity secondary to bleeding).

Adnexa
- 'Tubal ring' (extrauterine hypoechoic sac-like structure surrounded by a concentric ring)
- Extrauterine mass—could be a solid/complex adnexal mass, a gestational sac without live embryo, an embryonic heartbeat (pathognomonic), an echogenic 'tubal' mass (89–100%) or a corpus luteum within ovary on the side of ectopic pregnancy.

Cul-de-sac: Free fluid (40–83%). Color Doppler US features:
- High velocity low-impedance flow around extrauterine gestation
- Absence of peritrophoblastic flow after 36 days
- However, low-impedance flow can also be seen in corpus luteum cyst, tubo-ovarian abscess and fibroid.

Transvaginal probe is best for confirming the presence of an ectopic pregnancy as it can detect an intrauterine gestational sac within the choriodecidual mass as early as 4 to 5 weeks, much earlier than with abdominal US. In addition, the presence of adnexal mass associated with an ectopic pregnancy can be shown in great detail. With TVS, a yolk sac can be seen within a gestational sac of 8 to 10 mm or more; an embryo is sac of 10 to 15 mm. On TVS, an unruptured ectopic pregnancy typically appears as a rounded complex adnexal mass (10–30 mm diameter), which is in close proximity to, but separate from, the uterus and ovaries. Occasionally, the decidualized endometrium becomes necrotic and simulates sonographic appearance of a malformed gestational sac.

Although absence of intrauterine pregnancy, thickening of endometrium, decidual cast and pseudogestational sac are the USG features of ectopic pregnancy, acute abdomen with empty uterus and free fluid in cul-de-sac, i.e. pouch of Douglas (93% positive predictive value) suggests diagnosis of ectopic pregnancy.

On color doppler study **'Ring of Fire' appearance** is characteristic of ectopic pregnancy.

Molar Pregnancy

Molar pregnancy includes complete and partial molar pregnancy. The classic USG features of complete molar pregnancy are well-known and include enlarged uterus containing echogenic tissue that expands endometrial canal (snowstorm appearance). The USG feature of partial molar pregnancy overlap with other conditions (missed or incomplete abortion). Gestational trophoblastic disease includes the tumor spectrum of hydatidiform mole, invasive mole and choriocarcinoma. Although US is used for initial diagnosis of GTD and to exclude normal pregnancy, findings are nonspecific.

Gestational Trophoblastic Neoplasms

Theses include the tumor spectrum of hydatidiform mole, invasive mole (choriocarcinoma destruens) and choriocarcinoma. The US appearance of hydatidiform mole is most commonly the presence of a hyperechoic to moderately echogenic central uterine (soft tissue) mass distending the endometrial canal and punctated by multiple small hypoechoic cystic spaces—correspond to hydropic villi. In 25 percent cases atypical appearance in the form of central area of heterogeneous echotexture (snow-storm appearance) may be seen. No fetal parts or chorionic membrane visible. Bilateral theca lutein cysts, which may take 4 months to regress after evacuation of a molar pregnancy, can be a feature. Uterine enlargement is the most common CT feature of gestational trophoblastic neoplasms (GTD) (ECT shows heterogeneous uterine enhancement and focal enlargement or irregular hypodense regions within myometrium). Extrauterine findings in form of bilateral theca lutein cysts and locoregional spread may be seen.

GYNECOLOGY

Modalities for Detection of Gynecologic Lesions

USG

It is considered one of the most sensitive modalities for detection of gynecologic lesions and is the imaging modality of choice in the initial evaluation of a pelvic mass. Relative advantages of US include its ready availability, lower cost, lack of ionizing radiation, and ability to scan rapidly in multiple planes. Its disadvantages include operator dependency, inability to evaluate adjacent bony structures, inability to adequately characterize tissue, and limiting patient factors such as obesity or incomplete bladder filling. US limitations also include occasional difficulty in separating a pelvic mass from bowel loops and differentiating adnexal from uterine masses.

Sonographically, the lower uterine segment and cervix normally have a **Y-shaped** configuration.

In the normal population, the mean cervical length is greater than 3 cm.

With transabdominal ultrasound cervical canal width (diameter of internal os) of 8 mm or more is abnormal.

On transvaginal sonography, an anteroposterior diameter of the internal os of > 5 mm before 30 weeks gestation is regarded as significant dilatation.

CT

The major use of CT is in staging advanced pelvic malignancies. CT is superior to US in demonstrating tumor involvement of the parametrium, pelvic sidewall, adjacent bony structures, and pelvic and para-aortic lymph nodes. Limitations of CT include the use of ionizing radiation and contrast material, limited tissue contrast resolution, and image degradation by metallic clips or prostheses.

MRI

It is a promising imaging modality in the evaluation of pelvic neoplasia. It provides superior tissue contrast and delineation between tumor and normal tissue compared to US and CT. MRI adds only minor additional information over US in the evaluation of cystic lesions and fluid collections; therefore, US remains the initial imaging modality because of lower cost and easy availability. MRI is the imaging modality of choice when supplemental information is needed following initial US if the sonogram is inadequate, if the origin of the pelvic mass is not established, or when evaluation of the full extent of a noncystic lesion is desired. In the differential diagnosis of recurrent tumor versus fibrosis, MRI can offer tissue specificity.

CEMRI

Contrast enhanced magnetic resonance imaging (CEMRI) is now supposed to be investigation of choice for preoperative evaluation of endometrial and cervical cancer.

It is helpful in differentiating adenomyomatosis from uterine fibroids.

Imaging of Carcinoma Cervix

CT is not useful in evaluation of clinical stage I and II disease because the attenuation values of cervical carcinoma and normal cervix are similar. Contrast enhanced magnetic resonance imaging (CEMRI) is most useful investigation for the preoperative evaluation of cervical carcinoma. The normal cervix appears as two distinct zones, an inner high signal intensity zone (endocervical canal) and an outer low signal intensity zone (fibrous stroma). It may occasionally have three zones similar to those of the uterus. On axial images, the lower cervix normally is a complete, **low-intensity ring**. If disrupted, this may serve as an important landmark for the identification of parametrial tumor extension. MRI is quite accurate in detecting tumor involvement of the vagina, parametrium, pelvic sidewall, bladder, or rectum. However, MRI may underestimate the extent of very superficial disease and cannot detect carcinoma in situ reliably. It has similar constraints in the detection of lymph node enlargement as CT, namely, that it cannot depict microscopic tumor involvement of normal-sized nodes or differentiate benign nodal enlargement from malignant lymph node enlargement.

OVARIAN NEOPLASMS

Histological Types of Ovarian Malignancies

- Tumors of surface epithelium (60–70%)
- Germ cell tumors (15–30%)
- Sex cord-stromal tumors (5–8%).

Incidence of Malignant Ovarian Neoplasms

- Serous cystadenocarcinoma, 40 percent
- Mucinous cystadenocarcinoma, 12 percent
- Endometrioid carcinoma, 15 percent
- Undifferentiated adenocarcinoma, 15 percent
- Clear-cell carcinoma (mesonephroma), 6 percent
- Granulosa-theca cell tumor, 3 percent

- Dysgerminoma, 1 percent
- Malignant teratoma, 1 percent
- Metastatic carcinoma, 5 percent.

Omental Caking

The thickened omentum produced by "caking" appears as a large soft tissue mass with poorly defined edges. Fat planes are obscured.

Following diagnostic signs characterize the lesions of mesentery/omentum according to their appearance:
1. Rounded masses – NHL (most common), leukemia and ovarian tumor (rare)
2. Ill-defined masses – NHL, carcinoma ovary (most common), colon, pancreas, stomach (rarely)
3. Cake-like masses – Ovarian tumors, NHL and leukemia
4. Stellate pattern – All types of metastatic disease except lymphomas and leukemias.
   75 percent ovarian neoplasms are benign,
   21 percent are malignant, 4 percent are borderline malignant.

Features Favoring Tumors of Surface Epithelium
- Propensity for early peritoneal and lymphatic spread
- Peritoneal studding
- Omental cake
- Perihepatic diaphragmatic implants

Features Favoring Malignant Ovarian Tumors
- Several internal (papillary) excrescences protruding from the septa (Spokewheel-like septations suggest mucinous cystadenocarcinoma)
- Completely solid lesion
- Solid tissue on the inner cyst wall (mural nodule)
- Primarily solid with irregular cystic areas, or thick-walled with necrotic centers
- Free pelvic fluid.

Dermoid Cyst or Mature Cystic Teratoma
- It is congenital benign germ cell tumor containing mature tissues from all three germ cell layers with predominance of ectodermal component.

- It is most common ovarian neoplasm and accounts for 66 percent of pediatric ovarian tumors.
- About 80 percent present in reproductive life (20–40 years)
- If acute pain due to torsion or hemorrhage or rupture soft pelvic mass difficult to palpate malignant change in 1 to 3 percent cases.
- May be bilateral in 8 to 25 percent cases.
- Histopathologically contains mature epithelial elements (skin, hair, teeth, desquamated epithelial), bone, may contain struma ovarii carcinoid.

Plain Film (Diagnostic in 40 Percent Cases)

- Tooth/bone
- Fat density.

USG (77–87 Percent Sensitivity)

- Complex mass containing echogenic components
- May be purely cyst
- May be predominantly solid.

Specific Features

- Tip of Iceberg sign (echogenic mass with "dirty" acoustic shadowing in a predominantly cystic mass)
- Fat-fluid level or hair-fluid level
- Dermoid mesh
- Dermoid plug may be seen (Rokitansky nodule/protuberance in the form of solid round mural nodule seen projecting into cystic lumen)
- Tooth.

CT

- Rounded mass of fat in cystic lesion
- Dermoid plug
- Fat fluid level in cyst
- Rim of calcification
- Tooth.

Chapter 12

Breast Imaging

- Modalities available for breast imaging include:
  - Mammography (Screening > Diagnostic)
  - Xeroradiography (outdated)
  - USG (cyst, abscess)
  - CT (High radiation dose and poor tissue resolution)
  - MRI (for young females, for breast silicon implants and for dense breast)
  - FDG-PET scan (for cancer recurrence, bone and lymph node metastasis)
  - Mammoscintigraphy
- Hard lump is likely to be malignant, unless proved otherwise. Mammography is basically a screening tool.
- Although on USG malignant lesions show characteristic features, it may not be confirmatory.
- CT scan chest is useful to rule out lung metastasis, obvious axillary adenopathy and local spread of malignancy, but is not a primary tool for diagnosing carcinoma breast.
- Open biopsy is almost 100 percent specific and sensitive method to confirm carcinoma breast.

DIAGNOSTIC MAMMOGRAPHY VERSUS SCREENING MAMMOGRAPHY

- Diagnostic mammography should not be confused with screening mammography, which is performed after a palpable abnormality has been detected. Diagnostic mammography is aimed at evaluating the rest of the breast before biopsy is performed or occasionally is part of the triple-test strategy to exclude immediate biopsy.

- Subtle abnormalities (like clustered microcalcifications, densities (especially if spiculated), and new or enlarging architectural distortion) that are first detected by screening mammography should be evaluated carefully by compression or magnified views.

Indications for Mammography

- Before breast surgery, as it may avert an unnecessary biopsy demonstrating that the palpable mass has a characteristically benign appearance.
- Follow-up of breast cancer patients.
- Workup a patient with metastases from an unknown primary.
- Mammographic screening is best screening method for carcinoma breast (Flow chart 12.1).

Mammographic Findings in Various Breast Diseases

Ductal carcinoma *in situ* (DCIS): MRI more sensitive than mammography

Comedo type = "snake skin like" dotted casting calcifications

Noncomedo type = Fine granular "cotton-ball" calcifications common. However, coarse granular "crushed stone" or "broken needle lip" or arrowhead calcification can be seen.

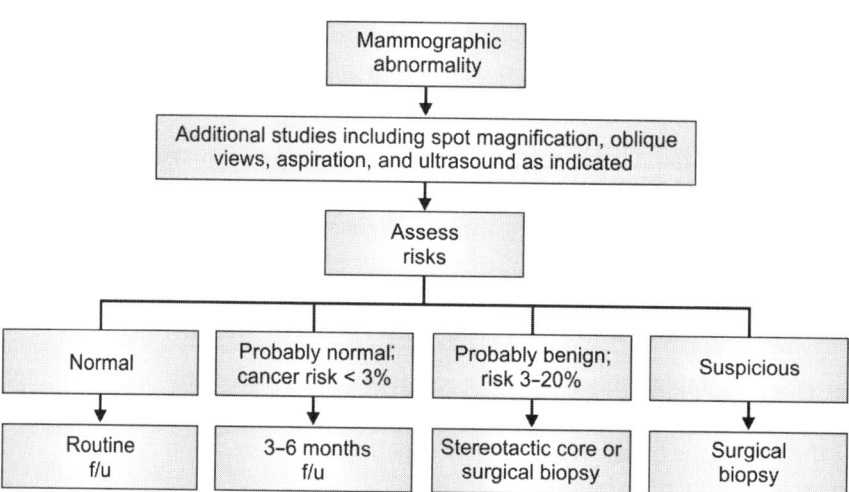

Flow chart 12.1: Mammography Algorithm

Carcinoma breast in all: The most common mammographic appearance of invasive carcinoma is a spiculated mass.
Other features are: Irregular border, microcalcification (30%), "sunburst" appearance, architectural distortion and high density mass.
Microcalcification represents the most sensitive mammographic sign of early breast cancer.
Cystosarcoma phylloides: Large noncalcified mass with fluid-filled clefts with smooth lobulated margins mimicking fibroadenoma.
Fat necrosis of breast: Ill-defined spiculated dense mass, and calcified only in 4 to 7 percent cases when it is called liponecrosis macrocystica calcifications (occasional eggshell/curvilinear calcification).
Fibroadenoma: Halo sign, "popcorn" type of calcifications (Pathognomonic) and on USG "hump and dip" sign.
Seborrheic keratosis is a cutaneous disease that can occur anywhere over the body with inframammary clefts being one of the known sites affected and on mammography one may see air lucencies trapped in the lesions.
Galactoceles are more frequently seen as mixed density lesions than radiolucent lesions. They may be managed by simple needle aspiration but in some cases this is difficult due to the thick consistency of the contents.

Radiographically, a galactocele is seen as single or multiple nodular lesions with a density equal to or less than that of the fibroepithelial tissue of the breast.

Mammographic Features of Breast Cancer

Sr No	Primary signs	Secondary signs
1.	High density irregular opacification	Disruption of architecture
2.	Microcalcification	Perifocal haziness
3.	Mammographic lesion less in size than physically seen	–
4.	Irregular (spiculated) margins	

- The most common mammographic appearance of invasive carcinoma is a "spiculated" mass.
- "Microcalcifications" may be seen in 30 percent cases of invasive carcinoma and 95 percent of cases of DCIS (granular and casting).
- Its "sunburst" appearance readily distinguishes it from benign breast masses.
- Often the tumor mass itself may not be visible, so that the only evidence of carcinoma is the presence of abnormal trabecular markings, i.e. "distorted architecture".

- Individual straight dense spicules with central solid mass which has little change in different views known as "white star" stellate or spiculated breast lesion favors malignancy.
- Well-defined nodules < 1 cm are of low risk for cancer.
- 'Halo' sign of apparent lucency due to optical illusion of Mach effect + true radiolucent halo is almost always benign.
- Fat containing lesions are never malignant.
- Granular calcification (amorphous, dot like/elongated, fragmented, grouped very closely to each other) and casting calcification (fragmented cast of calcification within ducts) favor malignancy.

Overall detection rate of carcinoma breast by mammography is 58 to 69 percent and 8 percent only if < 1 cm in size. Hence, mammography is a screening modality and not the best diagnostic measure.

The **BIRADS (Breast Imaging Reporting and Dictation System)** lexicon was developed by the American College of Radiology to provide a clear and concise way to report mammographic results:

1 = normal, 2 = benign finding, 3 = probably benign finding (6 months follow-up mammogram recommended); 4 = suspicious finding (biopsy recommended); 5 = high likelihood of malignancy (biopsy recommended); and 6 = confirmed malignancy.

Ultrasound Features of Breast Cancer

- Spiculations
- Taller than wide
- Angular margins
- Acoustic shadowing
- Branch pattern
- Markedly hypoechoic
- Calcifications
- Duct extension
- Microlobulation.

- **Lymphoma** is more common on right side presenting as mass with poorly defined borders but no calcification or spiculations seen, although bilateral axillary adenopathy is seen in 30 to 50 percent cases.
- **Phylloides** tumor is usually huge lobulated noncalcified mass.

MRI Breast

- **Magnetic resonance imaging (MRI)** appears to be very sensitive in the visualization of both invasive carcinoma and DCIS. Perhaps, most importantly, *MRI can detect invasive and noninvasive breast carcinoma that is both mammographically and clinically occult*, offering the potential for more accurate breast cancer staging and optimized treatment planning.
- **Magnetic resonance imaging (MRI)** is emerging as perhaps the most promising imaging investigation for breast cancer detection to date.
- **Positron emission tomography (PET)** may not yet be sensitive enough for small occult lesions mammographically detected by screening. However, it has been advocated as a means of staging larger tumors. It certainly should develop a major role in the difficult distinction between fibrotic disease and active tumor in the patient with abnormal anatomical features (on CT or MRI) after treatment.

Breast MRI–Key Indications

- It is 2nd choice in differentiation between postoperative scarring and local recurrence, provided enough time has elapsed to allow treatment-related enhancement to settle.
- It has an important role in the assessment of the indeterminate mass because of its very high sensitivity for malignancy, though at present, core biopsy is a more cost-effective approach.
- It is very accurate in the local staging of breast cancer in difficult cases (*very dense breasts, mammographically occult tumors, suspected multifocality or multicentricity and suspected chest wall involvement*).
- It is the technique of choice in the evaluation of implant integrity and detection of cancer in the augmented breast.
- It is also accurate in the differentiation of axillary recurrence and brachial plexopathy post-radiotherapy.
- Breast MRI appears highly accurate in the assessment of response to neoadjuvant and primary chemotherapy, predicting ultimate response before changes in tumor volume and differentiating between residual tumor and fibrosis.

Note: Fat within a breast lesion favors benignity!

Important Differential Diagnosis in Breast Diseases

Differential Diagnosis of Fat Containing Breast Lesions

- Lipoma
- Oil cyst

- Galactocele = fluid with high lipid content (last phase)
- Hamartoma
- Traumatic fat necrosis (cyst)
- Focal collection of normal breast fat.

Mixed Fat and Water-density Lesion

- Fibroadenolipoma/hamartoma
- Intramammary lymph node
- Galactocele
- Hamartoma = Lipofibroadenoma = Fibroadenolipoma
- Small superficial hematoma.

Breast Lesion with 'Halo Sign'

- High-Density Lesion (vessels + parenchymal elements not visible in superimposed lesion)
  - Cyst
  - Sebaceous cyst
  - Wart
- Low-Density Lesion (vessels + parenchyma seen superimposed on lesion)
  - Fibroadenoma
  - Galactocele
  - Cystosarcoma phylloides.

Differential Diagnosis of Radiolucent Lesions

- Lipoma
- Oil cyst
- Galactocele.

Differential Diagnosis of Mixed Density Lesions

- Adenolipoma/hamartoma
- Galactocele
- Hamartoma
- Lymph node.

Calcification in Few Breast Diseases, on Mammography

Sr No	Type of calcification	Breast disease
1.	Coarse irregular 'popcorn' calcification	Benign lesions like fibroadenoma
2.	Eggshell calcification	Traumatic fat necrosis
3.	Tentacles, spicules	Scirrhous Ca
4.	Fine, irregular, polymorphic microcalcifications	Ca breast (Scirrhous Ca, intraductal Ca)
5.	Needle shaped	Plasma cell mastitis
6.	Crescentic or 'tea cup' like	Microcysts
7.	Amorphous lumps	Fat necrosis and scars
8.	Fine, smooth, punctate, spherical	Papilloma, sclerosing adenosis, epithelial hyperplasia

Triple Assessment: It includes
- Clinical examination
- Radiological examination (mammography)
- Pathological examination (FNAC-cytology).

Section 2

Nuclear Medicine

Chapter 13

Radioactivity and Basics of Nuclear Medicine

WHAT IS RADIOACTIVITY?

What causes Radioactivity?

As its name implies, radioactivity is the act of emitting radiation spontaneously. This is done by an atomic nucleus that for some reason, is unstable; it "wants" to give up some energy in order to shift to a more stable configuration. During the first half of the twentieth century, much of modern physics was devoted to exploring why this happens, with the result that nuclear decay was fairly well understood by 1960. Too many neutrons in a nucleus lead it to emit a negative beta particle, which changes one of the neutrons into a proton. Too many protons in a nucleus lead it to emit a positron (positively charged electron), changing a proton into a neutron. Too much energy leads a nucleus to emit a gamma ray, which discards great energy without changing any of the particles in the nucleus. Too much mass leads a nucleus to emit an alpha particle, discarding four heavy particles (two protons and two neutrons).

How is Radioactivity Measured?

Radioactivity is a physical, not a biological, phenomenon. Simply stated, the radioactivity of a sample can be measured by counting how many atoms are spontaneously decaying each second. This can be done with instruments designed to detect the particular type of radiation emitted with each "decay" or disintegration. The actual number of disintegrations per second may be quite large. Scientists have agreed upon common units to use as a form of shorthand. Thus, a curie (abbreviated "Ci" and named after Pierre and Marie Curie, the discoverers of radium[87]) is simply a shorthand way of writing

"37,000,000,000 disintegrations per second," the rate of disintegration occurring in 1 gram of radium. The more modern International System of Measurements (SI) unit for the same type of measurement is the becquerel (abbreviated "Bq" and named after Henri Becquerel, the discoverer of radioactivity), which is simply a shorthand for "1 disintegration per second."

What is Radioactive Half-life?

Being unstable does not lead an atomic nucleus to emit radiation immediately. Instead, the probability of an atom disintegrating is constant, as if unstable nuclei continuously participate in a sort of lottery, with random drawings to decide which atom will next emit radiation and disintegrate to a more stable state. The time it takes for half of the atoms in a given mass to "win the lottery"—that is, emit radiation and change to a more stable state is called the half-life. Half-lives vary greatly among types of atoms, from less than a second to billions of years. For example, it will take about 4.5 billion years for half of the atoms in a mass of uranium 238 to spontaneously disintegrate, but only 24,000 years for half of the atoms in a mass of plutonium 239 to spontaneously disintegrate. Iodine 131, commonly used in medicine, has a half-life of only eight days.

What is a Radioactive Decay Chain?

Stability may be achieved in a single decay or a nucleus may decay through a series of states before it reaches a truly stable configuration, a bit like a Slinky toy stepping down a set of stairs. Each state or step will have its own unique characteristics of half-life and type of radiation to be emitted as the move is made to the next state. Much scientific effort has been devoted to unraveling these decay chains, not only to achieve a basic understanding of nature, but also to design nuclear weapons and nuclear reactors. The unusually complicated decay of uranium 238, for example—the primary source of natural radioactivity on earth proceeds as follows:

- U-238 emits an alpha
- Thorium 234 emits a beta
- Protactinium 234 emits a beta
- Uranium 234 emits an alpha
- Thorium 230 emits an alpha
- Radium 226 emits an alpha
- Radon 222 emits an alpha
- Polonium 218 emits an alpha
- Lead 214 emits a beta

- Bismuth 214 emits a beta
- Polonium 214 emits an alpha
- Lead 210 emits a beta
- Bismuth 210 emits a beta
- Polonium 210 emits an alpha
- Lead 206, which is stable.

How can Radioactivity be caused Artificially?

Radioactivity can occur both naturally and through human intervention. An example of artificially induced radioactivity is neutron activation. A neutron fired into a nucleus can cause nuclear fission (the splitting of atoms). This is the basic concept behind the atomic bomb. Neutron activation is also the underlying principle of boron-neutron capture therapy for certain brain cancers. A solution containing boron is injected into a patient and is absorbed more by the cancer than by other cells. Neutrons fired at the area of the brain cancer are readily absorbed (captured) by the boron nuclei. These nuclei then become unstable and emit radiation that attacks the cancer cells. Simple in its basic physics, the treatment has been complex and controversial in practice and after half a century is still regarded as highly experimental.

WHAT IS AN ELEMENT?

What are Atomic Number and Atomic Weight?

Chemical behavior is what originally led scientists to classify matter into various elements. Chemical behavior is the ability of an atom to combine with other atoms. In more technical terms, chemical behavior depends upon the type and number of the chemical bonds an atom can form with other atoms. In classroom, kits for building models of molecules, atoms are usually represented by colored spheres with small holes for pegs and the bonds are represented by the small pegs that can connect the spheres. The number of peg holes signifies the maximum number of bonds that an atom can form; different types of bonds may be represented by different types of pegs. Atoms that have the same number of peg holes may have similar chemical behavior. Thus, atoms that have identical chemical behavior are regarded as atoms of the same element. For example, an atom is labeled, "carbon atom" as if it can form the same number, types and configurations of bonds as other carbon atoms. Although the basics are simple to explain, how atoms bind to each other becomes very complex when studied in detail; new discoveries are still being made as new types of materials are formed.

What is Atomic Number?

An atom may be visualized as a miniature solar system, with a large central nucleus orbited by small electrons. The bonding capacity of an atom is determined by the electrons. For example, atoms that in their normal state have one electron, are hydrogen atoms and will readily (and sometimes violently) bond with oxygen. This bonding capacity of hydrogen was the cause of the explosion of the airship Hindenburg in 1937. Atoms that in their normal state have two electrons are helium atoms, which will not bond with oxygen and would have been a better choice for filling the Hindenburg.

We can pursue the question back one step further: What determines the number of electrons and the number of protons in the nucleus of the atom. Here, the analogy between an atom and the solar system breaks down. The force that holds the planets in their orbits, is the gravitational attraction between the planets and the sun. However, in an atom what holds the electrons in their orbit, is the electrical attraction between the electrons and the protons in the nucleus. The basic rule is that like charges repel and opposite charges attract. Although a proton has more mass than an electron, they both have the same amount of electrical charge but opposite in kind. Scientists have designated electrons as having a negative charge and protons as having a positive charge. One positive proton can hold one negative electron in orbit. Thus, an atom with one proton in its nucleus normally will have one electron in orbit (and be labeled a hydrogen atom); an atom with ninety-four protons in its nucleus will normally have ninety-four electrons orbiting it (and be labeled a plutonium atom).

The number of protons in a nucleus is called the atomic number and always equals the number of electrons in orbit about that nucleus (in a nonionized atom). Thus, all atoms that have the same number of protons--the atomic number--are atoms of the same element.

What is Atomic Weight?

The nuclei of atoms also contain neutrons, that help to hold the nucleus together. A neutron has no electrical charge and is slightly more massive than a proton. Since a neutron can decay into a proton plus an electron (the essence of beta decay), it is sometimes helpful to think of a neutron as an electron and a proton blended together, although this is at the best of an oversimplification. Since a neutron has no charge, it has no effect on the number of electrons orbiting the nucleus. However, because it is even more massive than a proton, a neutron can add significantly to the weight of an atom. The total weight of an atom is called the atomic weight. It is approximately equal to the number of protons and neutrons with a little extra added by the electrons. The stability of the nucleus and hence the atom's radioactivity, is heavily dependent upon the number of neutrons it contains.

What are Isotopes?

The isotopes of an element are all the atoms that have in their nucleus, the number of protons (atomic number) corresponding to the chemical behavior of that element. However, the isotopes of a single element vary in the number of neutrons in their nuclei. Since they still have the same number of protons, all these isotopes of an element have identical chemical behavior. But since they have different numbers of neutrons, these isotopes of the same element may have different radioactivity. An isotope that is radioactive is called a radioisotope or radionuclide. Two examples may help to clarify this.

The most stable isotope of uranium, U-238, has an atomic number of 92 (protons) and an atomic weight of 238 (92 protons plus 146 neutrons). The isotope of uranium of greatest importance in atomic bombs, U-235, though, has three fewer neutrons. Thus, it also has an atomic number of 92 (since the number of protons has not changed) but an atomic weight of 235 (92 protons plus only 143 neutrons). The chemical behavior of U-235 is identical to all other forms of uranium but its nucleus is less stable, giving it higher radioactivity and greater susceptibility to the chain reactions that power both atomic bombs and nuclear fission reactors.

Another example is iodine, an element essential for health; insufficient iodine in one's diet can lead to a goiter. Iodine also is one of the earliest elements whose radioisotopes were used in what is now called nuclear medicine. The most common, stable form of iodine has an atomic number of 53 (protons) and an atomic weight of 127 (53 protons plus 74 neutrons). Because its nucleus has the "correct" number of neutrons, it is stable and is not radioactive. A less stable form of iodine also has 53 protons (this is what makes it behave chemically as iodine) but four extra neutrons, for a total atomic weight of 131 (53 protons and 78 neutrons). With "too many" neutrons in its nucleus, it is unstable and radioactive with a half-life of eight days. Since it behaves chemically as iodine, it travels throughout the body and localizes in the thyroid gland just like the stable form of iodine. As it is radioactive, its presence can be detected. Iodine 131 thus became one of the earliest radioactive tracers.

USEFUL TERMINOLOGIES

Atomic number → number of protons in nucleus (Z)
Neutron number → number of neutrons in nucleus (N)
Atomic weight or Mass number → number of mass particles in nucleus (A) (A = N + Z)
Neutron excess → excess of neutrons over protons (N–Z).

Isotopes:	Atoms having same atomic numbers, different mass numbers (hence different neutron number), e.g. $_{17}Cl^{35}$, $_{17}Cl^{37}$
Isobars:	Atoms having same mass number, different atomic number (hence different neutron number), e.g. $_{28}Ni^{64}$, $_{30}Zn^{64}$
Isotones:	Atoms having same neutron number, different atomic mass number, e.g. $19K^{39}$, $20Ca^{40}$
Isomers:	Atoms having same atomic and mass numbers but different energy states in nucleus.

How can Different Isotopes of an Element be Produced?

How can isotopes be produced—especially radioisotopes, which can serve many useful purposes. There are two basic methods: Separation and synthesis.

Some isotopes occur in nature. If radioactive, these usually are radioisotopes with very long half-lives. Uranium 235, for example, makes up about 0.7 percent of the naturally occurring uranium on the earth. The challenge is to separate this very small amount from the much larger bulk of other forms of uranium. The difficulty is that all these forms of uranium as they all have the same number of electrons, will have identical chemical behavior: They will bind in identical fashion to other atoms. Chemical separation, developing a chemical reaction that will bind only uranium atoms, will separate out uranium atoms but not distinguish among different isotopes of uranium. The only difference among the uranium isotopes, is their atomic weight. A method had to be developed that would sort atoms according to weight.

One initial proposal was to use a centrifuge. The basic idea is simple: Spin the uranium atoms as if they were on a very fast merry-go-round. The heavier ones will drift toward the outside faster and can be drawn off. In practice, the technique was an enormous challenge: The goal was to draw off that very small portion of uranium atoms that were lighter than their brethren. The difficulties were so enormous that the plan was abandoned in 1942. Instead, the technique of gaseous diffusion was developed. Again, the basic idea was very simple: The rate at which gas passed (diffused) through a filter depended on the weight of the gas molecules: Lighter molecules diffused more quickly. Gas molecules that contained U-235 would diffuse slightly faster than gas molecules containing the more common but also heavier U-238. This method also presented formidable technical challenges but was eventually implemented in the gigantic gas diffusion plant at Oak Ridge, Tennessee. In this process, the uranium was chemically combined with fluorine to form a hexafluoride gas prior to separation by diffusion. This is not a practical method for extracting radioisotopes for scientific and medical use. It was extremely expensive and could only supply naturally occurring isotopes.

A more efficient approach is to artificially manufacture radioisotopes. This can be done by firing high-speed particles into the nucleus of an atom. When struck, the nucleus may absorb the particle or become unstable and emit a particle. In either case, the number of particles in the nucleus would be altered, creating an isotope. One source of high-speed particles could be a cyclotron. A cyclotron accelerates particles around a circular race track with periodic pushes of an electric field. The particles gather speed with each push, just as a child swings higher with each push on a swing. When traveling fast enough, the particles are directed off the race track and into the target.

A cyclotron works only with charged particles. However, another source of bullets are the neutrons already shooting about inside a nuclear reactor. The neutrons normally strike the nuclei of the fuel, making them unstable and causing the nuclei to split (fission) into two large fragments and two to three "free" neutrons. These free neutrons in turn make additional nuclei unstable, causing further fission. The result is a chain reaction. Too many neutrons can lead to an uncontrolled chain reaction, releasing too much heat and perhaps causing a "meltdown." Therefore, "surplus" neutrons are usually absorbed by "control rods." However, these surplus neutrons can also be absorbed by targets of carefully selected material placed in the reactor. In this way, the surplus neutrons are used to create radioactive isotopes of the materials placed in the targets.

With practice, scientists using both cyclotrons and reactors have learned the proper mix of target atoms and shooting particles to "cook up" a wide variety of useful radioisotopes.

BASIC ISOTOPE NOTATION

The atom may be thought of as a collection of protons, neutrons, and electrons. The protons and neutrons are found in the nucleus and shells of electrons orbit the nucleus with discrete energy levels. The number of neutrons is usually designated by N. The number of protons is represented by Z (also called the atomic number). The atomic mass number or the total number of nuclear particles is represented by A and is simply the sum of N and Z.

In this instance, 131 refers to the total number of protons and neutrons in the nucleus. By definition, all isotopes of a given element have the same number of protons and differ only in the number of neutrons. For example, all isotopes of iodine have 53 protons.

INSTRUMENTATION

The most widely used imaging devices in nuclear medicine are the simple gamma scintillation (Anger) camera, single-photon emission (SPECT) capable gamma cameras, and positron emission (PET) scanners. Several other instruments are commonly used in the nuclear medicine laboratory, including the dose calibrator, well counter and thyroid probe.

Gamma Scintillation Camera

A gamma camera converts photons emitted by the radionuclide in the patient into a light pulse and subsequently into a voltage signal. This signal is used to form an image of the distribution of the radionuclide (organ imaging).

The basic components of a gamma camera system are the collimator, the scintillation crystal, an array of photomultiplier tubes (PMTs), preamplifiers, a pulse-height analyzer (PHA), digital correction circuitry, a cathode ray tube (CRT), and the control console. A computer and picture archiving systems (PACs) are also integral parts of the system. Gamma cameras may be classified as either analog or digital.

Collimator

The collimator is made of perforated or folded lead and is interposed between the patient and the scintillation crystal. It allows the gamma camera to localize accurately the radionuclide in the patient's body. Thus, the collimator is the "rate limiting" step in the imaging chain of gamma camera technology.

- A well counter is a cylindrical sodium iodide crystal with a hole drilled in it and a PMT on the end.
- A thyroid probe has a single sodium iodide crystal, a PMT on the end and a single-hole collimator.
- The dose calibrator is a gas-filled ionization chamber.
- A gamma camera has a single large, flat sodium iodide crystal and multiple PMTs.
- A GM counter has a gas-filled probe and is used to perform low-level surveys to detect small amounts of contamination. For high activities or dose-rate surveys, an air-filled ionization survey meter is used.
- SPECT myocardial perfusion acquisition is usually done over 180 degrees; for most other studies, 360-degree acquisition is used.
- SPECT reconstruction uses the same basic Fourier transformation back-projection method as does CT.

RADIONUCLIDES

Unsealed Radionuclides used for Therapy

- Phosphorus-32
- Yttrium-90

- Gold-198
- Iodine-131
- Strontium-89
- Samarium-153
- Rhenium-186.

Photon-emitting Radionuclides for Imaging

- Technetium-99m
- Molybdenum-99
- Iodine-123
- Iodine-131
- Xenon-133
- Gallium-67
- Indium-111
- Indium-113 m
- Thallium-201
- Krypton-81 m.

Half-life of Important Radionuclides

- I^{131} — 8 days
- I^{132} — 2.3 hours
- Co^{60} — 5.2 years
- Tc^{99} — 6 hours
- P^{32} — 14 days
- Thallium — 3 days
- Gallium — 3 days
- Rn^{22} — 3-6 days
- Strontium-87m — 2.8 hours
- Strontium-89 — 50.5 days
- Technetium-99m — 6.03 hours
- Thallium-201 — 73 hours
- Xenon-127 — 36.4 days
- Xenon-I33 — 5.3 days

Nuclide	Half-life	Decay mode	Major emissions (MeV)
Carbon-11	20.3 min	β+	γ 0.511 (200%)
Cesium-137	30 years	β-	γ 0.660 (85%)
Chromium-51	27.8 days	EC	γ 0.320 (10%)
Cobalt-57	270 days	EC	γ 0.122 (86%)
			γ 0.136 (11%)
Cobalt-58	71.3 days	EC and β+	γ 0.811 (99%)
			γ 0.511 (31%)
Cobalt-60	5.26 years	β-	γ 1.173 (100%)
			γ 1.332 (100%)
Fluorine-18	109 min	EC and β+	γ 0.511 (194%)
Gadolinium-153	240 days	EC	γ 0.100 (55%)
			γ 0.040
			γ 0.0481
Gallium-67	78.1 hours	EC	γ 0.093 (38%)
			γ 0.184 (24%)
			γ 0.296 (16%)
			γ 0.388 (4%)
Gallium-68	68.3 min	EC and β+	γ 0.511 (178%)
			γ 1.077 (3%)
Indium-111	67 hours	EC	γ 0.1 (90%)
			γ 0.247 (94%)
Iodine-123	13 hours	EC	γ 0.159 (83%)
Iodine-125	60 days	EC	γ 0.027 (76%)
Iodine-131	8.06 days	β-	γ 0.284 (6%)
			γ 0.364 (82%)
			γ 0.637 (7%)
			β 0.192 (90%)
Krypton-81m	13 sec	IT	γ 0.191 (66%)
Molybdenum-99	66.7 hours	β-	γ 0.181 (8%)
			γ 0.740 (14%)
			γ 0.778 (5%)
Nitrogen-13	10 min	β+	γ 0.511 (200%)
Oxygen-15	124 sec	β+	γ 0.511 (200%)
Phosphorus-32	14.3 days	β-	β 0.695 (100%)
Rhenium-186	90 hours	EC	γ 0.137
			β 0.349
Rubidium-82	1.3 min	EC and β+	γ 0.511 (189%)
			γ 0.777 (13%)

NUCLEAR STABILITY AND RADIOACTIVE DECAY

A given element may have many isotopes and some of these isotopes have unstable nuclear configurations of protons and neutrons. These isotopes often seek greater stability by decay or disintegration of the nucleus to a more stable form. Of the known stable nuclides, most have even numbers of neutrons and protons. Nuclides with odd numbers of neutrons and protons are usually unstable.

Nuclear instability may result from either neutron or proton excess. Nuclear decay may involve a simple release of energy from the nucleus or may actually cause a change in the number of protons or neutrons within the nucleus. When decay involves a change in the number of protons, there is a change of element. This is termed as a *transmutation*.

Several mechanisms of radioactive decay to achieve stability include:
- Alpha decay
- Beta decay
- Electron capture
- Isomeric transition.

Alpha-particle Emission

Alpha particle, consisting of two protons and two neutrons, is released from the nucleus, with a resulting decrease in the atomic mass number (A) by four and reduction of both Z and N *by* two. The mass of the released alpha particles is so great that they travel only a few centimeters in air and are unable to penetrate even thin paper. These properties cause alpha-particle emitters to be essentially useless for imaging purposes.

Alpha-Particles (Helium Nuclei)

They have relatively large mass (two protons and two neutrons) and this together with their double charge means that they travel relatively slowly through matter.

They have least penetrating power and even a piece of paper is enough to protect against most alpha particles.

They have highest ionization potential and produce a relatively large amount of ionization per unit length of track.

They serve no useful purpose in diagnostic radiography.

Beta-particle Emission

It is another process for achieving stability and is found primarily in nuclides with a neutron excess. In this case, a beta particle (electron) is emitted from the nucleus accompanied by an antineutrino; as a result, one of the neutrons may be thought of as being transformed into a proton, which remains in the nucleus. Thus, beta particle emission decreases the number of neutrons (N) by one and increases the number of protons (Z) by one, so that A remains unchanged. When Z is increased, the arrow in the decay scheme points toward the right and the downward direction indicates a more stable state. The energy spectrum of beta-particle emission ranges from a certain maximum down to zero; the mean energy of the spectrum is about one third of the maximum. A 2-MeV beta particle has a range of about 1 cm in soft tissue and is therefore, not useful for imaging purposes.

In cases in which there are too many protons in the nucleus (a neutron-deficient nuclide), decay may proceed in such a manner that a proton may be thought of as being converted into a neutron. This results in *positron* (W) *emission,* which is always accompanied by a neutrino. This obviously increases N by one and decreases Z by one, again leaving A unchanged. The downward arrow in the decay scheme again indicates a more stable state and its leftward direction indicates that Z is decreased. Positron emission cannot occur unless at least 1.02 MeV of energy is available. When positron emission occurs, the positron usually travels only a short distance and combines with an electron in an annihilation reaction. When this happens, two photons of 511 keV are emitted in opposite directions (annihilation radiation). This radiation can be imaged and results from the conversion of the masses of the positron and electron to energy.

Electron Capture

It occurs in a neutron-deficient nuclide when one of the inner orbital electrons is captured by a proton in the nucleus, forming a neutron and a neutrino. This can occur when not enough energy is available for positron emission, and electron capture is therefore an alternative to positron decay. Because a nuclear proton is essentially changed to a neutron, N increases by one and Z decreases by one; therefore, A remains unchanged. Electron capture may be accompanied by gamma emission and is always accompanied by characteristic radiation, either of which may be used in imaging.

Isomeric Transition

If in any of these attempts at stabilization, the nucleus still has excess energy, it may be emitted as nonparticulate radiation, with Z and N remaining the same. Any process in which energy is given as gamma rays and in which the numbers of protons and neutrons are not changed is called *isomeric transition.* An alternative to isomeric transition is *internal conversion*. In internal conversion, the excess energy of the nucleus is transmitted to one of the orbital electrons; this electron may be ejected from the atom, which is followed by characteristic radiation when the electron is replaced. This process usually competes with gamma-ray emission and can occur only if the amount of energy given to the orbital electron exceeds the binding energy of that electron in its orbit.

In many instances, a gamma-ray photon is emitted almost instantaneously after particulate decay. If there is a measurable delay in the emission of the gamma-ray photon and the resulting decay process is an isomeric transition, this intermediate excited state of the isotope is referred to as *metastable*. The most well-known metastable isotope is ^{99m}Tc (the *m* refers to metastable). This isotope decays by isomeric transition to a more stable state.

RADIONUCLIDE PRODUCTION

Most radioactive material that does not occur naturally can be produced by particulate bombardment or fission. Both methods alter the neutron to proton ratio in the nucleus to produce an unstable isotope. Bombardment essentially consists of the irradiation of the nuclei of selected target elements with neutrons in a nuclear reactor or with charged particles (alpha particles, protons or deuterons) from a cyclotron.

Cyclotron-produced isotopes are usually neutron deficient and decay by electron capture or positron emission. Some common examples of cyclotron-produced isotopes include:
- Iodine-123 (123I)
- Fluorine-18 (18F)
- Gallium-67 (67Ga)
- Indium 111 (111In)
- Thallium-201 (201Th).

In general, cyclotron-generated radionuclides are more expensive than are those produced by neutron bombardment or fission, i.e. by *nuclear reactor*.

RADIOACTIVE DECAY

The amount of radioactivity present (the number of disintegrations per second) is referred to as *activity*. In the past, the unit of radioactivity has been the curie (Ci), which is 3.7×10^{10} disintegrations per second. Because the curie is an inconvenient unit, it is being replaced by an international unit called a becquerel (Bq), which is one disintegration per second. Conversion tables are found in Appendices B-1 and B-2. *Specific activity* refers to the activity per unit mass of material (mCi/g or Bq/g). For a carrier-free isotope, the longer the half-life of the isotope, the lower is its specific activity.

Radionuclides decay in an exponential fashion and the term *half-life* is often used casually to characterize decay. Half-life usually refers to the *physical half-life,* which is the amount of time necessary for a radionuclide to be reduced to half of its existing activity. The physical half-life (Tp) is equal to 0.693/A, where A is the decay constant. Thus, A and the physical half-life have characteristic values for each radioactive nuclide.

A formula that the nuclear medicine physician should be familiar with is the following:

$$A = A_o e^{-(0.693t/Tp)}$$

This formula can be used to find the activity (A) of a particular radioisotope present at a given time *(t)* and given a certain activity *(Ao)* at time O. For instance, if you had 5 mCi (185 MBq) of ^{99m}Tc at 9 am today, how much would it remain at 9 am tomorrow? In this case, Tp of ^{99m}Tc is 6 hours, *t* is 24 hours and *e* is a mathematical constant. Thus, after 24 hours, the amount of ^{99m}Tc remaining is 0.31 mCi (11 MBq).

Radioactivity is the property of an unstable isotope of emitting energetic particles and rays from its nucleus. The I^{125} used as radioactive labeled antigen in radioimmunoassay emits gamma rays (photons).

Besides technetium-99m, I-125, and thallium-201, other examples include iodine-131, used to measure thyroid activity; phosphorus-32, used to locate tumors and iron-59, used to measure the rate of formation of red blood cells.

The most commonly used radionuclides are–

- ^{32}P (phosphorus-32), ^{33}P (phosphorus-33), ^{3}H, ^{14}C, ^{35}S (sulfur-35), and ^{45}Ca (calcium-45). ^{125}I (iodine-125) is used for radioimmunoassay, protein metabolism, hormone, and anatomical imaging studies.
- Microspheres labeled with ^{46}Sc (scandium-46), ^{57}Co (cobalt-57), ^{85}Sr (strontium-85), ^{95}Nb (niobium-95), ^{113}Sn (tin-113), ^{153}Gd (gadolinium-153), and ^{141}Ce (cerium-141) are used for regional blood-flow studies.
- ^{60}Co (cobalt-60), ^{67}Ga (gallium-67), ^{99m}Tc (technetium-99m), ^{125}I, ^{123}I (iodine-123), ^{131}I (iodine-131), ^{192}Ir (iridium-192), and ^{201}Tl (thallium-201) are used in medical diagnosis and therapy.

Radioimmunoassay is a technique for analyzing blood and other body fluids for very small quantities of biologically active substances. The technique depends on the reversible binding of the substance to an antibody. Antibodies are produced in animals as protection against foreign substances. They protect by binding to the substance and countering its biological activity. Consider, *for example, the analysis for insulin in a sample of blood from a patient*. Before the analysis, a solution of insulin-binding antibodies has been prepared from laboratory animals. This solution is combined with insulin containing a radioactive isotope, in which the antibodies bind with radioactive insulin. Now the blood sample containing an unknown amount of insulin is added to the antibody-radioactive insulin mixture. The nonradioactive insulin replaces some of the radioactive insulin bound to the antibody. As a result, the antibody loses some of its radioactivity. The loss in radioactivity can be related to the amount of insulin in the blood sample.

Technetium-99m

Technetium-99m fulfills many of the criteria of an ideal radionuclide and is used in more than 70 percent of nuclear imaging procedures. It has no particulate emission, a 6-hour half-life and a predominant (98%) 140-keV photon with only a small amount (10%) of internal conversion.

Technetium-99m is obtained by separating it from the parent 91Mo (67-hour half-life) in a generator system.

In the alumina generator system, the molybdenum activity is absorbed on an alumina column. By passing physiologic saline over the column, ^{99m}Tc is eluted or washed off as *sodium pertechnetate*.

As pertechnetate, the technetium ion is a singly charged anion and is similar in size to the iodide ion. After intravenous injection, ^{99m}Tc pertechnetate is loosely bound to protein and rapidly leaves the plasma compartment. More than half lives, the plasma within several minutes and is distributed in the extracellular fluid. It rapidly concentrates in the salivary glands, choroid plexus, thyroid gland, gastric mucosa and functioning breast tissue; during pregnancy, it crosses the placenta.

Excretion is by the gastrointestinal and renal routes. Although ^{99m}Tc pertechnetate is excreted by glomerular filtration, it is partially reabsorbed by the renal tubules; as a result, only 30 percent is eliminated in the urine during the first day. The ion is also secreted directly into the stomach and colon, with a much smaller amount coming from the small bowel. The colon is the critical organ and receives 1 to 2 rad/10 mCi (0.02 mGy/MBq) of ^{99m}Tc pertechnetate administered. The principal emission (140-ke V photon) of ^{99m}Tc has a half-value layer (HVL) of 0.028 cm in lead.

67Ga Imaging

Sarcoidosis is suggested by the presence of the lambda sign (increased activity in the right paratracheal and bilateral hilar regions) and the panda sign (symmetrically increased activity in the lacrimal, parotid, and salivary glands). Diffuse lung activity on 67Ga scan is often due to PCP in patients with AIDS.

Acute fractures and hematomas can show mildly increased activity on leukocyte scans.

Focal activity in the abdomen on a leukocyte scan may be due to an abscess or inflammatory bowel disease (such as Crohn's disease). Activity in the colon can be seen in ulcerative colitis or cytomegalovirus.

Osteomyelitis in the axial skeleton (especially the spine) produces cold defects in up to half of the cases using labeled leukocytes. The scan may also have a normal appearance. Gallium is preferred to labeled leukocytes in the setting of suspected spinal osteomyelitis or discitis.

RADIOACTIVE ISOTOPES

A radioactive substance is one which is unstable and spontaneously decays to form a more stable substance, giving out electromagnetic rays.

DIAGNOSTIC USES

- The radioactive isotope may be given *to define an organ* such as the thyroid.
- To test for *selective uptake in an organ* by scanning the whole body.
- To determine the presence of uptake in organs suspected of being the site of *metastases*.
- To *estimate the activity of an organ* such as the thyroid so that an assessment of the degree of thyrotoxicosis may be made.
- Some tumors of the thyroid-follicular carcinomas may produce functioning secondary deposits and if radioactive iodine is given these may be detected, and also *treated by* larger doses of iodine.

Chapter 14

Nuclear Scans

RADIONUCLIDE SCANS

Radiopharmaceutical	Critical organ/Disease (imaged)
Salivary gland	^{99m}Tc pertectinate
PET-sestamibi fusion scan	Parathyroid
^{99m}Tc-sestamibi	
^{99m}Tc-thalium^{201} subtraction scan	
^{131}I, ^{125}I, ^{123}I	Thyroid
^{99m}Tc-MDP	Bone
^{99m}Tc pertechnetate	Meckel's diverticulum, gastric mucosa, Intestine, thyroid, choroid plexus
^{99m}Tc DTPA	Renal GFR
^{99m}Tc DMSA	Renal cortical function
Xe-127, Xe-133, Kr-81m	Lung (VP scan), trachea
Tc-tagged RBCs	Spleen, GI bleeding
^{99m}Tc HMPAO	Brain scan
Stress induced thalium-201	Reversible myocardial ischemia
^{99m}Tc Stannous pyrophosphate > Tetrofosmin	Acute myocardial infarction (Heart)
HIDA/DISIDA	Biliary scintigraphy
^{99m}Tc sulfur colloid	Liver pathologies
Ga^{67}/Indium^{111} labeled WBC	Intra-abdominal abscess and inflammatory bowel disease

DOPA-PET > MIBG/MRI
Selenium methionine
SRS (Octreoscan)

Extra-adrenal pheochromocytoma
Pancreas
Pancreatic neuroendocrine tumors

SINGLE PHOTON EMISSION COMPUTED TOMOGRAPHY

- Three-dimensional images
- Axial, coronal and sagittal slices
- Gamma camera is rotated around the patient in all three anatomical planes
- Competing signal from overlying structures is eliminated
- Accurate detection of subtle signal changes and better spatial resolution of signal changes
- Mainly used for brain, liver, heart and bone scan.

BRAIN SCAN

Brain Tumors

In the differentiation of recurrent malignant glioma from radiation necrosis, ^{99m}Tc-HMPAO (hexamethylpropyleneamine oxime) images generally show a focal defect in the region of abnormality, whether containing necrotic tissue, recurrent tumor or both.

In conjunction with Thallium-201, single photon emision computed tomography (SPECT) brain perfusion imaging may be valuable in distinguishing between radiation necrosis and tumor recurrence in patients with malignant gliomas treated with high-dose radiation. The study may also localize suspected recurrences for biopsy. Thallium-201 activity, however, is a marker of viability, localizing in living tumor cells but not in nonviable tumor cells or necrotic tissue. A high degree of increased thallium activity in the region of a ^{99m}Tc-HMPAO defect is indicative of tumor recurrence, whereas a low degree is consistent with postradiation necrosis.

Positron emission tomography (PET) using fluorine-18 deoxyglucose also permits the differentiation of recurrent hypermetabolic neoplasm from hypometabolic radiation necrosis by using a single radiopharmaceutical. The study may occasionally be affected by therapy with corticosteroids because steroids have been shown to decrease glucose metabolism in the brain.

Yet, *PET is the best investigation helpful in differentiating tumor recurrence from radiation necrosis in a patient of brain tumor treated with radiation.*

Epilepsy

Patients with partial (focal) epilepsy refractory to therapy may benefit from surgical ablation of the seizure focus. The most common pathology at these foci is mesial temporal sclerosis (gliotic temporal scarring). Although most complex partial seizures arise from epileptic foci in the temporal lobes, they also may arise from other cortical areas. If seizure foci can be localized to the temporal lobes, about 70 percent of patients undergoing partial temporal lobectomy experience amelioration or eradication of seizures. The value of SPECT and PET imaging in this setting is well established.

The primary nuclear imaging techniques used for seizure localization have been those that attempt to localize the seizure foci based on their metabolic or perfusion status. Seizure foci may exhibit hyperperfusion and hypermetabolism during seizures (ictal studies), hypometabolism and hypoperfusion between seizures (interictal studies). PET imaging using IBFDG is the method of choice for evaluating metabolism, whereas SPECT imaging with ^{99m}Tc perfusion agents, such as HMPAO or ECD, appears to be the method of choice for evaluation of perfusion status.

Ictal SPECT Imaging: By using ^{99m}Tc-HMPAO or ^{99m}Tc-ECD, which do not significantly redistribute, patients can be injected during the seizure or within 30 seconds after its completion. To obtain ictal studies, the patient may be hospitalized and monitored with electroencephalography. The radiopharmaceutical is kept at the bedside until a seizure occurs, at which time it is injected. Other times the studies are obtained inadvertently while an intended interictal study is being performed. Epileptogenic foci appear as areas of increased activity (hyperperfusion) and may involve the entire temporal lobe or only a small mesial focus.

Interictal SPECT Imaging: Because interictal SPECT perfusion studies are performed between seizures, blood flow to epileptic foci is normal or reduced. To be detected on SPECT imaging, these must be seen as areas of decreased activity (hypoperfusion).

The common indications for brain imaging are perfusion abnormalities (stroke), dementia (Alzheimer's or multi-infarct), epilepsy, brain death and distinguishing recurrent tumor from radiation necrosis.

The radiopharmaceuticals ^{99m}Tc-HMPAO (SPECT), ^{99m}Tc-ECD (SPECT) and nitrogen-13 (C3N)-ammonia (PET) are perfusion agents.

The radio pharmaceuticals ^{99m}Tc-HMPAO and ^{99m}Tc-ECD are lipophilic, extracted on the first pass and reflect perfusion. Their uptake is highest in the cortical and subcortical gray matter. On imaging, the central area of decreased activity is primarily white matter and should not be mistaken for dilated lateral ventricles.

The radiopharmaceuticals 201Th (SPECT) and 18FDG (PET) are metabolic agents that show activity in viable recurrent or persistent tumors but not in areas of radiation necrosis.

Multi-infarct dementia presents with multiple asymmetric cortical perfusion defects. Multiple small perfusion defects can also occur from cocaine abuse or vasculitis.

Alzheimer's dementia classically presents with symmetrically decreased activity in the posterior parietal-temporal lobes with preserved activity in the calcarine cortex and basal ganglia. This is not pathognomonic and can be seen in other entities, including Parkinson's dementia. About 30 percent of Alzheimer's patients have asymmetrically decreased activity.

Herpes encephalitis can be seen as increased activity in the temporal lobe.

Epileptic seizure foci show increased perfusion ^{99m}Tc-HMPAO or ^{99m}Tc-ECD and metabolism C8FDG) during seizure activity but decreased or normal activity interictally.

A normal radionuclide angiographic examination of the brain presents a trident appearance of intracranial flow in the anterior cerebral and right and left middle cerebral territories. In brain death, there is no obvious arterial phase (the trident is absent) and only scalp activity is seen, which is often accompanied by a hot-nose sign. These studies can also be performed by using ^{99m}Tc-HMPAO or ^{99m}Tc-ECD (SPECT or planar).

A Diamox challenge study evaluates cerebral vascular reserve. It is analogous to use of dipyridamole in myocardial perfusion studies.

In areas of vascular disease, regional perfusion worsens after Diamox compared with perfusion without Diamox.

Cerebrospinal Fluid Imaging

Common indications for cerebrospinal fluid (CSF) imaging are for evaluation of a CSF leak or for differentiating normal-pressure hydrocephalus from other causes of hydrocephalus. These studies are done with intrathecal administration of ^{111}In-DTPA.

SALIVARY GLAND SCAN

Evaluation of suspected mass lesions of the salivary glands is best done by using computed tomography. Salivary glands are usually seen on ^{99m}Tc pertechnetate scan unless the patient has Graves' disease. They are not seen on an ^{123}I scan. Use of ^{99m}Tc-pertechnetate scans is generally reserved for functional evaluation, although most mass lesions, including primary tumors and metastases, are seen as areas of decreased activity. The exception to this is Warthin's tumor, which usually appears as a focal area of increased uptake. Warthin's tumors are benign parotid gland lesions, which predominate in elderly men and are frequently bilateral.

THYROID SCAN

Two isotopes of iodine ^{123}I and ^{131}I are clinically useful for imaging and may be administered as iodide.

Iodine-123 has a 13.3-hour half-life and decays by electron capture to tellurium-I 23 *C23Te)*. The photons emitted are 28-keV (92%) and 159-keV (84%) gamma rays. Iodine-123 is usually produced in a cyclotron by bombardment of antimony-I 2 I (I2ISb) or tellurium-l22. The cyclotron production and short half-life make it expensive and its distribution on a nationwide basis difficult. Iodine-123 has a whole body dose of 0.04 rad/mCi (0.01 mGy/MBq) and a thyroid dose of 16 rad/mCi (4.3 mGy/MBq).

Iodine-131 is a much less satisfactory isotope from an imaging viewpoint because of the high radiation dose to the thyroid and its relatively high photon energy. However, it is widely available, is relatively inexpensive and has a relatively long shelf life. Iodine-131 has a half-life of 8.06 days and decays predominantly by beta-particle emission to stable 131Xe.

Iodine-131 gives a whole-body dose of 0.5 to 3.5 rad/mCi (0.14 to 0.95 mGy/MBq) and a thyroid dose of 1000 to 2000 rad/mCi (270 to 540 mGy/MBq).

Common indications for radionuclide thyroid imaging are to differentiate between various types of hyperfunction (Graves' disease, toxic multinodular goiter, or autonomous adenoma) and to assess nodularity (cold or hot) and ectopic tissue.

A lingual thyroid is usually located in the midline at the base of the tongue, with no thyroid seen in the normal location. The ectopic gland is often hypofunctional.

A thyroid gland with an organification defect is usually seen as a normal gland on a ^{99m}Tc pertechnetate scan but manifests no activity on an iodine scan in a child with a high thyroid-stimulating hormone (TSH) level.

A large gland with intense homogeneous activity is usually Graves' disease. A pyramidal lobe is commonly associated with Graves' disease.

A large gland with patchy activity is usually a multinodular goiter but could also be chronic thyroiditis or an infiltrative process.

Most hot nodules are benign hyperfunctioning adenomas. They can be single or multiple and can suppress the normal portions of the gland.

Chronic thyroiditis can mimic numerous thyroid conditions but on imaging is usually patchy and decreased in activity.

Subacute thyroiditis classically presents with a markedly depressed radioiodine uptake and nonvisualization of the gland in a patient with thyrotoxicosis and a tender, swollen thyroid.

Thyroid cancer is usually a single focal cold lesion and only rarely is seen to be diffuse or multifocal on thyroid scans.

Thyroid cancers may concentrate ^{99m}Tc-sestamibi and persist on delayed images. They are typically "cold" on ^{99m}Tc-pertechnetate scans.

If there is a rising serum Tg and a negative whole body iodine scan, thyroid cancer can sometimes be visualized on a ^{99m}Tc-sestamibi or 18FDG PET scan.

Whole-body thyroid scans may be performed with ^{123}I rather than ^{131}I. The ^{123}I scans have better resolution and may cause less stunning.

Most patients with Graves' disease are treated with about 10 to 15 mCi (370–555 MBq) of ^{131}I, and most with toxic multinodular goiter are given about 15 to 29 mCi (555 MBq-1.1 GBq) of ^{131}I.

Cancer treatment doses depend on the size and stage of disease but most patients receive about 100 to 150 mCi (3.7-5.5 GBq) of '311.

After successful radioiodine ablation of residual thyroid tissue, serum Tg measurements are a sensitive method to detect recurrent thyroid cancer.

Iodine-131 treatment doses for thyroid cancer have been shown to be effective when using the following schedule:

Functioning tissue in the thyroid bed: 50 to 100 mCi (1.85-3.7 GBq) of ^{131}I
Cervical node metastases: 150 mCi (5.5 GBq) of ^{131}I
Lung or skeletal metastases: 200 mCi (7.4 GBq) of ^{131}I

Hot nodule — Adenoma and thyroid carcinoma (extremely rare)
Cold thyroid nodule - Inflammatory mass, benign tumor and malignant tumor.

PARATHYROID SCAN

Radionuclide scintigraphy with ^{201}T$_1$ (Technetium thallium) or ^{99m}Tc-MIBI (Technetium–99m sestamibi), using a subtraction technique whereby the image of thyroid gland as shown by ^{99m}Tc or ^{123}I is removed, is thus a noninvasive and other best technique for tumor and other lesions localization of **parathyroid gland. Presently,** Technetium–99m sestamibi is the best agent for parathyroid scanning.

The most common indication for parathyroid imaging is to localize the hyperfunctioning gland (adenoma) either in the thyroid bed or in an ectopic location (lower neck or mediastinum).

Parathyroid adenomas are usually single.

Parathyroid imaging is usually performed by using ^{99m}Tc-sestamibi with sequential images over 2 hours. Normal thyroid tissue and thyroid adenomas usually fade over 2 hours, whereas parathyroid adenomas usually hyperconcentrate ^{99m}Tc-sestamibi and persist over time.

Decreased salivary uptake on a ^{99m}Tc pertechnetate scan can be caused by the thyroid taking most of the activity (e.g. Graves' disease) or by a salivary problem (Sjögren's disease).

V/Q SCAN

Unless it is completely and absolutely normal, never interpret a ventilation-perfusion scan without a recent chest radiograph.

A normal perfusion lung scan essentially excludes clinically significant pulmonary emboli.

In addition to pulmonary embolism, other causes of perfusion defects are chronic obstructive pulmonary disease (COPD), pneumonia, asthma, tumor, mediastinitis, mucous plug, fat emboli, and vasculitis.

In the interpretation of V/Q lung scans, an *unmatched difeit* refers to one that is seen on the perfusion scan without an accompanying ventilation abnormality. It does not refer to a defect on the ventilation scan when the perfusion scan is normal.

Even a low probability scan has a 15 percent to 20 percent probability of pulmonary embolism. A very low probability scan has a positive predictive value of less than 10 percent.

A scan with a combination of findings that does not clearly fit a defined category is most likely an intermediate probability scan.

Asthma, mucous plugs and COPD can cause segmental perfusion defects but they should not have normal ventilation scans.

Currently computed tomography angiography computed tomography angiography (CTA) is considered to be the best diagnostic investigation for pulmonary embolism.

While over 90 percent of pulmonary embolism studies are now performed by CT-angiography, V/Q scans remain useful in patients with renal failure, contrast allergies or other situations in which CT is difficult or not available.

MYOCARDIAL SCAN

Myocardial ischemia and viability can be studied–
Directly with myocardial perfusion imaging by
- Thallium–201 chloride SPECT imaging
- Tc-99m sestamibi/tetrofosmin SPECT imaging
- Tc-99m stannous pyrophosphate scan (Acute myocardial infarct scintigraphy)
- PET (Best).

Indirectly with ventricular function imaging by–
Multigated acquisition scan (**MUGA**)
First pass radionuclide coronary angiography

Simultaneous assessment of myocardial perfusion + ventricular function by First pass radionuclide angiography + gated SPECT perfusion imaging

Relative Advantages of Thallium 201 and Technetium 99m		
Thallium	–	Lower radiopharmaceutical cost
	–	Measurement of increased pulmonary uptake
	–	Less hepatobiliary and bowel uptake
	–	Detection of resting ischemia (hibernating myocardium)
Technetium *(tetrofosmin and sestamibi)*		
	–	Better image quality (particularly in obese patients)
	–	Ventricular function assessment (gated SPECT)
	–	Shorter imaging time
	–	Shorter imaging protocols (patient/scheduling convenience)
	–	Acute imaging in myocardial infarction and unstable angina
	–	Superior quantification

Thus, **direct** measure in the form of Thallium scan will **best** tell about reversibility of myocardial ischemia and viability. Tc-99m stannous pyrophosphate scan and more so PET scan is best for myocardial infarct imaging, i.e. to differentiate salvageable from nonsalvageable myocardium.

MYOCARDIAL PERFUSION STUDIES

The common indication for myocardial perfusion studies is to determine whether there is normal perfusion, ischemia or infarction. The images obtained represent relative, not absolute blood flow.

Technetium-99m sestamibi and tetrophosmin have a higher photon energy (140 keV) than do the mercury daughter X-rays (69 to 81 keV) from 201Tl. As a result, there is less soft tissue attenuation with ^{99m}Tc-labeled radiopharmaceuticals than with thallium.

Myocardial uptake of 201Tl-chloride and ^{99m}Tc sestamibi or tetrofosmin is proportional to regional blood flow and requires cell viability.

Thallium is actively taken up by the Na^+-K^+ pump in the cells, whereas ^{99m}Tc sestamibi and tetrofosmin passively diffuse across the membrane and localize primarily in cytoplasmic mitochondria.

Infarcts and hibernating myocardium produce perfusion defects on the rest images.

Stress images are needed to elucidate ischemia with lesser degrees of stenosis (50 to 90%). Stenoses less than 50 percent in diameter are not detected at rest and are variably diagnosed with gated equilibrium radionuclide angiograms (MUGA scans) are performed with ^{99m}Tc red blood cells. Common indications include assessment of LVEF and regional wall motion. The normal LVEF is 50 to 65 percent. The lower limit is 50 percent in older people. Ejection fractions higher than 70 percent may reflect hypertrophy, valvular regurgitation or idiopathic hypertrophic subaortic stenosis (IHSS). The normal right ventricular ejection fraction is 40 to 50 percent.

MULTIPLE GATED ACQUISITION SCAN

In multiple gated acquisition (**MUGA**) for cardiac imaging, gated equilibrium images depict average cardiac contraction by summation over several minutes.

Recording of ejection fraction of left ventricle before and after exercise, regional wall motion of ventricular chambers and regurgitant index is done.

Advantages of MUGA Scan

- Higher information density than 1st pass method
- Assessment of pharmacological effect possible
- "Bad beat" rejection possible.

Disadvantages of MUGA Scan

- Significant background activity
- Inability to monitor individual chambers
- Plane of AV valve difficult to identify.

Hibernating myocardium is a chronically hypoperfused area that has reduced cellular metabolism. This area has decreased contractility. Revascularization is usually needed.

Stunned myocardium is due to an acute occlusion with relatively rapid perfusion return. These areas have normal or near-normal perfusion and decreased contractility. Revascularization is not usually needed.

LIVER SCAN

In colloid liver imaging, the photopenic lesions in the liver can be due to anything that does not have reticuloendothelial activity (cyst, hematoma, abscess, fatty).

Focal nodular hyperplasia can accumulate ^{99m}Tc sulfur colloid but hepatic adenomas and other tumors do not.

Blood pool imaging of the liver is commonly performed to differentiate cavernous hemangioma from other focal liver lesions seen on ultrasound or CT.

Hemangiomas are not seen to be hypervascular on early arterial images. On late blood pool images, a hemangioma usually shows activity that is more intense than the normal liver.

Hypovascular tumors are photopenic on early and late images, and hypervascular tumors are usually increased in activity on early images but may be hot or cold on delayed images.

Although hemangiomas and cysts are usually occult, asymptomatic lesions, ultrasound can reliably distinguish between cysts (which are hypoechoic) and hemangiomas (which are hyperechoic). CT with intravenous contrast is more specific, usually demonstrating characteristic progressive enhancement toward the center of a hemangioma.

Cavernous hemangioma is highly likely when a defect seen with ^{99m}Tc sulfur colloid imaging shows increased activity after administration of a ^{99m}Tc blood pool agent, such as ^{99m}Tc red blood cells, owing to labeling of the blood pool in the lesion. To allow equilibration of the hemangioma blood pool with the labeled red blood cells, delayed imaging (sometimes over several hours) may be necessary when planar imaging is used. Dynamic or blood flow images frequently show normal or decreased perfusion of the lesions. Use of SPECT in the setting of suspected hepatic hemangioma increases the sensitivity of the study, especially when lesions are deep or less than 5 cm in diameter. SPECT provides nearly 100 percent sensitivity for detection of hemangiomas larger than 1.5 cm in diameter; sensitivity is 50 percent or less for lesions smaller than 1.0 cm in diameter.

Applications of Hepatobiliary Scintigraphy in Liver Diseases

- Assessment of regional liver function
- Demonstration of bile leaks in liver trauma
- Differential diagnosis of hepatocellular tumors.

BILIARY SCINTIGRAPHIC SCAN

The most common indications for a hepatobiliary study are to differentiate between acute or chronic cholecystitis, to look for suspected bile leaks or biliary obstruction and in the setting of neonatal jaundice, to differentiate neonatal hepatitis from biliary atresia.

Phenobarbital augmented cholescintigraphy is 90 to 97 percent sensitive, 60 to 94 percent specific and 75 to 90 percent acurate for diagnosis of EHBA. It reveals no visualization of bowel on delayed images at 6 and 24 hrs. It is impossible to differentiate it from neonatal hepatitis in absence of small bowel activity and requires liver biopsy.

Hepatic iminodiacetic acid scan (**HIDA scan**) is a biliary scintigraphic scan. Its applications and indications include:
- Acute cholecystitis (**investigation of choice**)
- Congenital biliary atresia
- Biliary leak evaluation
- Biliary–enteric fistula
- Chronic GB dysfunction.

Others

- Biliary obstruction
- Choledochal cyst and other congenital anomalies of biliary tract
- Detection of abnormalities of bile flow in gastrointestinal tract (GIT)
- Demonstration of gallbladder (GB) function (including obstruction of cystic duct as in acute cholecystitis)
- Biliary dyskinesia
- Sphincter of oddi dysfunction.

MECKEL'S DIVERTICULUM IMAGING

These scans are performed with ^{99m}Tc pertechnetate, which concentrates in normal and ectopic gastric mucosa.

Most Meckel's diverticula do not contain ectopic gastric mucosa but the ones that bleed almost always do.

Look for a focus of activity in the mid-abdomen or right lower quadrant. It should increase in activity similar to the stomach mucosa and should remain in a fixed spot.

GASTROINTESTINAL BLEEDING STUDIES

Usually these are performed with ^{99m}Tc-labeled red blood cells, but ^{99m}Tc sulfur colloid can also be used.

If bleeding is intermittent, use ^{99m}Tc-labeled red blood cells. If bleeding is active, either ^{99m}Tc labeled red blood cells or ^{99m}Tc sulfur colloid can be used.

The sensitivity of angiography for detecting GI bleeding is about 10 to 20 percent less as compared to nuclear imaging.

The *^{99m}Tc-RBC scan* will image bleeding at rates as low as 0.05 to 0.1 mL/min.

Angiography can image bleeding at a rate of 0.5 to 1.0 mL/min or less.
Angiography will detect bleeding only if extravasation is occurring during the injection of contrast.

RENAL SCAN

^{131}I OIH (Orthoiodohippurate)

Largely replaced by Tc –99m MAG3 used for evaluation of renal tubular function/effective renal plasma flow.

^{99m}Tc DTPA (Diethylene Triamine Penta-acetic Acid)

It is agent of choice for assessment of
- Perfusion
- GFR
- Obstructive uropathy
- Vesicoureteral reflux.

^{99m}Tc DMSA (Dimercoptosuccinic Acid)

It is suitable for imaging of functioning cortical mass pseudotumor versus the lesion.

^{99m}Tc Mercaptoacetyltriglycine (MAG3)

True renal plasma flow detected.
Replacing DTPA.

Diuretic renal scans	– These are primarily done to rule out obstruction at pelvi-ureteric or vesico-ureteric junction in a child with hydronephrosis.
	– Additionally, information about the function of each kidney can be gathered.
	– There are three agents which can be used for a diuretic renal scan-DTPA or MAG3 or LLEC.
	– All three are good but LLEC is supposed to be the best as the image quality is the best.
DMSA scan	– This scan is done to ascertain whether the kidney is involved in urinary infection or done to look for any scarring of the kidney post infections.
	– This test also gives a very precise idea about the relative kidney function on either side.
Direct radionuclide cystogram (DRCG)	– This test is done to diagnose vesico-ureteral reflux (VUR) in a child.

ACE Inhibitor Scintigraphy

- It is for screening of renovascular hypertension, used as 2nd line study
- No anatomic detail other than renal size is provided by the captopril renogram.

ADRENAL SCAN

NP-59 is an adrenal cortical imaging agent with imaging performed at 4 to 5 days. Unilateral adrenal uptake is usually an adenoma and bilateral uptake is usually due to adrenal hyperplasia.

Metaiodobenzylguanidine (MIBG) is a medullary adrenal imaging agent which effectively localizes in pheochromocytoma and neuroblastoma. It may also localize in carcinoid, medullary thyroid carcinoma and paraganglioma.

TESTICULAR SCAN

Common indications are to differentiate between epididymitis and acute or delayed torsion.

The initial problem is to determine whether blood flow is increased or decreased. The best way to determine which side is abnormal is to obtain a patient history. If this is not available, the abnormal side is usually obvious on the blood pool and delayed images.

Epididymitis should be diffusely hot on all images and frequently focally hot in the region of the epididymis.

Acute torsion should have decreased or absent testicular flow.

Increased flow to one hemiscrotum and a rim of testicular activity with a cold center (halo sign).

BONE SCAN

The technetium-99m (^{99m}Tc) labeled polyphosphates and pyrophosphates are the radionuclides most commonly used for skeletal scintigraphy. Skeletal radionuclide scintigraphy usually becomes abnormal very early in the course of osteomyelitis and is highly sensitive from 24 to 72 hours after the onset of symptoms.

The three-phase skeletal scintigraphy technique apparently augments the specificity of skeletal scintigraphy for suspected osteomyelitis. Three-phase skeletal scintigraphy consists of a radionuclide angiogram (perfusion phase) scan during injection, immediate postinjection "blood-pool" images, and 2 to 3-hour delayed (bone uptake) images. This method makes it easier to discriminate between soft tissue infections, septic arthritis, noninfectious skeletal disease, and osteomyelitis.

Radionuclides Considered for Bone Scanning

- 45Ca Calcium
- 85Sr Strontium
- 131Ba Barium
- 157Dy Dysprosium
- 67Ga Gallium
- 32P Phosphate
- 18F Fluorine
- Technetium ^{99m}Tc
- Technetium-Snippy
- Technetium-Sn-MDP
- Ga is not suitable for diagnostic scanning of skeletal diseases as number of chemical-biological phenomenon, including variation or organ distribution, colloid formation and soft tissue uptake occur and this has prevented adoption as a bone scanning agent.
- Technetium-Sn-MDP is most rapidly cleared ^{99m}TcPh and is the most useful radiopharmaceutical in skeletal scanning.

Bone Lesions Showing No Osteoblastic Activity, i.e. No Tracer Uptakes
- Fibrous cortical defect
- Bone island
- Osteopoikilosis
- Osteopathia striata
- Nonossifying fibroma.

Bone Lesions Showing Increased Tracer Uptake
- Fibrous dysplasia
- Paget's disease
- Osteoid osteoma
- Eosinophilic granuloma
- Melorheostosis
- Enchondroma
- Exostosis.

Tumors on Bone Scans
Intense
  Fibrous dysplasia
  Giant cell tumor
  Aneurysmal bone cyst
  Osteoblastoma
  Osteoid osteoma
Moderate
  Adamantinoma
  Chondroblastoma
  Enchondroma
Mild or Isointense
  Fibrous cortical defect
  Bone island
  Cortical desmoid
  Nonossifying fibroma
  Osteoma
Cold
  Bone cyst without fracture
  Multiple myeloma
Variable
  Hemangioma
  Multiple hereditary exostosis

Common Indications for Bone Scans

Include evaluation of primary osseous or metastatic neoplasms, a vascular necrosis of the hips or shoulders, trauma, infection and less commonly, arthritis or reflex sympathetic dystrophy (RSD) in the peripheral skeleton.

A lesion that is hot on all three phases of a bone scan can be osteomyelitis but also may be an acute fracture, hypervascular tumor, neuropathic joint or RSD.

Most osseous metastases begin in the red marrow and therefore are predominantly located in the skull, ribs, spine, pelvis, and proximal extremities.

In a patient with known metastases, an increasing apparent number and intensity of lesions compared with prior bone scans can indicate more disease or may indicate the flare phenomenon from recent treatment. A flare phenomenon is most likely seen within 1 to 3 months of therapy completion.

Not all multifocal hot lesions are metastases; also consider hyperparathyroidism, fractures, multifocal osteomyelitis, multiple enchondromas, polyostotic fibrous dysplasia or Paget's disease.

Paget's disease is commonly seen as intense activity in the skull, femur, vertebral body or half of the pelvis. It is usually polyostotic (80%) but it may be monostotic and may cause bowing of a femur.

Good visualization of the bones and not of the kidneys may indicate a *superscan* due to *diffuse metastases or hyperparathyroidism*. If the skull is hot and the distal extremities are well seen, it is probably the latter.

Focal hot lesions in multiple adjacent ribs are essentially always due to fractures. Long lesions running along the length of a rib are not usually fractures.

Stress fractures usually occur in the pelvis and below the knees. They can be seen as focal or fusiform, primarily cortical activity.

Bilaterally increased activity along the cortex of the tibias may be due to shin splints, hypertrophic osteoarthropathy or periosteal reaction of other causes.

Osteomyelitis, acute fractures, vascular tumors, such as Ewing's sarcoma and RSD are hot on angiographic, blood pool, and delayed bone scan images.

Cellulitis is hot on the first two phases but fades on delayed images.

Osteomyelitis usually does not cross joints. Increased activity seen on both sides of a joint is more likely the result of septic arthritis.

Cold lesions can be due to poor perfusion of an area of bone, lack of bony matrix (aggressive tumor), overlying attenuating material or gamma camera dysfunction, such as a bad photomultiplier tube.

Multiple sequential cold vertebral bodies are almost always due to radiation therapy.

Tumors that commonly cause cold (photopenic) metastatic lesions include kidney, lung, thyroid, and breast tumors.

In multiple myeloma, ^{99m}Tc products do not localize well in the destructive/ lytic lesions (no osteoblastic activity, hence no uptake - *cold spots*). Positive areas of augmented uptake are reported only in 24 percent to 44 percent of patients with radiographically apparent lytic areas. Although the isotope bone scan is far less reliable in multiple myeloma than in metastatic disease, occasionally scan findings will precede roentgen changes. Bone scan is not useful in evaluating multiple myeloma.

Summary
- A distinct advantage of nuclear imaging over X-ray techniques is that both bone and soft tissue can be imaged very successfully and there is good contrast between bone and soft tissues.
- The most useful radiopharmaceutical for skeletal imaging is technetium-99m linked to methylene disphosphonate (^{99m}Tc-MDP).

- The mean effective dose is 4 mSv per bone scan, compared to 5.3 mSv per CT scan (all examinations).
- The mean effective dose per bone scan is equivalent to 200 chest X-rays.

SCINTIGRAPHIC SCAN FOR NEUROENDOCRINE TUMORS

Radionuclide scan (**somatostatin receptor scintigraphy and MIBG scan**) have major role in localization of pancreatic islet cell tumors and their metastases and also investigation of gastrointestinal carcinoids, apudomas and related neuroendocrinotumors and their metastases.

MISCELLANEOUS

Gallium-67 scans for inflammatory lesions are performed 24 hours after injection; for tumors, they are usually done at 48 to 72 hours.

Lymphoma and hepatoma are particularly gallium-avid tumors. Other tumors (such as lung cancer) also accumulate gallium.

If a lymphoma accumulates gallium initially but not on a post-therapy scan, there is probably a favorable therapeutic response. If on subsequent follow-up scans, gallium again accumulates, the probability of tumor recurrence is high. 18F-FDG PET/CT scans are preferred for staging and restaging lymphoma.

A gallium scan can most often be recognized by noting activity in the lacrimal glands, nasopharynx, liver, bowel and skeleton. The images are usually count-poor (coarse).

Gallium-67 may localize in the parotid glands after radiotherapy and the thymus after chemotherapy, especially in children and young adults. Reactive thymic changes should not be mistaken for recurrent mediastinal lymphoma.

Thallium-201 and 18F-FOG accumulate nonspecifically in many tumors, including recurrent brain tumors.

Many breast cancers, parathyroid adenomas and metastatic thyroid cancers accumulate the cardiac agent ^{99m}Tc-sestamibi. Some benign breast conditions accumulate this agent.

Indium-111 octreotide is accumulated by tumors with somatostatin receptors, including pheochromocytoma, carcinoid, neuroblastoma, gastrinoma, islet cell tumors, pituitary adenomas, medullary thyroid cancer and small-cell lung cancer.

MIBG is accumulated by pheochromocytomas and neuroblastomas.

Kaposi's sarcoma is thallium-avid but does not accumulate gallium. Lymphoma concentrates both agents.

Lymphoscintigraphy is performed with intradermal or peritumoral injection of filtered ^{99m}Tc-sulfur colloid. The purpose is to identify the sentinel node which is the lymph node most likely to be involved with metastatic tumor.

THERAPEUTIC USES

Role of Radionuclides in Radiotherapy

Those used therapeutically (either in tele or brachy or in both)

Bismuth-213, Cobalt-60, Dysprosium-165, Erbium-169, Holmium-166, Iodine-125, Iodine-131, Iridium-192, Lutetium-177, Palladium-103, Phosphorus-32, Rhenium-186, Rhenium-188, Samarium-153, Strontium-89, Yttrium-90, Cesium, Gold and Ruthenium (Radium outdated) (Table 14.1), etc.

Precursors

Molybdenum-99, Ytterbium-177, Strontium-92, etc.

Table 14.1: Some useful radionuclides used in clinical radiotherapy

Sr No	Radionuclide	Energy	Half-life	Medical uses
1.	Radium-226	0.83 MV	1625 years	For brachytherapy but not used nowadays
2.	Cobalt-60	1.25 MV	5.4 years	Teletherapy and brachytherapy (T > B)
3.	Caesium-137	0.666 MV	30 years	Teletherapy and brachytherapy
4.	Iridium-192	0.380 MV	72 days	Brachytherapy only
5.	Iodine-125	0.030 MV	60 days	Brachytherapy
6.	Iodine-131	0.61 MV	8 days	Unsealed radioiodine for thyroid cancer Rx
7.	Gold-198	0.412 MV	2.7 days	Brachytherapy
8.	Strontium-90	2.24 MV	30 years	For shield (mold) in eye tumors
9.	Phosphorous-32	1.71 MV	14 days	Intraperitoneal

- By replacing existing radiation sources—for example, radium has been replaced by Co 60, gold grains have replaced radon seeds.
- By providing large sources which previously were unobtainable or difficult to obtain because of scarcity or high cost, for example, the use of *radioactive cobalt*, which can be obtained in large quantities relatively easily, for teletherapy machines.
- To obtain shapes and sizes of applicators which were previously difficult to make for example, a *strontium applicator* for beta-ray application, whole-body strontium machines using a large source, or tantalum wire which can be cut to the right length and molded for any particular situation.

- To treat by selective uptake, for example, the treatment of thyrotoxicosis by radioactive iodine or polycythemia rubra vera by radioactive phosphorus.
- To treat malignant effusions in the chest or the abdomen. Radioactive colloidal gold applied to the serous lining of the cavity and as a result of the radiation, the fluid does not collect as rapidly as before and repeated tappings are not necessary. This is, of course, a palliative treatment.
- A radioactive fluid may be inserted into a balloon within the bladder to treat superficial tumors of the mucosa.
- The characteristics of a certain isotope may be exploited; thus, radioactive yttrium is a beta-emitter of high energy and may be inserted into the pituitary gland so that this structure is destroyed but practically no radiation is received outside the fossa.

More Example of Therapeutic Uses

- ^{131}I decays by beta particle emission and a principle gamma ray energy. Its beta emission makes it therapeutically useful. Nonmalignant condition like thyrotoxicosis and well-differentiated thyroid tumors and their metastases are treated by ^{131}I.
- ^{125}I emits X-rays by electron capture. It is mainly useful for diagnostic imaging and in radioimmunoassay (RIA) but therapeutic use in prostatic cancer (permanant source) with ^{125}I seeds is effective.
- **Cesium** emits gamma rays.
- **Phosphorus**-32 is pure beta particle emitter. It is normally administered intravenously and used in the treatment of polycythemia vera and related blood disorders.
- **Yttrium-90** is also pure beta emitter used in intra-articular treatment of arthritis and intrapleural or intrapulmonary treatment of malignant effusions.
- **Strontium-89** decays by beta particle emission, administered 150 MBq intravenously for the palliation of pain from bone metastases secondary to prostate and breast cancer.
- Co60, an artificial radioactive source (Co59 → Co60 → Ni) is widely used in teletherapy.

Section 3

Radiotherapy and Radiation Oncology

Chapter 15

Radiation Oncology

AN OVERVIEW

The various modes of treating a tumor include:
- Surgery
- Chemotherapy
- Radiotherapy
- Ablation: Physical (Hyperthermia, Hypothermia, Laser, Photodynamic therapy, etc.) and chemical
- Immunoradiotherapy
- Embolization.

WHAT ARE ELECTROMAGNETIC RAYS?
- Electromagnetic waves are forms of energy and constitute a spectrum of decreasing wavelength from radiowaves to infrared rays to visible light to ultraviolet-light down to the smaller wavelength of ionizing radiations. Thus, the ionizing rays, X- and gamma, have no mass but are pockets of available energy which may be released by collision with a substance.
- The energy of the gamma-rays will depend on the substance whose breakdown or decay results.
- The energy of X-rays will vary according to the energy applied to the machine to produce them. Essentially X-rays are produced when a stream of electrons, accelerated by a high voltage applied between the filament and the target, strikes the target, the electrons give up their energy, There is a limit to the initial power that can be applied to the electrons because very high voltages cannot be

produced by transformers and cables will not carry them without serious breakdown and loss of insulation.
- X-rays and gamma rays are similar; the former are produced in X-machines and the latter from the breakdown of certain radioactive elements, but both are *electromagnetic rays,* Having a wave formation with wavelength and frequency.
- The *alpha* and beta rays previously described are formed of particles, respectively helium nuclei and electrons, and a beam of radiation can also be composed of neutrons-all these are particles and have a mass and are, therefore, called *particulate radiations.*
- **Ultraviolet rays** are electromagnetic radiations having wavelength less than 400 nm are not ionizing radiations, but they do affect the skin.

WHAT IS IONIZING RADIATION?

What is Radiation?

Radiation is a very general term, used to describe any process that transmits energy through space or a material away from a source. Light, sound, and radiowaves are all examples of radiation. When most people think of radiation, however, they are thinking of ionizing radiation–radiation that can disrupt the atoms and molecules within the body. While scientists think of these emissions in highly mathematical terms, they can be visualized either as subatomic particles or as rays. Radiation's effects on humans can best be understood by first examining the effect of radiation on atoms, the basic building blocks of matter.

What is Ionization?

Ionization is the process where a charged portion (usually electron) of an atom or molecule is given enough kinetic energy to dissociate. Atoms consist of comparatively large particles (protons and neutrons) sitting in a central nucleus, orbited by smaller particles (electrons): a miniature solar system. Normally, the number of protons in the center of the atom equals the number of electrons in orbit. An ion is any atom or molecule that does not have the normal number of electrons. Ionizing radiation is any form of radiation that has enough energy to knock electrons out of atoms or molecules, creating ions.

How is Ionizing Radiation Measured?

Measurement lies at the heart of modern science, but a number by itself conveys no information. Useful measurement requires both an instrument for measurement (such as a stick to mark off length) and an agreement on the units to be used (such as inches, meters, or miles). The units chosen will vary with the purpose of the measurement. For example, a cook will measure butter in terms of tablespoons to ensure the meal tastes good, while a nutritionist may be more concerned with measuring calories, to determine the effect on the diner's health.

The variety of units used to measure radiation and radioactivity at times confuses even scientists, if they do not use them every day. It may be helpful to keep in mind the purpose of various units. There are two basic reasons to measure radiation: the study of physics and the study of the biological effects of radiation. What creates the complexity is that our instruments measure physical effects, while what is of interest to some are biological effects. A further complication is that units, as with words in any language, may fade from use and be replaced by new units.

Radiation is not a series of distinct events, like radioactive decays, which can be counted individually. Measuring radiation in bulk is like measuring the movement of sand in an hourglass; it is more useful to think of it as a continuous flow, rather than a series of separate events. The intensity of a beam of ionizing radiation is measured by counting up how many ions (how much electrical charge) it creates in air. The Roentgen (named after Wilhelm Roentgen, the discoverer of X-rays) is the unit that measures the ability of X-rays to ionize air; it is a unit of exposure that can be measured directly. Shortly after World War II, a common unit of measurement was the Roentgen equivalent physical (rep), which denoted an ability of other forms of radiation to create as many ions in air as a Roentgen of X-rays. It is no longer used, but appears in many of the documents examined by the Advisory Committee.

What are the Basic Types of Ionizing Radiation?

There are many types of ionizing radiation, but the most familiar are alpha, beta, and gamma/X-ray radiation. Neutrons, when expelled from atomic nuclei and traveling as a form of radiation, can also be a significant health concern.

Alpha particles are clusters of two neutrons and two protons each. They are identical to the nuclei of atoms of helium, the second lightest and second most common element in the universe, after hydrogen. Compared with other forms of radiation, though, these are very heavy particles—about 7,300 times the mass of an electron. As they travel along, these large and heavy particles frequently interact with the electrons of atoms, rapidly losing their energy. They cannot even penetrate a piece of paper or the layer of dead cells at the surface of our skin. But if released within the body from a radioactive atom inside or near a cell, alpha particles can do great damage as they ionize atoms, disrupting living cells. Radium and plutonium are two examples of alpha emitters.

Beta particles are electrons traveling at very high energies. If alpha particles can be thought of as large and slow bowling balls, beta particles can be visualized as golf balls on the driving range. They travel farther than alpha particles and, depending on their energy, may do as much damage. For example, beta particles in fallout can cause severe burns to the skin, known as beta burns. Radioisotopes that emit beta particles are present in fission products produced in nuclear reactors and nuclear explosions. Some beta-emitting radioisotopes, such as iodine 131, are administered internally to patients to diagnose and treat disease.

Gamma and X-ray radiation consists of packets of energy known as photons. Photons have no mass or charge, and they travel in straight lines. The visible light seen by our eyes is also made up of photons, but at lower energies. The energy of a gamma ray is typically greater than 100 kiloelectron volts (keV-"k" is the abbreviation for kilo, a prefix that multiplies a basic unit by 1,000) per photon, more than 200,000 times the energy of visible light (0.5 eV). If alpha particles are visualized as bowling balls and beta particles as golf balls, photons of gamma and X-radiation are like weightless bullets moving at the speed of light. Photons are classified according to their origin. Gamma rays originate from events within an atomic nucleus; their energy and rate of production depend on the radioactive decay process of the radionuclide that is their source. X-rays are photons that usually originate from energy transitions of the electrons of an atom. These can be artificially generated by bombarding appropriate atoms with high-energy electrons, as in the classic X-ray tube. Because X-rays are produced artificially by a stream of electrons, their rate of output and energy can be controlled by adjusting the energy and amount of the electrons themselves. Both X-rays and gamma rays can penetrate deeply into the human body. How deeply they penetrate depends on their energy; higher energy results in deeper penetration into the body. A 1 MeV ("M" is the abbreviation for mega, a prefix that multiplies a basic unit by 1,000,000) gamma ray, with an energy 2,000,000 times that of visible light, can pass completely through the body, creating tens of thousands of ions as it does.

A final form of radiation of concern is neutron radiation. Neutrons, along with protons, are one of the components of the atomic nucleus. Like protons, they have a large mass; unlike protons, they have no electric charge, allowing them to slip more easily between atoms. Like a Stealth fighter, high-energy neutrons can travel farther into the body, past the protective outer layer of the skin, before delivering their energy and causing ionization.

Several other types of high-energy particles are also ionizing radiation. Cosmic radiation that penetrates the Earth's atmosphere from space consists mainly of protons, alpha particles, and heavier atomic nuclei. Positrons, mesons, pions, and other exotic particles can also be ionizing radiation.

How does Radiation Affect Humans?

Radiation may come from either an external source, such as an X-ray machine, or an internal source, such as an injected radioisotope. The impact of radiation on living tissue is complicated by the type of radiation and the variety of tissues. In addition, the effects of radiation are not always easy to separate from other factors, making it a challenge at times for scientists to isolate them. An overview may help explain not only the effects of radiation but also the motivation for studying them, which led to much of the research examined by the Advisory Committee.

What Effect can Ionizing Radiation have on DNA?

Ionizing radiation, by definition, "ionizes," that is, it pushes an electron out of its orbit around an atomic nucleus, causing the formation of electrical charges on atoms or molecules. If this electron comes from the DNA itself or from a neighboring molecule and directly strikes and disrupts the deoxyribonucleic acid (DNA) molecule, the effect is called direct action. This initial ionization takes place very quickly, in about 0.000000000000001 of a second. However, today it is estimated that about two-thirds of the damage caused by X-rays is due to indirect action. This occurs when the liberated electron does not directly strike the DNA, but instead strikes an ordinary water molecule. This ionizes the water molecule, eventually producing what is known as a free radical. A free radical reacts very strongly with other molecules as it seeks to restore a stable configuration of electrons. A free radical may drift about up to 10,000,000,000 times longer than the time needed for the initial ionization (this is still a very short time, about 0.00001 of a second), increasing the chance of it disrupting the crucial DNA molecule. This also increases the possibility that other substances could be introduced that would neutralize free radicals before they do damage.

Neutrons act quite differently. A fast neutron will bypass orbiting electrons and occasionally crash directly into an atomic nucleus, knocking out large particles such as alpha particles, protons, or larger fragments of the nucleus. The most common collisions are with carbon or oxygen nuclei. The particles created will themselves then set about ionizing nearby electrons. A slow neutron will not have the energy to knock out large particles when it strikes a nucleus. Instead, the neutron and the nucleus will bounce off each other, like billiard balls. In so doing, the neutron will slow down, and the nucleus will gain speed. The most common collision is with a hydrogen nucleus, a proton that can excite or ionize electrons in nearby atoms.

What Immediate Effects can Ionizing Radiation have on Living Cells?

All of these collisions and ionizations take place very quickly, in less than a second. It takes much longer for the biological effects to become apparent. If the damage is sufficient to kill the cell, the effect may become noticeable in hours or days. Cell "death" can be of two types. First, the cell may no longer perform its function due to internal ionization; this requires a dose to the cell of about 100 gray (10,000 rad). (For a definition of gray and rad, see the section below titled "How Do We Measure the Biological Effects of Radiation?") Second, "reproductive death" (mitotic inhibition) may occur when a cell can no longer reproduce, but still performs its other functions. This requires a dose of 2 gray (200 rad), which will cause reproductive death in half the cells irradiated (hence such a quantity is called a "mean lethal dose"). Today we still lack enough information to choose among the various models proposed to explain cell death in terms of what happens at the level of atoms and molecules inside a cell. If enough crucial cells within the body totally cease to function, the effect is fatal. Death may also result if cell reproduction ceases in parts of the body where cells are continuously being replaced at a high rate (such as the blood cell-forming tissues and the lining of the intestinal tract). A very high dose of 100 gray (10,000 rad) to the entire body causes death within twenty-four to forty-eight hours; a whole-body dose of 2.5 to 5 gray (250 to 500 rad) may produce death within several weeks. At lower or more localized doses, the effect will not be death, but specific symptoms due to the loss of a large number of cells. These effects were once called nonstochastic; they are now called deterministic. A beta burn is an example of a deterministic effect.

What Long-term Effects can Radiation have?

The effect of the radiation may not be to kill the cell, but to alter its DNA code in a way that leaves the cell alive but with an error in the DNA blueprint. The effect of this mutation will depend on the nature of the error and when it is read. Since this is a random process, such effects are now called stochastic. Two important stochastic effects of radiation are cancer, which results from mutations in nongerm cells (termed somatic cells), and heritable changes, which result from mutations in germ cells (eggs and sperm).

How can Ionizing Radiation cause Cancer?

Cancer is produced if radiation does not kill the cell but creates an error in the DNA blueprint that contributes to eventual loss of control of cell division, and the cell begins dividing uncontrollably. This effect might not appear for many years. Cancers induced by radiation do not differ from cancers due to other causes, so there is no simple way to measure the rate of cancer due to radiation. During the period studied by the Advisory Committee, great effort was devoted to studies of irradiated animals and exposed groups of people to develop better estimates of the risk of cancer due to radiation. This type of research is complicated by the variety of cancers, which vary in radiosensitivity. For example, bone marrow is more sensitive than skin cells to radiation-induced cancer.

Large doses of radiation to large numbers of people are needed in order to cause measurable increases in the number of cancers and thus determine the differences in the sensitivity of different organs to radiation. Because the cancers can occur anytime in the exposed person's lifetime, these studies can take seventy years or more to complete. For example, the largest and scientifically most valuable epidemiologic study of radiation effects has been the ongoing study of the Japanese atomic bomb survivors. Other important studies include studies of large groups exposed to radiation as a consequence of their occupation (such as uranium miners) or as a consequence of medical treatment. These types of studies are discussed in greater detail in the section titled "How do scientists determine the long-term risks from radiation?"

How can Ionizing Radiation Produce Genetic Mutations?

Radiation may alter the DNA within any cell. Cell damage and death that result from mutations in somatic cells occur only in the organism in which the mutation occurred and are therefore termed somatic or nonheritable effects. Cancer is the most notable long-term somatic effect. In contrast, mutations that occur in germ cells (sperm and ova) can be transmitted to future generations and are therefore called genetic or heritable effects. Genetic effects may not appear until many generations later. The genetic effects of radiation were first demonstrated in fruit flies in the 1920s. Genetic mutation due to radiation does not produce the visible monstrosities of science fiction; it simply produces a greater frequency of the same mutations that occur continuously and spontaneously in nature.

Like cancers, the genetic effects of radiation are impossible to distinguish from mutations due to other causes. Today at least 1,300 diseases are known to be caused by a mutation. Some mutations may be beneficial; random mutation is the driving force in evolution. During the period studied by the Advisory Committee, there was considerable debate among the scientific community over both the extent and the consequences of radiation-induced mutations. In contrast to estimates of cancer risk, which are based in part on studies of human populations, estimates of heritable risk are based for the most part upon animal studies plus studies of Japanese survivors of the atomic bombs.

The risk of genetic mutation is expressed in terms of the doubling dose: the amount of radiation that would cause additional mutations equal in number to those that already occur naturally from all causes, thereby doubling the naturally occurring rate of mutation.

It is generally believed that mutation rates depend linearly on dose and that there is no threshold below which mutation rates would not be increased. Spontaneous mutation (unrelated to radiation) occurs naturally at a rate of approximately 1/10,000 to 1/1,000,000 cell divisions per gene, with wide variation from one gene to another.

Attempts have been made to estimate the contribution of ionizing radiation to human mutation rates by studying offspring of both exposed and nonexposed Japanese atomic bomb survivors. These estimates are based on comparisons of the rate of various congenital defects and cancer between exposed and nonexposed survivors, as well as on direct counting of mutations at a small number of genes. For all these endpoints, no excess has been observed among descendants of the exposed survivors.

Given this lack of direct evidence of any increase in human heritable (genetic) effects resulting from radiation exposure, the estimates of genetic risks in humans have been compared with experimental data obtained with laboratory animals. However, estimates of human genetic risks vary greatly from animal data. For example, fruit flies have very large chromosomes that appear to be uniquely susceptible to radiation. Humans may be less vulnerable than previously thought. Statistical lower limits on the doubling dose have been calculated that are compatible with the observed human data. Based on our inability to demonstrate an effect in humans, the lower limit for the genetic doubling dose is thought to be less than 100 rem.

CANCER BIOLOGY

Cell Cycle (G_1, S, G_2 and M)

- Cell cycle
    - A normal cell cycle consists of five stages—**G_2, M, G_1, S, and G_0**.(ALL INDIA 2003)
        i. **M**—is mitotic phase
        ii. **S**—is synthetic phase (DNA Synthesis)
        iii. **G_1** and **G_2**—are growth phase
        iv. **G_0**—is resting phase (i.e. gap-phase).
    - The continuously dividing human cell takes approximately 22 hours to divide.
    - Normally **times required** for different phases are as follows:
        i. G_2 takes five hours
        ii. M-phase takes one hour
        iii. S-phase takes eight hours, and
        iv. G_1 phase takes eight hours.
    - However, the time required for G_1 and G_2 phase are characteristically variable.
    - Most normal cells are in G_0 phase and rapidly dividing cells have shorter G_1 phase.
    - It is notable that tumor cells can no longer enter G_0 phase.
    - The cells in G_2M, especially in M-phase, are most radiosensitive.
    - The cells in S-phase are radioresistant
- Growth of human tumors
- Polypeptide and neuropeptide growth factors

- Chemical carcinogenesis
- *Chromosomes and cancer:* Chromosomal abnormalities—myeloid leukemia, malignant diseases affecting lymphocytes
- *Physical carcinogenesis:* Ionizing radiation-Ionizing radiation and cancer—physical factors—Ultraviolet radiation and carcinogenesis
- Genetics and familial cancer
- Pathogenesis of metastasis (Mechanism).

PRINCIPLES OF RADIATION THERAPY

General Considerations

Radiosensitivity is the sensitivity of a particular tissue to irradiation *(growth* which is killed by a small dose of radiation is said to be *radiosensitive).* Radiosensitivity can also be applied to normal tissues.

Radiation techniques vary according to the nature of the tumor, its history, site, the age of the patient and so on, but there are certain basic principles of radiotherapy, which are applicable to all treatments.

Physical Considerations

- Electromagnetic radiation
- Ionizing and nonionizing radiations
- Particulate and nonparticulate beams
- Low and high LET rays.

Biological Considerations

- Interaction of radiation with biologic materials
- Cell survival considerations.
- Repair of radiation damage,
- Oxygen enhancement ratio (OER)
- Variation of radiation response during the division cycle
- Linear energy transfer
- Relative biologic effectiveness (RBE)
- Adverse effects of radiation
- Acute and late normal tissue effects
- Fractionation
- Definition of radiosensitivity.

Simplified Medical Physics

To understand radiotherapy it needs to understand the basic principles of radiation and its interaction with matter. Basically, radiation is produced by the decay of an unstable radionuclide from its nucleus as either α, β, or γ-rays. Thus γ-rays are produced intranuclearly.

While, X-rays are produced extranuclearly. In case of linear accelerator, very high speed electrons strike at a target material which in turn produce X-rays. The above process removes inner cell electron of the target element, so that there are reshuffling of the other shell electrons, leading to X-ray production. The X-rays are either of low energy (KeV) or high-energy (MeV) beams depending upon the capacity of the X-ray generator.

The most commonly used radiation for the medical purposes are either of X-ray or of γ-ray, in the biological system both radiations have similar properties. They can be thought of as packets of energy, or photons. Sometimes β-rays and electrons (e^-) are used for the treatment of superficial tumors. However, the use of heavy ions, particles, proton beams, neutron beams and π-mesons are used in research set up only. The radiations are further classified as electromagnetic radiation (X-ray, gamma ray) or particulate radiation (electron, proton, alpha particles, neutrons, negative pi-mesons, and heavy charges particles).

The interaction of the radiation to the biological system is very interesting. Low energy radiations (KeV) interact with the inner shell electron (bound electron) leading to removal of latter called photoelectric effect. This effect depends upon the atomic number of the material; therefore, bone can absorb low energy photons better than soft-tissue. This effect predominates in diagnostic radiology.

When a high energy beam (MeV) interacts with outer shell electron (free electron), results in removal of above electron called Compton effect. This is a common interaction in the biological system and this interaction does not depend upon the atomic number. Hence, high-energy beams can pass through bones to the deep-seated tumor, in contrast to low energy beams. This effect predominates in therapeutic radiology.

Every radionuclide has a specific half-life. The term half-life is defined as the time taken by a given radionuclide to reduce to half of its activity. The radionuclide having long half-life is hazardous for the protection of medical personnel. The radiation can be shielded in its path by metals of higher atomic number (lead (Pb), tin (Sn), copper (Cu), aluminum (Al), or tungsten). These metals have specific shielding properties expressed as half value layer **(HVL)**. Many beam-modifying devices are used to skew or shield sensitive tissues from the path of radiation beam called shielding, wedges, compensators or filters during radiotherapy.

Basic Radiobiology

The radiation used in medicine we mean ionizing radiation. X-rays, and gamma-rays are commonly used radiations, described as pockets of energy called *photons*. The other rare radiations are pi-mesons, heavy ions, protons, and neutrons. The radiation can pass through muscles, bones, skin, blood and lungs, etc. by different biological interactions. The radiations are invisible, intangible, tasteless and odorless; while passing through the human body produce ionization of the tissues along its path.

Law of Radiobiology

Bergonie and Tribondeau's law of radiobiology states that the sensitivity of cells to irradiation is inversely proportional to degree of differentiation and directly proportional to their reproductive activity.

The changes induced in living tissues by irradiation are highly complex, being mainly physical and chemical in nature. These changes are roughly proportional to the energy absorbed from the radiation within the cell. All living tissues, whether malignant or normal, are vulnerable to radiation damage but individual cells are more sensitive during the stage of cell division. Malignant lesions are specifically so because they have a greater proportion of dividing cells than the adjacent normal tissues and so are more likely to show a greater response to irradiation. In addition, more actively dividing tumors—anaplastic—are likely to show greater effect than more slowly growing tumors—differentiated because they contain a greater proportion of cells in mitosis. The ideal in radiotherapy would be to kill off all the tumor cells without causing any damage to normal cells; however, this is not possible and we have to compromise by causing as little damage as possible to normal cells.

The cell is vulnerable to radiation in the stage of mitosis, less so during synthesis and relatively insensitive during the resting periods.

Molecular Mechanism of Action of Ionizing Radiations

- Action on enzymes
- Direct DNA damage
- Indirect injury by free radical injury (80%)
- Linear energy transfer (LET).

The ultimate target of the ionizing radiation is nucleus-containing DNA. The radiation can interact with the cells in two distinct fashions. The predominant mechanism is indirect mechanism through hydrolysis of water. The radiation inside the cytoplasm causes hydrolysis of water (H_2O) to H^+ and OH ions. The free radical (OH ion) can penetrate the nuclear membrane and induce damage to the cellular DNA in presence of nascent oxygen by cross-linking. Oxygen is the ultimate radiation sensitizer and help radiation damage to tumor cell DNA by cross-linking. The second mechanism is called direct interaction. Direct interaction occurs when the non-ionizing/or ionizing beams strike directly to the DNA. The ultimate damage to DNA leads to reproductive death of the cell or apoptosis. *The radiation* damage may be sub-lethal (SLD), potentially lethal (PLD), or lethal (LD) damage. These radiation injuries can be repaired efficiently in normal cells by the presence of enzyme *ribonuclease*, but the same enzyme is deficient in cancer cells. The above differentiating properties result in sterilization of cancer cells and preservation of normal cells.

The arrangement of appropriate number of fractions over a time depends upon the **4-R's of radiobiology**, i.e. *repair* of sublethal damage, *repopulation* of tumor clonogens, *redistribution* of cells in different phases of cell cycle and *reoxygenation* of tumor ball after every fraction of radiotherapy. It takes approximately 4 to 6 hours for normal tissues to repair any radiation damage, whereas malignant tissues take a much longer time for the same repair. Over a course of treatment, multiple sublethal injuries accumulate in tumor tissues. During this period of time malignant tissues cannot recover from this injury but normal tissues can repair this damage. *This is how radiation can specifically damage cancer cells, but spares normal cells.* Radiation mediated cell kill is more marked during G2 and M phase of the cell cycle, with G2M interphase being most radiosensitive phase, followed by M and then G2. Radiation while shrinking the cancer cells by killing, at the same time tumor clonogens start dividing by the influence of radiation called re-population. These cells rearrange themselves to M and G2 phases of the cell cycle to be killed effectively by radiation called redistribution.

The radiation can kill cancer cells better in the presence of oxygen molecule. In the anoxic and hypoxic medium, radiation is least effective leading to suboptimal control of cancer. Radiation delivered in divided dose can induce gradual tumor debulking thereby improve oxygenation. Cancer patients whose hemoglobin levels are less than 10 gm/dl have lower levels of tumor sterilization than patients do with hemoglobin levels more than 10 gm/dl. Hence, all the patients with low hemoglobin levels are advised to receive blood transfusion before starting radiotherapy. Each radiation has a particular value of *radiobiological equivalence (RBE)*. The deep X-ray (250 KeV) beam is considered as one and comparatively other radiation are categorized as 0.85 for X-ray or X-rays and 4 in case of proton beam. Hence, radiations with higher RBE (i.e. proton, neutron, pi-meson, heavy ions, etc.) are more lethal to the nucleus than the X-ray or X-rays. Moreover, some radiations are thickly ionizing (e.g. proton beam) than X-rays (thinly ionizing) along the track of radiation expressed as linear energy transfer (LET). *There is a linear relation between radiobiological efficiency (RBE) and the linear energy transfer (LET).*

Low LET radiations	*High LET radiations*
X-rays	Beta particles
Gamma-rays	Proton
Electrons	Neutron
	Pi-meson
	Heavy ions

Relation between LET and RBE of different radiation		
Radiation	LET in keV/length	RBE
X-ray and γ-ray	0.3–11	
Beta-radiation	0.5–15	1–2
Neutrons	20–50	2–5
Alpha-radiation	80–250	3–20

RADIOSENSITIZER AND RADIOPROTECTOR

Many chemical agents are now available which can interact with radiation to improve cell kill induced by radiation therapy. Nitrosoimidazole group of compounds can mimic oxygen molecule and enhanced radiation damage like oxygen fixation, thereby enhance radiation damage at the DNA level. The useful nitrosoimidazole compounds are *metronidazole, misonidazole, etanidazole, and pimonidazole*. These drugs are now on extensive clinical research trials and their peculiar neurological toxicities prevent them to be used in routine practice. Other agents like pyrimidine analogues (*Idoxuridine IUdR, Bromodeoxyuridine BUdR*) can interlink with DNA and make the DNA chain unstable to be damaged by the radiation.

Many thiol [SH] groups of compounds like *amifostine* are used to protect normal cells from the harmful side effects of radiation. The agent amifostine is used commonly in clinical practice to protect from toxicities of chemoradiotherapy.

Radiosensitizers/Radiomimetics

Drugs which enhance radiation effect by sensitizing the cell:
- Hyperbaric oxygen
- Cisplatin
- 5-FU
- Hydroxyurea
- Metronidazole, Misonidazole, Pimonidazole (Nitroimidazoles)
- Vincristine
- Bleomycin
- Gemcitabine
- Cytofluor
- Sr2508 (Etanidazole).

Radioprotectors

Drugs which protect the cell from radiation injury:
- Amifostine
- Sodium butyrate
- Zinc oxide
- Pentoxifylline
- Estramustine
- Antioxidants (Vitamin C, E, A)
- Chlorhexidine (*for stomatitis*)
- Potassium iodide (*for thyroid against radioactive iodine*)
- Melatonin (*for skin mitotic cells against chromosomal damage*).

Amifostine

- **Amifostine** has emerged as a *pancytoprotectant* shown protection against **nephrotoxicity, neurotoxicity and ototoxicity** in preclinical studies.
- With administration of a cytoprotective agent, the timing relative to the administration of the cytotoxic drug is crucial.
- Amifostine has a very short half-life (of the order of minutes) and must be given within 30 minutes of cisplatin administration for effective cytoprotection.
- Amifostine and glutathione have been found to **diminish sensory neuropathies** caused by cisplatin.
- Preclinical studies have demonstrated that the administration of amifostine can protect against the **nephrotoxic effects** of cisplatin.
- Studies have shown impressive radioprotection at bone marrow and mucosal sites, particularly the **salivary glands**, with the use of amifostine.
- It does not cross blood brain barrier (BBB).

Radiopotentiators (Radiation Recall Reactions)

Drugs that flare up dermatitis or esophagitis in areas previously treated by radiation:
- Doxorubicin
- Dactinomycin

Summary
One of the major limitations of radiotherapy is that the cells of solid tumors become deficient in oxygen. This is because solid tumors usually outgrow their blood supply, causing a low-oxygen state known as hypoxia. The more hypoxic the tumors are the more resistant they are to the effects of radiation because oxygen "fixes" or makes permanent the radiation damage to DNA. Much research has been devoted to overcoming this problem including the use of hyperbaric oxygen, blood substitutes that carry increased oxygen, erythropoietin, hypoxic cell radiosensitizers such as misonidazole and metronidazole and hypoxic cytotoxins, such as tirapazamine. Interestingly, recent data has indicated that patients ingesting excess amounts of antioxidant vitamins (such as C or E) may actually diminish the effectiveness of the radiation treatment.

Chapter 16

Radiotherapy

Radiotherapy is the medical use of ionizing radiation, generally as part of cancer treatment to control or kill malignant cells. It works by damaging the DNA of cancerous cells. This DNA damage is caused by one of two types of energy, photon or charged particle. This damage is either direct or indirect ionization of the atoms which make up the DNA chain. Indirect ionization happens as a result of the ionization of water, forming free radicals, notably hydroxyl radicals, which then damage the DNA.

SCHEDULE OF RADIOTHERAPY

Fractionation Schedules

Many radiotherapy techniques are aimed at increasing this difference increasing the vulnerability of the tumor cells or decreasing that of the normal cells. Fractionation of the treatment over a period, for example, giving relatively small treatments for 4 or 6 weeks, will allow some recovery of the cells after each dose; this recovery is likely to be greater for normal cells than for the malignant cells. In addition, repeated small courses of radiation at daily intervals will find a greater proportion out cancer cells than normal cells in a-stage of division.

Following an exposure of radiation to a given tumor, a particular proportion or fraction of tumor cells are killed (sterilized), but the cell-killing rate is never zero. Subsequent to a radiation injury, the cells recover within 4 to 6 hours. Hence radiation is usually delivered in multiple fractions (fractionation) than in single treatment. *Hence all over the world majority of radiations are given at a dose rate of around 200 cGy (2 Gy) per day, treating 5 days a week (Monday-Friday) except some variation in few places.* The total duration of radiotherapy course varies from 5 to 7 weeks depending upon individual cases.

Fractionation Radiotherapy

It refers to the division of the total dose into a number of separate fractions, conventionally given on a daily basis, usually 5 days a week (Monday to Friday).

Types
- Conventional fractionation
- Hyperfractionation RT
- Accelerated RT
- CHART (Continuous Hyperfractionated Accelerated Radiotherapy) regimen for lung cancer and head and neck malignancies
- Hypofractionation RT.

Hyperfractionation

Instead of giving once a day radiation therapy, multiple doses of radiation (b.i.d or t.i.d) can be given to exploit the radiobiological advantages. Firstly, by giving multiple fractions per day (hyperfractionation), higher radiation dose can be delivered to the tumor. Secondly, hyperfractionation results in 15 percent higher local control and survival rates than conventional radiotherapy with very minimal late complications. This approach has been explored in tumors where conventionally fractionated RT has often failed cure tumors, e.g. cerebral gliomas and advanced head and neck cancer. The most encouraging results of hyperfractionation radiotherapy have been found in localized head and neck cancers and small cell carcinoma of lung. The rationale for giving more than one fraction per day is based on the 4 Rs of radiobiology:

1. *Dose per fraction:* As the dose per fraction decreases the oxygen enhancement reaction decreases
2. *Morbidity:* Small field size is used, as it is associated with more severe acute reactions.

Hypofractionation schedule: When radiotherapy is used for palliation of advanced cancers, the duration is very short (5 to 10 days only) and dose per fraction is more concentrated. It is more logical in treating tumors with higher capacity for repair, e.g. melanomas, soft tissue sarcomas and in palliative RT (bone metastases and non-small cell lung cancers).

Continuous Hyperfractionated Accelerated Radiotherapy (CHART)

Continuous hyperfractionated accelerated radiotherapy (CHART) is characteristically used in treatment of lung carcinoma.

MODES OF RADIOTHERAPY

- Brachytherapy
- Teletherapy (including newer techniques)
- Systemic radiotherapy.

Brachytherapy

Brachy means '*short range*' in Greek language. When the radiation source (sealed radionuclides as tube, seeds, needles) is placed close to the tumor it is called brachytherapy.

Brachytherapy, also known as sealed source radiotherapy or endocurietherapy, is a form of radiotherapy where a radioactive source is placed inside or next to the area requiring treatment. Conversely, external beam radiotherapy, or teletherapy, is the application of radiation that has been externally produced, usually by a linear accelerator.

Brachytherapy is commonly used to treat localized prostate cancer and cancers of the head and neck.

In short, the ideal brachytherapy source of γ-ray emitters should be of medium energy (0.2–0.4 MeV) and monoenergetic to simplify the dosimetry.

Thus,
- The source used is inside the body, source is implanted in the body cavity or tumor itself.
- The main advantage is a required very high dose can be given to the limited and only required volume of tissue.
- But the tumor have to be assessable and size must be accurately definable
- Brachytherapy is a type of radiation therapy, which uses sealed sources placed within or near to the tumor for therapy, i.e. short distance therapy.

There are four subtypes of brachytherapy

1. When the radionuclide is placed on the surface of the skin (mould or plaque) is called plesiocurietherapy.
2. When placed inside the natural body cavity, it is called intracavitary brachytherapy.
3. When the radionuclide is implanted (needled) into the substance of the tumor, it is called interstitial brachytherapy.
4. Lastly when a catheter with the radionuclide (sources) is inside the vasculature it is called intravascular brachytherapy.

- Molds [used in skin cancer, carcinoma of pinna of ear, and hard palate]
- Intracavitary brachytherapy [Cancer cervix, cancer endometrium, cancer nasopharynx]
- Interstitial brachytherapy [Cancers of tongue, cheek, breast, prostate and everywhere]
- Intraluminal brachytherapy [endobronchial cancer, esophageal cancer]
- Intravascular brachytherapy [intracoronary irradiation to prevent re-occlusion of stent]

- **Mold brachytherapy:** Superficial tumors can be treated using sealed sources placed close to the skin. Dosimetry is often performed with reference to the Manchester system; a rule-based approach designed to ensure that the dose to all parts of the target volume is within 10 percent of the prescription dose.
- Surface applicator is usually called strontium plaque therapy and is used for very superficial lesions less than 1 mm thick. The plaque is a hollow, thin silver casing that encloses a radioactive Strontium-90 powdered salt. The beta (electron) particles produced from Strontium's radioactive decay have a very shallow penetration. Typically the Sr 90 plaque is placed on the bed of a resected pterygium. A stat dose of around 10 to 12 Gy is delivered by timing the contact. As the electrons only penetrate a few mm of air, radiation protection issues are slightly less but very different to other radiation sources. Cleaning the plaques that are placed on the eye sclera is required but must be gentle because the silver casing is thin and easily damaged. Strontium belongs to the same chemical class as calcium, i.e. an alkaline earth metal, and so will co-locate in the bone if any strontium salt makes contact with the eye and is absorbed. Operators can prevent exposure to the beta rays by holding the applicator to face away from their bodies.
- **Intracavitary brachytherapy** places the sources inside a pre-existing body cavity. The most common applications of this method are gynecological in nature, although it can also be performed on the nasopharynx.
- **Interstitial brachytherapy:** Here the sources are inserted into tissue. The first treatments of this kind used needles containing Radium-226, arranged according to the Manchester system, but modern methods tend to use Iridium-192 wire. Iridium wire can be arranged either using the Manchester or the Paris system; the latter was designed specifically to take advantage of the new nuclide. Prostate cancer treatment with Iodine-125 seeds is also classified as interstitial brachytherapy. For details of the gamma emitters please see commonly used gamma emitting isotopes.
- **Intravascular brachytherapy** places a catheter with the sources inside the vasculature. The most common application of this method uses Strontium-90 in the Novoste Beta-Cath System (now offered by Best Vascular), is the treatment of coronary in-stent restenosis, although the therapy has also been investigated for use in the treatment of peripheral vasculature stenoses. Its use in treatment of painful bone metastases is also promising.

Radiotherapeutic Treatment of Painful Bone Metastasis

Therapies with intravenously administered radionuclides are directed at palliation of pain (not at cure), decreased need for opiates, and improved quality of life. With most of the methods, the patient may have a transient increase in pain beginning 2 to 3 days after treatment and lasting for several days due to transient swelling of the treated lesions. Palliative symptomatic improvement usually begins 7 to 20 days after treatment and often lasts 3 to 6 months. Pain will not be relieved if it is caused by a pathological fracture or is of nonosseous origin (such as epidural metastases with pressure on the spinal cord or soft tissue masses pressing on nerves).

External beam teletherapy is recommended if there are only one or two lesions causing the patient's pain or if there is impending spinal cord compression.

The most commonly used radionuclide is strontium-89 (H9Sr) chloride (Metastron). The radionuclide decays by beta emission with a physical half-life of 50.5 days. The maximum range of the beta emission in tissue is 8 mm. After intravenous administration, localization in bone occurs in areas of active osteogenesis. Metastases with a blastic response have significantly more concentration and longer retention than does normal bone. Excretion is primarily urinary and to a lesser extent fecal. For the first week, medical staff handling these items should wear gloves and follow local disposal regulations.

Strontium-89 therapy depresses the bone marrow and should not be used if the leukocyte count is below 2400/l L or if the platelets are below 60,000/l L. The typical dose is 40 to 60/lCi/kg (1.5 to 2.2 MBq/kg) up to 4 mCi (148 MBq) given by slow (l to 2 minutes) intravenous injection using syringe shielding (especially plastic) appropriate for a beta emitting radionuclide. After administration, peripheral leukocyte counts are usually obtained every 2 weeks until marrow recovery occurs. Repeated doses are usually not given at intervals of less than 3 to 4 months, and it is unusual to give more than three doses without being cautious about bone marrow reserve. Because excretion is primarily urinary, 89Sr therapy should be used advisedly in patients with decreased renal function.

Pain relief typically takes 1 to 3 weeks to become apparent, and generally this therapy should not be used in patients with a life expectancy of less than 3 months. In addition, issues relative to handling of a deceased patient recently treated with H9Sr need to be addressed. Many states have regulations prohibiting cremation in this setting, and some have allowed only certain funeral homes to service these patients.

Other radiopharmaceuticals have been developed and used with some success. These are rhenium-186 (186Re), HEDP or etidronate, and samarium-153 (153Sm) EDPMT, also known as 153Sm lexidronam (Quadramet).

Samarium-153 EDPMT has many of the advantages of rhenium, including a short half-life (46 hours) and, in addition to beta rays, a gamma photon (103 keV, 30% abundance) that can be imaged. Imaging is usually done at 6 hours after administration. There may be an initial increase in bone pain within 72 hours, which usually responds to analgesics. Pain relief may begin at about 1 week and reaches a maximum in about 3 weeks. About 70 percent of patients report pain relief, and about 35 percent report to be "much better" or "completely improved." No additional advantage is obtained by dose escalation. There can be bone marrow suppression, and about 95 percent of patients will have a nadir of white blood cell counts and platelets to about 40 to 50 percent of baseline at 3 to 5 weeks. As a result, it should not be given concurrently with radiation therapy or chemotherapy unless marrow status has been adequately evaluated. The recommended dose is 1.0 mCi/kg (37 MBq/kg) administered intravenously over a period of 1 minute followed with a saline flush. Hydration following injection is recommended to reduce bladder dose because about one third of the administered activity is eliminated in the urine in the first 6 hours. Precautions should be in place *for* 12 hours by using a toilet instead of urinal and flushing several times.

The radionuclides like radium, cesium, cobalt, iridium, tantalum, iodine, strontium, palladium, etc. are commonly used for the brachytherapy purpose. Almost all radionuclides produce γ-rays, but some radionuclides produce exclusive β-rays for short-range radiotherapy alike electron beam. The least important radiation is α-rays, which is more lethal to nucleus but due to their heavy weight, they are least penetrating and less useful in clinical radiotherapy.

Due to the difficulty in radiation protection, the use of radium, cobalt and cesium are gradually unpopular. instead, newer radionuclides with good safety profile and adequate specific activity, i.e. iridium-192, iodine-125, palladium-103, etc. are used commonly for brachytherapy. *A safe principle called afterloading method is used to improve the safety in the brachytherapy.*

In past, the understanding about radiation safety was not clear. Peoples used radiation casually to treat patients with cancers and noncancerous conditions. Radiation sources were used widely over several years for brachytherapy purpose until the introduction of radiation safety principles in 1950s. From the experiences of radiation hazard, *afterloading systems for brachytherapy* evolved, making the radiation therapy a safe specialty without the fear of exposure to the medical personnel.

In brachytherapy, various types of rules or systems of arrangement of radionuclides are described. The most popular principles of brachytherapy are Paris system, Manchester system, Stockholm system, Quimby system and Patterson and Parker rule. Nevertheless, at present the help of sophisticated computers can individualize all the brachytherapy dose calculations. The treatment time for brachytherapy depends upon the dose rate, which in turn, depends upon the source strength. Typically, in low dose system, treatment time may be 2 to 4 days, whereas in high dose system, treatment time is usually a few hours.

Brachytherapy includes the following:

Interstitial radiations

1. Removable/temporary sources or implants
   - Radium
   - Tantalum
   - Iridium
   - Cesium (^{137}Cs)
   - Cobalt (^{60}Co)
   - Californium
2. Permanent sources or implants
   - Iodine
   - Gold
   - Radon

Intracavitary radiations

1. Removable:
   - Radium
   - Cesium
   - Cobalt
2. Permanent
   - Colloidal radioactive gold
   - Yttrium
   - Radioactive iodine (^{131}I)

Clinical, e.g.

1. ^{192}Iridium wires: Ca breast
2. ^{137}Cesium: Ca cervix
3. Strontium: Ca tongue

At present radioactive **cobalt**, **gold** and **iridium (instead of radium)** are being employed in small sources used in body cavities or implanted directly into tissues (the brachytherapy).

Remote and Manual Afterloading Machines

Afterloading machines as they are called are the machines that perform brachytherapy treatments.

Manual Afterloading Machines

In the early days of brachytherapy (Ca 1920), the only way to place the radioactive material into the hollow tubes or hollow body cavities was for someone to carry the source up to the patient's bedside (room or operating theater) in a safe, take it out and place it inside the hollow destination. By necessity, the staff member (usually the doctor) undertaking this received some radiation dose. *This was manual loading.*

In cases such as cervix brachytherapy where a Heyman capsule was used, radiation exposure from manual loading could be appreciable as all the sources had to be placed individually while the patient was anesthetized on the operating bed. It was not long before the doctors who were exposed reasoned that their exposure could be lessened by placing metal tubes first, and then placing the radioactive sources inside metal tubes at a later time. The metal tubes allowed the development of standard sizing and strength sources so that source numbers could be calculated first, and then prepared to facilitate a single step procedure to manually afterload.

Manual afterloading machines could not be activated from outside the room, as the source had to be manually inserted. The source would have been prepared in a hot lab as a source train and inserted in a theater or ward. The source could not be unloaded for nursing visits.

Remote Afterloading Machines

Although manual afterloading reduced exposures, the guiding principle of radiation protection is to keep exposures as low as reasonably achievable (ALARA) given prevailing economic, political and societal factors. *The move to reduce exposures even further led to the introduction of remote afterloading.* This technique relies on the use of hollow tubes that are connected to a safe containing a small radioactive source welded to a wire that is driven out by a stepping motor to predetermined positions to deliver radiation dose.

These machines deliver their treatment remotely. A plan is produced that describes the patterns of the stepping motor (distance and well time). The motor is only engaged when all staff have left the shielded room that holds the patient for the duration of the treatment.

This means that the nurse or therapeutic radiographer that administers can leave the room (located either in theater or ward) and start the treatment outside. Empty catheters are placed into the patient and the 'live' source is entered at a later date. This means that the nonactive dummy guides can be repositioned and checked. In other words, the source is not placed into the guides until the positioning is acceptable. The machine then runs a pneumatic drive wire through the catheters and guidewires to check that there are no obstructions and the source can safely run through the course of it. After this the check has been performed the source leaves it secure safe and the treatment begins. The development of the remote afterloading machines is a benefit to the many radiation safety issues surrounding manual afterloading machines, but they are *expensive and more prone to error.*

Advantages of Remote over Manual

- No radiation exposure in patient transit
- No exposure to theater or ward staff.

Teletherapy

Teletherapy in radiation oncology means a source of radiation coming from a distance. It is also called percutaneous radiotherapy. It is the most commonly used type of radiotherapy. About 60 percent of cancer patients referred for radiotherapy are treated with external beam radiotherapy or teletherapy equipment.

External Beam Therapy Machines (Teletherapy Machines)

The name of few teletherapy units are as follows:
- Deep X-ray units [DXT]
- Radium bomb
- Telecesium unit
- Telecobalt unit
- Linear accelerator (Linac)
- Betatron
- Neutron generator [d,T generator]
- Microtron
- Cyclotron
- Synchrotron
- Gamma knife unit.

Out of the above 11 teletherapy units, we commonly use linear accelerators [linacs], telecobalt units, betatrons, gamma knife unit and occasionally deep X-ray (DXR), in clinical practice. The remaining teletherapy units are obsolete, rarely being used or for experimental treatments only.

The telecobalt units produce γ-rays while linear accelerators produce X-rays for the treatment. The X-rays are originated from the outer shell of an atom whereas the γ-rays are produced from the nucleus itself. A high energy X-ray unit with all mechanical parts to produce X-rays and electrons for treatment. Thus, besides high-energy photons (X-ray), linear accelerators can produce electron beams too for the treatment of superficial cancers. High-energy radiation beams are more penetrating, thereby cause less complications.

Radioactive Cobalt (^{60}Co) Machines

These are perhaps the most widely used sources of megavoltage irradiation. The gamma rays from cobalt are approximately equivalent to X-rays produced with energy of about 1.3 million volts. Essentially machine is a large "block of shielding material, usually lead, with a hole in one side. The source is contained within the shield and when required is moved to a position opposite the hole to give radiation externally to the patient. The size of the field to be irradiated is determined by two pairs of moveable thick diaphragm set at right angles so that rectangular fields varying from 4×4 cm to 20×20 cm may be used.

The cobalt is measured in curies and the amount used in machines will vary up to several thousand curies. Radioactive cobalt is continuously decaying and the output of such a machine decreases by 10 percent per year; thus, output charts need to be changed as time goes on and it becomes necessary to replace the cobalt source after about 4 or 5 years if the treatment time is not to be too long. The advantage of this type of megavoltage machine is that there are no complicated electronics to go wrong and the periodic replacement of cobalt is practically the only servicing needed. This type of machine is therefore eminently suitable for the department with limited physical and technical resources.

Radioactive cesium 137 Co may also be used in teletherapy machines; these machines are designed to operate much closer to the patient than the cobalt machines. The amount of stray radiation outside the primary beam is greater and they thus have certain limitations in use.

Linear Accelerators

Following world war-II, from the experience of radar system, the concept of *linear accelerator* evolved. More and more refined X-ray generators (Van de Graaff generator and linear accelerators) have developed afterwards to make radiation more penetrating than the previously available low energy X-ray generators. *Artificially prepared radionuclides* such as cobalt-60 (^{60}Co) and Cesium-137 (^{137}Cs) are being used as a source of radiation since last 7 decades. At present in some developing countries, *telecobalt units* are still in use for cancer treatment.

These machines produce X-rays at very high energies—in clinical practice most machines operate at between 4 and 10 million volts. Many models can also produce an electron beam for external use.

Over the past 20 years, considerable advances have been made in the design of the machines and consequently they have become smaller and more mobile while still providing X-rays at the same energy.

Linear accelerators are so called because they accelerate a stream of electrons down an evacuated tube to hit the target and produce X-rays: The advantage of electron-beam therapy is that at practically all the energy of electrons is expelled in the tissue, depending on the voltage used to produce the electrons, and there is little spread beyond the target.

Thus they have distinct advantages when it is desirable to reduce the dose of radiation to deeper lying tissues; for example, in the treatment of the buccal aspect of the cheek or the scalp, a high dose can be given to the tumor but the mouth and brain receive very low doses.

Cyclotrons

In these machines, the electrons instead of traveling down a straight tube, are accelerated in circular orbits within an evacuated circular area. They can thus be accelerated along much longer path, which is possible with a straight tube, and very high energies can be obtained. These machines will produce neutron beams for therapy, which have distinct radiobiological advantages. Cyclotrons can also be used to produce certain isotopes (especially the positron emitters), which are not available from a nuclear reactor.

Betatrons

These machines are designed specifically to produce beams of electrons, and may have variable-energies of up to 40 million volts. With low energies there is a sharp cut-off of dose in tissue but disadvantage is its loss of energies above 20 million volts when the isodose distribution becomes somewhat smaller to that from a linear accelerator.

Fast Neutrons Generators

In recent years, new machines have become available for the production of neutrons but the output of these machines is at present too low for general therapeutic use.

- The dose rate at any practical distance from the source in air can be calculated by *inverse square law*.

Inverse Square Law

It states that the intensity of radiation is inversely proportional to the square of distance of the source from target.

Applications of inverse square law

In radiotherapy, the dose rate at any practical distance from a gamma ray emitting point source in air can be obtained by means of inverse square law.

In radiography to calculate mA at a given film focal distance.

In radiation protection to calculate safer distance from the source of radiation, especially when operating mobile units in wards.

Beams Commonly used for External Radiotherapy

- X-ray beams
  - Conventional
    i. Superficial: 40 to 120 kV
    ii. Orthovoltage: 250 to 400 kV
  - Supervoltage: 2, 4, 6, 12 and 35 MeV
  - Megavoltage: >10 MeV
- Gamma ray beams
  - Cobalt 60 beam
  - Cesium 137 beam
- Particle beams
  - Electrons
  - Protons
  - Neutrons.

Forms of X-ray Therapy

Kilovoltage range
- Low voltage range
- Not preferred commonly
- Useful in Ca lip and skin (50–100 kV)
- Useful in palliative treatment of bone metastasis and chest lesions (200–250 kV)

Supervoltage range
- High voltage range between 2 and 10 MeV
- Preferred commonly due to less scatter radiation and high absorption, accuracy of dosimetry and sharpness of beam.
- Linear accelerator is used as a source for supervoltage range of radiation (4–10 MeV)

Orthovoltage range
Megavoltage: Megavoltage X-ray therapy (>1 MeV) has following advantages over orthovoltage therapy (150 to 400 kV):
- Skin-sparing effect
- Very low lateral scatter
- Homogeneous distribution of the radiation energy
- Greater deposit of the energy in the tumor, or in the target volume.

Cobalt-60

A commonly used radioisotope for external beam irradiation in treating cancer patients is Cobalt–60. It emits two gamma rays per disintegration. It is *artificial radioactive material* having a half-life of 5.3 years. It is used as a teletherapy source as well as in tubes and needles for interstitial and intracavitary brachytherapy. It decays (into nickel), and during decay it emits beta and gamma rays and it has to be replaced at regular intervals of about 4–5 years.

Teletherapy: Clinical, e.g. Cervical Cancer

- External beam via cobalt or linear accelerator and brachytherapy (e.g. radium, cobalt or cesium) are used in the treatment of carcinoma cervix.
- The radium dosage is calculated with respect to the amount of irradiation received at 2 theoretical points A and B
- **Point A** lies 2 cm above and 2 cm lateral to the base of the radium tube in the cervical canal. It approximates to the position in the pelvis where the uterine artery and ureter cross. Dose: 5000–8000 rads.
- **Point B** lies 3 cm lateral to point A and roughly corresponds to the position of obturator nodes. Dose: 3000–5000 rads.
- The Manchester method of radiotherapy for a Ca cervix is a variation of the Stockholm technique and uses rubber avoids loaded with radium in plate of the platinum boxes for vaginal vault.

Thus,
- In teletherapy the source used is outside the body and thus the beam of photon is given from outside
- 4-linear accelerator is most widely used equipment for external source radiation therapy (preferred in Ca breast, head and neck malignancies)
- External beam radiotherapy machines are mainly of two types:
  1. **X-ray machine**: In which X-rays are produced only when current is switched on.
  2. **Teletherapy apparatus**: In which a source of radioactive material (natural or artificial) gives out X-rays all the time.

Summary

RT is delivered by one of the *three* methods: brachytherapy, teletherapy, and systemic radiotherapy.

In teletherapy, the ionizing radiation produced by a machine (cobalt-60, linear accelerator) is directed at the tumor and its surrounding region to include potential areas of locoregional spread. The region to be irradiated is defined using clinical, endoscopic, imaging and other methods.

During EBRT, certain normal structures and organs are likely to be irradiated along with the locoregional volume of the tumor.

Brachytherapy, where radioactive isotopes are directly inserted into the tumor tissue, lumen or body cavity, is sparingly utilized for GI malignancies (e.g. anal canal, esophagus). However, brachytherapy forms an integral component of RT practice in certain pelvic neoplasms (e.g. cervix). The advantages of brachytherapy are its ability to deliver a concentrated dose of RT to the tumor region, to spare the normal tissues/organs substantially, and a shorter duration of treatment compared to EBRT.

The radiation dose, whether by EBRT or brachytherapy, is calculated for the irradiated volume by the unit of Gray (Gy, 1 Gy = 100 cGy). When the intent of therapy is curative, irradiation is delivered by radical RT or chemoradiotherapy or as an adjuvant (preoperative or postoperative). In these situations, the RT dose is usually 50–80 Gy, except for certain neoplasms. This dose is delivered over 5–8 weeks, conventionally at 5 fractions per week @ 180–200 cGy per fraction daily. Palliative RT is of a shorter duration with variable doses and is used to achieve palliation of symptoms and restrict tumor growth.

Temporary brachytherapy sources	Permanent brachytherapy sources	Sources of teletherapy	Sources of systemic RT
Cs 137	– Cs 131	– 4 MV and 10 MV linear accelerator (Main source)	– I 131
Ir 198	– Yttrium		– Strontium 89
	– Gold		– Samarium 138
	– Radium–226 (Outdated)	– 137Cs teletherapy	– Yttrium
	– I 125	– ^{60}Co teletherapy	– Rhenium
	– Palladium	– 150-440 KVp X-ray therapy	– Phosphorus 32
		– Cyclotron	
		– 20–24 MV Betatron	

Steps Of Radiotherapy

During planning a case of solid tumor, many factors are taken into consideration. They are types of histology of tumor, location inside the body, relation of the tumor to adjacent viscera.

Step-1: Patient Selection

Not all patients who are referred for radiotherapy are suitable for radiation therapy. Some early stage cancers are suitable for a protracted course of radical radiotherapy. In case of advanced cancer, with very short life expectancy are offered a short and simple course of palliative radiotherapy. In very advanced and flail patients with very poor performance status, radiotherapy is not useful, rather they are advised to undergo supportive care in palliative care units or hospice. The contraindications for giving radiotherapy are undiagnosed cancers, no histopathology or cytological proof of cancer, unlocalized tumor, previous history of radiotherapy to the same site and comatose patients are contraindications to deliver radiotherapy. Last but not least, all cancers must be staged with a convenient (TNM staging) system before offering treatment.

Step-2: Tumor Volume Delineation

The exact tumor volume location is very important for proper planning of radiotherapy. The tumor location information can be obtained from clinical palpation, surgeon's description in operation notes, CT scan, MRI scan and from the radioopaque markers in the residual tumor bed. A radiation oncologist can, with his remarkable accuracy, place marks on the patients' skin over the underlying disease. This is done by the help of radiological investigations and surface anatomical landmarks. The position of the tumor has to be ascertained in relation to the normal sensitive viscera, i.e. brain, eye, spinal cord, lungs, heart, kidney, liver, etc. as each structure has separate tolerance dose of radiation.

Step-3: Simulation

Radiation oncologists usually use a special type of moving (360°) diagnostic X-ray machine called simulator. Simulator is thus an X-ray machine with monitor, which simulates exactly like a teletherapy machine. Radiation oncologist for planning patients uses it. This machine can revolve 360° around a center called *isocenter*. An ideal field on the simulator should cover the tumor volume information obtained from step-2 and the various anatomical sites are localized by the use of image intensifier and monitor. The simulator exactly simulates as if the patient is lying in the actual radiation unit (teletherapy unit). After proper X-ray checking, patient's X-ray record (marker films) are kept for future record.

Step-4: Immobilization

In the radiotherapy of mobile part (i.e. breast, hand, leg, head, tongue, etc.) of the body, it has to be stabilized by the help of immobilization device. Any change in position beyond 2 to 3 mm can result in significant error to deliver radiation dose to the tumor. Commonly plaster of Paris, BDS (thermoplastic) material and Perspex materials are used to make immobilization shell. Other useful devices are headrest, mouth bite, head fixation device, etc. are used to keep the part stable for daily positioning and reproducibility. Sometimes semipermanent and permanent tattoos are put over the covered part of the body for day-to-day set up and future reference.

Step-5: Dose calculation (Dosimetry and Optimization)

The simulator plan from step-3 is fed to a treatment-planning computer. These computers have very sophisticated software, which display the body images in 2 or 3 dimensions. The radiation dose levels, homogeneity, and differential dose around the tumor volume are checked. The radiation dose, time and frequency of treatment and use of radiation accessories are decided in this step.

Step-6: Treatment Verification

After dose calculation, a verification film is taken on the teletherapy unit to check treatment plan before starting actual radiotherapy. There should not be any difference between the marker (simulator) film and the verification film (port film). In some teletherapy units the electronic portal imaging (EPI) system are in-built to take care of day-to-day reproducibility of set-up for radiotherapy.

Step-7: Actual Treatment

After verification of a particular treatment plan, patients are treated by actual teletherapy machine. Each field is usually treated daily to a radiation dose of 200 cGy (or rads) treating 5 times a week (Monday through Friday) for 5 to 7 weeks. This treatment policy is called conventional fractionation followed worldwide. Each time the radiation technologist tries to match the field outlines as simulated for a greater duplication of set-up.

TYPES OF RADIOTHERAPY TREATMENT

Radical Radiotherapy [Organ Preservation, Function Preservation Techniques]

Used when radiotherapy is the only option available. Here the radiation is given as the main treatment. The doses of radiation given are 7000–8000 cGy depending on the site and stage of the disease.

Radical radiotherapy is used in early stages of cancers at an aim to cure. The radiation oncologist takes a lot of time to accurately delineate the tumor volume, analyze image data, simulate, perform dosimetric analysis of a plan and actual radiation dose delivery. It usually takes about 6–8 weeks to complete a course in multiple sequential phases called *shrinking field technique*. The common tumors treated by radical radiotherapy are *vocal cord cancer of larynx, nasopharynx, cancer of uterine cervix, skin cancers, bladder cancers, breast cancers, and prostate cancers*, etc.

Palliative Radiotherapy

In very advanced cancers, there are poorly defined generalized symptoms, which are difficult to manage. In this situation, cure is not possible and the concern is with the issues of quality of life. The aim is therefore for minimizing discomfort called palliative treatment. This form of therapy should be simple, should not produce morbidity, and improve quality of life and without prolongation of life expectancy. Palliation involves *surgical diversion procedure, nerve block, analgesic medication, transcutaneous electrical nerve stimulation [TENS] and radiotherapy*. Chemotherapy is rarely utilized for palliation in chemosensitive tumors.

Most of the times cancers in developing countries are advanced. They need symptom control by the use of radiation or other modalities. A short and sharp course of radiation for 1 to 2 weeks is delivered to suppress malignant tumor and symptom control.

The Lesions which are Best Palliated by Radiotherapy Include
- Multiple brain metastases (Whole brain irradiation- Usually 30–37.5 Gy is administered in 10–15 fractions)
- Painful bone metastases (Systemic RT with Sr89–8Gy in single fraction)
- Uncontrolled bleeding from vagina due to gynecological cancers, and
- Superior vena cava obstruction due to nonsmall cell lung carcinoma.

Pain is the major morbidity of advanced cancers. Besides radiotherapy, supplemental analgesic administration is quite necessary for the control of cancer pain. World Health Organization (WHO) has recommended "WHO three-step ladder pattern" for the prescription of analgesics in cancer related pain. The use of morphine sulfate tablets (MST) should be freely used in higher doses according to the necessity for adequate pain control without fear of addiction.

Bone Metastases

Palliation of metastatic disease is a substantial component of radiation oncology, and a vital aspect of cancer. Patient care in general; severe pain and debilitation resulting from untreated metastases not only have a significant impact on the patients' quality of life, but on health care and economics as well. Standard treatment was 30 Gy in 10 fractions. However, there are recent trials, which have found 8 Gy in single fraction to be as effective, and this is standard today. Thus, although to control pain of bone metastases different fractions are given. 8 Gy single fraction produces equally good results as 30 gy/10 fracture or 20 Gy/5 fracture but the duration of pain relief is relatively shorter. Preferred institutional practice is 8 Gy in single fraction.

Brain Metastases

- Radiation is primary treatment for brain metastases
- It gives better quality of life to patients with brain metastases

- It reduces the intracranial edema and controls the growth of tumor
- Whole brain irradiation is usually used
- Usually 30–37.5 Gy is administered in 10–15 fractions. At times 20 Gy/5 fracture are also given
- Stereotactic radiosurgery is of benefit in patients with four or less metastases demonstrable by MRI.

Difference between radical radiotherapy and palliative radiotherapy	
Radical radiotherapy	*Palliative radiotherapy*
Treatment is aimed at complete eradication of cancer	The aim of palliation to induce temporary halt of the cancer growth, control symptoms, and improve general well-being
Radical radiotherapy is intended to give maximum possible dose (up to 70 Gy), up to the tolerance of normal tissues. The dose per fraction is less (usually < 200 cGy) to avoid long-term complications	All care taken to minimize acute side-effects of radiotherapy, radiotherapy is given quickly, at concentrate dose (300–500 cGy), due to short patient survival, less concern about long-term side-effects
Patient expects and accepts some extent of acute and chronic complications if he bargains for cure	Toxicity is not acceptable as the palliation is aimed at improvement in quality of life, not to worsen it
Patient often needs prolonged time to deliver high radiation dose up to tolerance	Patient prefers short or brief treatment (1 or 5 fractions) and few hospital visits

Adjuvant Radiotherapy

The word adjuvant is derived from the Latin verb called '*adjuvere*' meaning to help. In situation where radiotherapy is utilized for the improvement of results of another modality (usually surgery) is called adjuvant radiotherapy. Radiotherapy can be delivered before surgery (preoperative radiotherapy), after surgery (postoperative radiotherapy), during surgery (intraoperative radiotherapy and combination of preoperative and postoperative radiotherapy (sandwich radiotherapy). When radiation therapy is administered during surgery, the microscopic and minimal macroscopic disease in the tumor bed is sterilized and thereby improves local control and ultimately survival. The commonly encountered cancers requiring adjuvant radiotherapy are rectal cancers, head and neck cancers, breast cancers, and brain tumors, etc. Radiotherapy is however, most frequently used in postoperative set-up. Surgeons feel difficulty in excising an infiltrating tumor, because his excision may not be pathologically free. He likely leaves residual disease, spill tumor to the adjacent areas during handling of the tumor. In this situation radiotherapy frequently helps surgeons to circumscribe the tumor and overcome above difficulties. Radiotherapy usually fails at the tumor center, which contains radioresistant tumor *clonogens*. In contrast, radiotherapy is efficient in eradication small number of well-vascularized tumor cells at the resection margin. Hence combination of radiotherapy and surgery sounds logical. The brightest example of postoperative radiotherapy is demonstrated in *stage-I seminoma of the testis*. By giving prophylactic postoperative radiotherapy, the relapse reduces from 15 percent to near zero percent. The other example is in *postexcision breast cancer*. In this situation the breast relapse reduces from 35 percent to less than 10 percent after postoperative radiotherapy. Colonic cancer is also a good example.

Adjuvant chemotherapy is suited for treating:
- Lymphomas
- Wilms' tumor (kidney)
- Seminomas
- Ewing's sarcoma.

In *neoadjuvant chemotherapy*, the chemotherapy is used before radiotherapy or surgery with the intention of down-staging the tumor, i.e. reducing the size of tumor, e.g. carcinoma breast.

Concurrent Chemoradiotherapy

Sometimes antineoplastic drugs like cisplatinum, 5FU and hydroxyurea when given in conjunction with radiotherapy, enhance the efficacy of radiation. When radiation given **concurrently** with chemotherapy the cancer cell kill increases by two fold. These principles are used in the organ preservation techniques in *anal canal cancer, bladder cancer, esophageal cancer, cervical cancers, and head and neck cancers*.

Intraoperative Radiotherapy

Radiation can be delivered during operation resulting in sterilization of the malignant cells in the tumor bed. The irradiation of tumor in this technique is superior to percutaneous external beam radiotherapy in multiple doses. Sometimes, electron beam irradiation and interstitial brachytherapy is used to improve local control. Radiation is given to the operative bed in the operation theater. This requires a very specialized setting where the radiation machine is in the operation theater. *Electrons are used in the treatment.* After surgical excision is completed, the organs at risk are packed away from the radiation field and the treatment given. This is not a commonly followed practice as the set up required is extensive and the modality is still in the experimental stages. Intraoperative radiotherapy has higher incidence of neuropathy as side effect.

This principle of radiotherapy is used in:
- Soft tissue sarcoma
- Pancreatic cancers
- Stomach cancer
- Retroperitoneal sarcomas.

Preoperative Radiotherapy

In this setting, when the primary tumors are bulky or show borderline operability, preoperative radiation is given in
- Carcinoma of the cervix
- Rectal cancers
- Inoperable nonsmall cell carcinoma of lung.

Advantages

- Increases tumor respectability.
- Eliminates potential seeding of tumor during surgery.
- Avoids complications of postoperative radiation.
- Treating a well-oxygenated area renders the tumor more radiosensitive.

Disadvantages

- Pathological extent of the disease cannot be assessed.
- Pathological downstaging of disease influencing the adjuvant treatment.
- Limitation of total dose of radiation.
- Increases incidence of wound dehiscence.

Postoperative Radiotherapy

This is, as the name suggests, is given following surgery.

Indications

- Poorly differentiated tumors
- Depth of infiltration more, e.g. >4 mm (tongue Ca), >1/2 thickness of myometrium (endometrial Ca), full thickness of wall (esophagus, rectum), etc.
- Positive cut margins (R1 resection)

- Multifocal tumors
- Nodal positivity
- Presence of lymphovascular embolization
- Gross disease left behind (R2 resection).

Application in

- Breast postoperative
- Soft tissue sarcoma
- Ca endometrium
- Ca urinary bladder
- Ca rectum
- Ca lung
- Seminoma testis.

Combined Modality Approach

- Certain cancers are better managed by combining surgery and radiation.
    - For example, breast cancer is usually managed with resection followed by radiation.
      For example, sarcoma is usually managed with radiation followed by resection.
      In both above settings, chemotherapy is used to give better overall survival by decreasing the metastatic potential.
    - Large tumor for which resection is expected to result in poor local control or the respectability of which is marginal should be considered for prospective irradiation.
- After resection, any one or more of the following adverse factors should, at least, lead to consideration of postoperative irradiation.
    - Microscopically positive resection margins
    - Microscopically close margins (<5 mm)
    - Large primary tumors (T3/T4)

    Regardless of margin status
    - Tumors that invade beyond the capsule of their organ of origin.
    - Tumors with extensive lymph node involvement or extranodal extension.
    - Tumors with lymphatic permeation; with perineural invasion and tumor with bone invasion.
- Chemoradiotherapy.
  Increasingly radiotherapy is being given with concurrent chemotherapy especially in squamous cell carcinoma and adenocarcinoma, e.g. site:

- Carcinoma anal canal
- Carcinoma cervix
- Head and neck cancers
- Carcinoma esophagus
- Carcinoma rectum.

Concomitant chemoradiation: It appears to improve overall survival and progression-free survival in locally advanced cervical cancer. It also appears to reduce local and distant recurrence suggesting concomitant chemotherapy may afford radiosensitization and systemic cytotoxic effects. Some acute toxicity is increased, but the long-term side effects are still not clear. It is useful in treatment of:
- Head and neck cancer (especially nasopharyngeal Ca)
- Ca and canal (**nigro regimen**)
- Carcinoma cervix stage IIb/IIIa onwards.

Multimodal (Holistic) Approach

Due to volume effect of the tumor and proportion of cancer cells removed at a time, many anticancer treatments are joined together to attack cancer cell in many ways called multi-modal (holistic) approach in cancer treatment.

One kilogram of cancer contains about 10^{12} number of cancer cells.

If such tumor were removed totally by surgery, the remaining tumor load would be only 10^9, which may not be visible (microscopic). Radiation therapy if given to that area can reduce that tumor burden to 10^6 or below. In this low tumor cell load, they can be easily controlled by hosts own immune defense or immunotherapy. Chemotherapy can also decrease proportional amount of cell burden in chemosensitive tumor alike radiotherapy. In a combined modality policy, radiotherapy and surgery interval should be kept between 4 to 6 weeks except for Wilms' tumor where radiotherapy should be started on 10th day. If the interval is prolonged beyond stipulated period, resistant clonogens grow and make the tumor more difficult to control by radiotherapy. The best example of combined modality therapy in cancer is in the management of Wilms' tumor. The above tumors are managed with initial nephrectomy then local radiotherapy (10.8 Gy) on the 10th day and subsequently chemotherapy (VAC) for 12 to 24 months. The other examples are management of:

- Locally advanced breast cancer
- Cancer endometrium
- Soft tissue sarcoma.

Note: Indications for postoperative radiotherapy in a case of carcinoma endometrium include myometrial invasion of more than half-thickness, positive lymph nodes, and endocervical involvement.

High Dose Rate and Pulsed Dose Rate Brachytherapy

Traditionally radium-226 was the radionuclide of choice for brachytherapy used since last half a century. The dose rate of 54 cGy/ hour at a reference point was the most optimum dose rate for tumor control and low tissue complications; hence called "gold standard" for low dose rate brachytherapy.

However, due to its prolonged half-life (1625 years) and difficulty in protection, newer radionuclides like cobalt-60, iridium-192, cesium-137, iodine-125 are used with good safety profile. But, the dose rates of the above radionuclides are higher than radium dose rate. Hence, ICRU-38 in 1985 has recommended the outlines the dose rates for International comparison.

They are high dose rate[**HDR**] > 12 Gy per hour, medium dose rate [**MDR**] 2–12 Gy/hour and low dose rate [**LDR**] 0.4–2 Gy/hour at the point of dose calculation. Recently high dose rate equipments are being used due to its short duration of therapy and patient convenience.

HDR Brachytherapy

High dose rate (HDR) brachytherapy is a common brachytherapy method. Applicators in the form of catheters are arranged, usually according to the Manchester or Paris system on, or in the patient. A high dose rate source (often iridium 192) is then driven along the catheters on the end of a wire by a machine while the patient is isolated in a room. The source dwells in a preplanned position for a preset time before stepping forward along the catheter and repeating, to build up the required dose distribution. The advantage of this treatment over implanting radioactive sources directly is that there is lower staff exposure and the source can be more active due to low staff exposure, thus making treatment times quicker.

LDR Brachytherapy

Low dose rate (LDR) brachytherapy with a machine works in a similar way. Another variant is the sources being in the form of active and inactive balls which are again driven into the patient using a machine.

There are some drawbacks of the HDR system. Hence, in pulsed dose rate source the high dose sources are exposed to the tumor in a pulse of 1 hour to simulate like LDR brachytherapy. Many early stages of cancers are being treated with brachytherapy using HDR or PDR brachytherapy technique. Brachytherapy using HDR and PDR is used in many cancer sites as a primary treatment alone, along with external beam radiotherapy or with surgery. Often HDR is used for palliative treatment of *endobronchial cancer* with good palliation.

Endocavitary Radiotherapy

In case of *small superficial tumors of the rectal wall* especially if they are small in size (2–4 cm), exophytic tumor, well-differentiated histology, and within the reach of the sigmoidoscope can be effectively treated with this technique. A contact X-ray unit (50 kVp) is kept in contact with the rectal tumor under vision and a very high dose of radiation [10 Gy/minute] is delivered to the tumor base. This treatment is repeated every 3-weeks for 3–4 treatments. A cure rate up to 80 percent is possible in this condition popularized by Pappillon, hence named as Papillon's technique.

Intracoronary Brachytherapy

Intracoronary stent is the treatment of choice in coronary vascular disorders. But the major problem of the above procedure is re-occlusion due to endothelial cell proliferation. Currently thin radionuclide source (iridium-192) is inserted into the lumen of the affected coronary artery to deliver precise dose of radiation to prevent re-occlusion of the stent in ishemic heart disease.

Intraoperative Radiotherapy

This is a very simple technique where radiation from a deep X-ray machine or electron beam from a dedicated linear accelerator is delivered to the tumor bed after the removal of the tumor. This procedure is done under the supervision of radiation oncologist. The tumor bed is considered to harbor microscopic or gross residual tumor cell seedlings, which are difficult to control, by external beam radiotherapy.

This is most required in the abdominopelvic sites. Following surgical excision of the abdominal tumor, a single large dose of radiation (usually 20 Gy) is delivered to the precise area under observation by an electron applicator. Intraoperative Radiotherapy (IORT) seems to improve local control figures in *retroperitoneal soft tissue sarcomas, pancreatic cancers, and other abdominopelvic tumors* where external radiation is not feasible in view of higher normal tissue complications.

Craniospinal Irradiation (Prophylactic)

Lung cancer, breast cancer, leukemias, NHT, gartrointestinal malignancies and melanoma are common tumors that metastasize to brain.

By contrast prostate and overian cancer and Hodgkin's disease (HD) rarely metastasize to brain. Radiation is the primary treatment for brain metastases.

Thus prophylactic craniospinal irradiation is useful in lung cancer, ALL and NHL but not in HD.

RECENT ADVANCES IN RADIOTHERAPY

- 3 DCRT
- IMRT
- IGRT
- 4D arc modulation RT
- Stereotactic RT
- Immunoradiotherapy
- Proton beam therapy.

Conformation Therapy

During usual external radiotherapy the radiation is delivered by square or rectangular-shaped fields according to the shape of the collimator. In such geometric portals (fields) many normal tissues are irradiated unnecessarily in addition to tumor volume. Recently modern linear accelerators are available which can shield normal tissues individually, that conform the outline of the irregular tumor volume only, by the help of a multileaf collimator (MLC). This technique substantially cuts down normal tissue irradiation and thereby reduces morbidities. Conformation therapy found useful in early stage prostate cancer, intracranial tumors and the tumors of the head and neck. 3D CRT and IMRT are two main varieties.

What is 3D Conformal Radiotherapy?

Conformal radiotherapy uses a different way of planning and giving radiotherapy. Planning radiotherapy in the standard way is done using X-rays. X-rays give images of tumors in two dimensions (2D)—width and height. With computer technology it is now possible to see the tumor in three dimensions (3D)—width, height and depth using CT scan or MRI scan.

The information from these scans feeds directly into the radiotherapy planning computer. So we can see the treatment area in three dimensions. The computer program then designs radiation beams that 'conform' more closely to the shape of the tumor and avoid healthy tissue as far as possible. This is called '3D conformal radiotherapy' (3DCRT).

The main benefit with using conformal radiotherapy is that it allows to plan in 3D so is more precise. Conformal radiotherapy can give a better chance of killing the cancer by delivering a higher dose of radiation straight to it. As less healthy tissue is included in the radiotherapy field it is likely to has fewer long-term side effects.

Planning Conformal Radiotherapy

Planning conformal radiotherapy treatment is very similar to planning other types of external radiotherapy. But planning for conformal radiotherapy may take longer. For instance, patient has to have a CT scan first, to help plan CRT.

Planning involves several steps, which usually begin with a 'virtual simulation' session. This session involves:
- Planning the radiotherapy to make sure that all the tumor is inside the radiotherapy beams (or 'fields')
- Making marks on the skin to make sure the same area is treated each session (see skin markings)
- Making molds to stop certain parts of your body moving during treatment.

An X-ray machine called a 'simulator' is used to plan radiotherapy treatment. It is called a simulator because it is built to be like (or simulate) a radiotherapy machine, but without giving the treatment. The specialist uses the pictures it produces, along with any scans, to draw on the treatment area. Conformal radiotherapy is sometimes planned entirely by CT scanning. The specialist may also use information from MRI scans or PET scans to refine the treatment plan even further.

If CRT is being given to the head or neck area, patient may need to wear a 'perspex' mold (sometimes called a 'shell' or 'mask') during treatment. Some types of masks are seen through, others are not. Patient can have a mold for other parts of the body, such as the breast, limbs and sometimes the whole body. The mold keeps the area completely still. So treatment will be as accurate as possible. This also means that patient can have any markings made on the mask, instead of on your skin.

Which Types of Cancers are Treated with Conformal Radiotherapy?

Conformal radiotherapy is most useful for tumors that are close to important organs and structures in your body. This is because it helps to avoid radiation damage to healthy body tissues and organs.

Specialists often use conformal radiotherapy to treat prostate cancer. It can lower the number of men who have long-term side effects of straining and bleeding from the back passage (proctitis) after radiotherapy. Conformal radiotherapy is the best way to give radiotherapy for prostate cancer. It also allows them to use a higher dose of radiotherapy.

Other cancers where CRT may be used are esophageal cancer, some types of lung cancer, bladder cancer, pancreatic cancer, liver cancer, head and neck cancers and brain tumors.

What are the Side Effects of 3D Conformal Radiotherapy?

Because conformal radiotherapy means that less normal tissue will be in the field of the radiotherapy, the risk of side effects is lower. As always, this is a bit of a balancing act. If too much of the surrounding area out of the radiotherapy treatment field is taken, there is a chance that cancer cells may be missed.

Intensity Modulated Radiotherapy

Nowadays it is possible to modulate a given radiation beam accurately, which can fit to the tumor shape. Modern linear accelerators are attached with multileaf collimator to alter the quality of radiation beam and to modify dose distribution. It eliminates the need for traditional wedged beams. Like conformal radiotherapy, IMRT shapes the radiation beams to closely fit the area where the cancer is. But it also alters the radiotherapy dose depending on the shape of the tumor. This means that the central part of the cancer receives the highest dose of radiotherapy and a surrounding area of tissue gets lower doses. A machine called a linear accelerator (LINAC) delivers the radiotherapy. The LINAC has a special device called a *multileaf collimator* (MLC) that moves around the patient and shapes the beams of radiotherapy to fit the tumor.

Intensity modulated radiotherapy (IMRT) found useful in the treatment of prostatic cancer, small brain tumors, and head and neck cancers. It is most suitable for prostatic cancer. Also, the clinical trials using IMRT in breast cancer and cancer of the larynx are in progress.

Summary: IMRT
It is advanced technique of radiotherapy.

Computer, multileaf collimators (MLC), and highly controlled X-ray accelerators are required.

It is an iteration of 3D CRT that employs dynamic multileaf collimation to shape profile of beam and vary the intensity over its area, allowing greater conformality than standard 3D CRT.

It is an aggressive therapy that requires fractionated treatment sessions typically 5 days a week for 6 to 10 weeks.

It is being used to treat cancer of prostate, head and neck, breast, thyroid and lung.

Stereotactic Radiotherapy [Gamma-knife, X-knife]

This is a relatively new technique used primarily in the early intracranial neoplasms. Stereotactic radiotherapy is broadly divided into X-knife or γ-knife (radiosurgery). X-knife or stereotactic multiarc radiotherapy **(SMART) technique** involves multiple precise narrow beams of radiation (X-rays) in arcs cross firing to a high dose point called isocenter. This high dose point is precisely focused to the tumor nidus by the help of 3-dimensional treatment planning computer and a linear accelerator. The gamma-knife or radiosurgery involves a comprehensive unit containing 201 cobalt-60 sources focused to single point. Both X-knife and γ-knife need a head fixation device called Leksell's apparatus, before delivery of radiation therapy. Stereotactic radiotherapy found useful in the treatment of *arteriovenous malformation (AVM) of brain, acoustic neuromas, small [<4 cm] intracranial gliomas, trigeminal neuralgia, and thalamectomy in psychiatric conditions*.

Focused megavoltage irradiation is achieved by
- Precise MRI localization
- High-voltage linear accelerator
- Accurate isocentric rotational arcing.
  Stereotactic radiosurgery delivers a large single high-energy dose from:
- Cobalt–60 source (gamma-knife),
- Linear accelerator (X-ray knife), or
- Cyclotron (High-energy proton beam).

Thermoradiotherapy

Temperature nearly to 43° can kill cancer cells in synthetic and interphase stage of the cell cycle. This principle was used in the past by using therapeutic pyrexia to treat malignant disease. Radiation related cellular death is encountered during the mitotic and G2 phase of the cell cycle. Intratumoral hyperthermia could be possible by the use of interstitial microwave antenna [400–2450 MHz]. Hence, simultaneous use of hyperthermia followed by radiation enhanced the cancer cell sterilization. This thermoradiotherapy is found useful in the management malignant melanoma of skin and chest wall recurrence of breast cancer patients.

Image-guided Radiation Therapy

Image-guided radiation therapy (IGRT) is the use of frequent imaging during a course of radiation therapy to improve the precision and accuracy of the delivery of the treatment.

In IGRT, machines that deliver radiation, such as a linear accelerator, are equipped with imaging technology so that the physician can image the tumor immediately before or even during the time radiation is delivered, while the patient is positioned on the treatment table. Using specialized computer software, these images are then compared to the images taken during simulation. Any necessary adjustments are then made to the patient's position and/or radiation beams in order to more precisely target radiation at the tumor and avoid healthy surrounding tissue.

Computed tomography (CT), magnetic resonance imaging (MRI), positron emission tomography (PET), ultrasound (US) and X-ray imaging may be used for IGRT.

IGRT is used to treat tumors in areas of the body that are prone to movement, such as the lungs (affected by breathing) and prostate gland, as well tumors located close to critical organs and tissues. It is often used in conjunction with intensity-modulated radiation therapy (IMRT), an advanced mode of high-precision radiotherapy that utilizes computer-controlled X-ray accelerators to deliver precise radiation doses to a malignant tumor or specific areas within the tumor.

Proton Beam Therapy

Proton beam therapy uses a special machine called a cyclotron or a synchrotron to generate and accelerate protons. The protons leave the machine and are steered by magnets toward the tumor. Other pieces of equipment are used to modify the range of the protons, shape of the beam, and to compensate for organ location.

Proton therapy is being used to treat tumors in these areas of the body with encouraging early results:
— Lung
— Prostate
— Brain
— Spinal or vertebral body tumors
— Skull base sarcomas
— Pediatric brain tumors
— Head and neck
— Eye melanomas.

Targeted Radiotherapy (Metabolic Radiotherapy)/Immunoradiotherapy

Some tumors can selectively concentrate some radionuclides due to their specific metabolic properties. Neural tumors like pheochromocytomas and neuroblastomas can concentrate meta-iodo-benzyl-guanidine (MIBG) more efficiently. Hence, MIBG tagged with iodine-131 when injected parenterally, specifically concentrate in the diseased site and deliver significant radiation dose to the tumor. Usually a dose of 200 mCi of I-131 tagged MIBG is required for the treatment of neuroblastoma. The other novel principles of selective radiotherapy is metabolic radiotherapy of I-131 in thyroid cancer and monoclonal antibody (MAb) tagged I-131 therapy in colorectal cancers and hepatocellular carcinoma.

Ibritumomab is a protein that specifically targets white blood cells (lymphocytes) in the body. When ibritumomab is attached to a radioactive chemical, such as indium-111 and yttrium-90, the radiation is delivered directly to the sites of the lymphoma. Ibritumomab is a protein that specifically targets white blood cells (lymphocytes) in the body. When ibritumomab is attached to a radioactive chemical, such as indium-111 and yttrium-90, the radiation is delivered directly to the sites of the lymphoma.

Ibritumomab is used in a regimen with rituximab and a radioactive chemical in the treatment of non-Hodgkin's lymphoma.

Contraindications: Previous allergic reaction to ibritumomab, rituximab (Rituxan), radioactive chemicals, mouse protein, or other medicines, liver disease, renal disease, bleeding or blood clotting problems, hypotension, history of heart disease, heart attack, angina (chest pain), or irregular heart beats, pregnancy.

Rituxan® (Rituximab) is an inactive treatment of B-cell non-Hodgkin's lymphoma (NHL). Rituxan is for people who have relapsed or refractory low-grade or follicular, CD20+, B-cell non-Hodgkin's lymphoma. Rituxan effectively works with your immune system and targets the cells involved in B-cell NHL.

Gleevec (Imatinib mesylate) is a man-made drug currently used for the treatment of patients with certain types of leukemia (most commonly chronic myeloid leukemia) and a rare type of cancer known as gastrointestinal stromal tumor (GIST). It may also be used to treat other types of cancers as part of a research trial. Imatinib works by blocking (*inhibiting tyrosine kinase*) signals within cancer cells and preventing a series of chemical reactions that cause the cell to grow and divide.

High-Yield Facts
- For radiotherapy various modifications are made to minimize radiation to surrounding tissues while maximizing radiation to cancer like **3D conformal radiation therapy (3DCRT) and intensity modulated radiation therapy (IMRT)** improved outcomes have been shown for prostate cancer patients receiving IMRT.
- *Gamma knife radiosurgery:* Brain metastases
- *Accelerated fraction radiation:* Head and neck cancer; lung cancer

- *Chemoradiation:* Rectum
- *Concurrent radiation and chemotherapy:* Cancer H and N
- *Electron beam therapy:* Superficial skin tumors.
- *Radiolabeled ablation (Ibritumomab, tiuxetan and tositumomab):* Low-grade NHL
- Radiotherapy is used with curative intent for:
  - Larynx
  - Oral cavity
  - Pharynx
  - Esophagus
  - Vagina
  - Prostate
  - Skin
  - HD
  - Some tumors of brain and spinal cord.
- *Resection of isolated metastasis:* Mainly used for carcinoma breast with single brain/liver/lung lesion. Also effective for carcinoma of colon.

RADIATION PORTALS

Various types of radiation fields are prepared for each individual case. The shape and size of the radiation field depends upon the site and volume of the tumor. According to the International Commission on Radiation Units (ICRU) report number-50, the various tumor volumes have to be defined for radiotherapy treatment planning. The various tumor volumes are gross tumor volume (GTV), clinical target volume (CTV), and planning target volume (PTV), etc. defined by the radiation oncologist. The most popular radiation fields used in clinical radiotherapy are *mantle field* and *total axial nodal irradiation* (TANI) portal for Hodgkin's lymphoma, and *spade technique* for sacral plexus irradiation, *whole body irradiation* for mycosis fungoides and before bone marrow transplant, *whole brain irradiation* for cerebral metastases, and *craniospinal irradiation* (CSI) technique for medulloblastomas, NHL, small cell carcinoma of lung, and leukemias (Acute leukemic leukemia).

COMPLICATIONS OF RADIOTHERAPY

Radiotherapy is not free of side effects. It is usual to see some percentage of radiation complications if treated in curative intent; hence it is called "radiation accompaniment" or radiation morbidities.

The incidence of systemic symptoms of radiotherapy depends upon the field size, fraction size and the total dose of radiation. Radiation injury to the cells can induce change in rapidly dividing cells (early reacting tissues) and slowly dividing cells (late reacting tissues). The rapidly dividing cells are usually present in mucosa and hematopoietic cells those have greater potentiality to regenerate and repair after a given radiation damage called sublethal radiation damage. However, stable cells like kidney, and brain cannot regenerate after a given radiation damage and the effects of radiation damage are permanent. The change in the early reacting tissues is seen during or immediately after radiotherapy, whereas the late effects are seen 6 months to years following radiotherapy. The common acute reactions are radiation sickness, mucositis and sore throat, diarrhea, cystitis, vomiting and fall in blood counts. The late-effects of radiation appear 6 months to years following radiotherapy. If the radiation treatment dose exceeds a particular threshold dose, the latter induces permanent damage due to fibrosis. The common late effects are rectal bleeding, hematuria, osteoradionecrosis, radiation nephritis, square pneumonia, etc.

Growth retardation is a significant problem in pediatrics age group of patients who receive radiotherapy to the axial skeletons (skull and spine). The decrease in the sitting height up to 20 percent at 10-year is noted among patients who received radiotherapy to their axial skeleton. Similarly pediatric leukemia patients received prior cranial irradiation prophylaxis show signs of 10 to 20 percent decrease in the IQ level compared to controls. Facial asymmetry, chest deformity, aplasia of breast and endocrinological alterations are a few morbidities encountered after radiotherapy. The late side effects are sometimes proportionate to the dose (non-stochastic effect, e.g. cataract) or irrespective of dose (stochastic, e.g. second cancer). The commonest neoplasm induced by radiation is development of osteosarcoma in retinoblastoma patients received radiotherapy in the past and leukemia in total axial nodal irradiation for Hodgkin's lymphoma.

Radiosensitive Tissues

- Bone is among the most **radioresistant** organs, radiation effects being manifested mainly in children through premature fusion of the epiphyseal growth plate.
- Organs with less need for cell renewal, such as heart, skeletal muscle, and nerves, are more resistant to radiation effects.
- In radiation-resistant organs, the vascular endothelium is the most sensitive component.

Radioresistant Tissues

- By contrast, the male testis, female ovary, and bone marrow are the most sensitive organs. Any bone marrow in a radiation field will be eradicated by therapeutic irradiation.

- Organs with more self-renewal as a part of normal homeostasis, such as the hematopoietic system and mucosal lining of the intestinal tract, are more sensitive.

Acute Effects of Total Body Irradiation

At the human level the effects of radiation are studies and conclusions drawn from the nuclear accidents, e.g. **nuclear survivors of Hiroshima and Nagasaki, Marshallese accident** in 1954, **Chernobyl** reactor accident.

Sr No	Dose (cGY)	Time of post-exposure to death	System affected	Presentation
1.	250–500	Weeks	*Hemopoietic syndrome*	Mitotically active precursor cells are sterilized by radiation. This prevents replenishment of these cells. Time of crisis is seen after all the circulating cells in the body reach the minimum value. **Prodromal symptoms:** Nausea and vomiting. Infection and chills, fatigue, petechial hemorrhages and ulceration of mouth These symptoms are the manifestation of depression of blood elements
2.	500–1200	Days	*Gastrointestinal syndrome*	*Nausea, vomiting and prolonged diarrhea. Loss of appetite, sluggishness and lethargy* Symptoms and death are due to depopulation of the epithelial lining of the GIT
3.	>10,000	24–48 hrs	*Cerebrovascular syndrome*	*No prodromal symptoms* • Severe nausea and vomiting within minutes • Disorientation • Loss of coordination of muscular movement • Respiratory distress • Diarrhea • Convulsions • Coma and finally *death*. At this dose all other systems are also seriously damaged. But cerebrovascular damage brings death so fast, that the failure of the other systems does not become obvious.

Hemopoietic and *gastrointestinal syndromes* are reversible with good symptomatic and supportive care.

Late Effects of Radiation

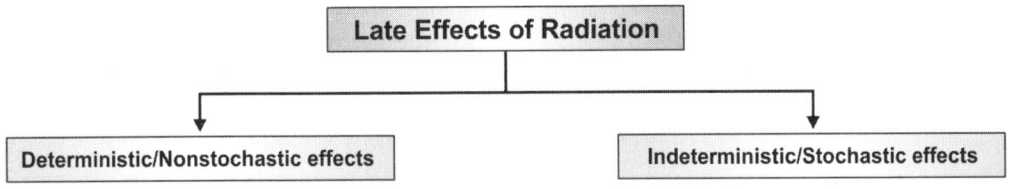

Deterministic/Nonstochastic effects
- Depend on the total dose of the given radiation. Chances of the occurrence increase as the dose given increases
- Example: Alopecia in the irradiated portal

Indeterministic/Stochastic effects
- Independent of the total dose of radiation. It is an "ALL OR NONE" type of a phenomenon.
- Example: Genetic mutations

BENIGN DISEASES THAT CAN BE TREATED WITH RADIOTHERAPY

Eye
- Pterygium
- Exophthalmos
- Macular degenerations.

Skin
- Keloids
- Plantar warts
- Keratoacanthoma.

Hemangiomas (cutaneous, CNS and spinal cord, vertebral hemangiomas, etc.)
Prevention of **vascular restenosis** after angioplasty

Bone
- Ameloblastoma
- Aneurysmal bone cyst
- Plantar fascitis.
  (also to prevent recurrent myositis ossificans)

Glandular tissues
- Gynecomastia
- Ovarian ablation
- Parotitis.

Total lymphoid irradiation before organ transplant.
Especially bone marrow transplant, bone marrow ablation.

Radiotherapy in Graves' Disease

I-131 is used in the treatment of Graves' disease in the dose of 5 to 15 mCi. I-131 therapy is designed to administer a sufficient radiation dose to partially destroy the thyroid parenchyma. Biologic effects of I-131 include pyknosis and necrosis of the follicular cells and, later, vascular and stromal fibrosis. The studies directed at evaluating the safety of radioiodine therapy have failed to show any significant carcinogenic, leukemogenic or teratogenic effect in doses used to treat hyperthyroidism.

Formula tried to calculate an optimal dose of radioiodine that achieves euthyroidism, without a high incidence of relapse or progression to hypothyroidism:

I-131 dose (in mCi): Weight of gland (gm) × Dose (mCi/gm)/Uptake (%)

A practical strategy today is to give a fixed dose based on clinical features, like the severity of thyrotoxicosis, the size of goiter, and the level of radioiodine uptake. The dose of I-131 that is used for treatment of Graves' disease may range from 70 to 215 mCi/gm. However, **I-131 dosage** generally **ranges between 5 mCi to 15 mCi**, i.e. 185 MBq to 555 MBq.

Tumors and their Treatments of Choice

Surgery Alone: Treatment of Choice

- Lower esophagus, stomach, colon
- Pancreas
- Kidney
- Thyroid
- Melanoma
- HCC
- Keratoacanthoma

Radiotherapy: Treatment of Choice

- Oral cavity, lip, tongue, cheek
- Nasopharynx, oropharynx and hypopharynx
- Nasal cavity
- Larynx
- Skin cancers (except melanoma)

Cervix
Bladder (except T1)
Testis—seminoma
Hodgkin's disease—early disease
NHL—early disease
Medulloblastoma (following surgical resection)
Astrocytomas (grade 3 and 4)
Retinoblastoma

Chemotherapy–Treatment of Choice

Acute and chronic leukemias
HD (advanced)
NHL (advanced)
Testicular teratoma
Choriocarcinoma
Small cell lung cancer
Rhabdomyosarcoma
Neuroblastoma

Radiosensitivity of different tumors			
Highly radiosensitive	*Moderately radiosensitive*	*Relatively resistant*	*Highly resistant*
Lymphoma	Small cell lung cancer	Squamous cell carcinoma of lung	Melanoma
Seminoma	Breast cancer	RCC	Osteosarcoma
Myeloma	Basal cell carcinoma	Rectal carcinoma	Pancreatic carcinoma
Ewing's sarcoma	Medulloblastoma	Bladder carcinoma	HCC
Wilms' tumors	Teratoma	Sift tissue sarcoma	Malignant fibrous
	Ovarian cancer	Cervical cancer	Histiocytoma

Type of RT	*Indications*
Whole body RT	– Mycosis fungoides
	Before bone marrow transplant
Mantle RT	– Hodgkin's lymphoma

Prophylactic craniospinal RT	– ALL
	– Small cell lung cancer
	– NHL
CHART	– Nonsmall cell lung cancer
Accelerated RT	– Head and neck cancer
Hyperfractionated RT	– Lung cancer
	– Head and neck cancer
Emergency RT	– SVC obstruction due to lung cancer
	– Cardiac temponade due to pericardial invasion by malignancy
	– Spinal cord compression by metastases
Intraoperative RT (electrons > X-rays)	– Breast cancer
	– Pancreatic cancer
	– Lung carcinoma
	– Skull base
	– Melanoma
Postoperative RT	– Tumor margins positive
	– Tumor margins within 5 mm
	– LN metastases
	– Peritumoral invasion
	– Deep lobe involvement of parotid
	– Endocervical involvement
	– More than 50% of uterine wall involved
	– Recurrent tumor
	– High grade malignancies
IMRT	– Ca prostate
	– Head and neck cancer
	– Oral cancers
3D CRT	– Head and neck cancer
	– Lung cancer
	– Thyroid cancer
	– Breast cancer
Sterotactic radiosurgery	– Brain metastases (<4 in number)
– Co-60 (Gamma-knife)	– AVMs
– Linear accelerator (X-ray knife)	– Small meningioma
– Cyclotron (Proton beam)	– Small acoustic neuroma
	– Pituitary adenoma

Neutron therapy	– Salivary gland tumor – Cystic gliomas of brain
Proton therapy	– Stereotactic RT – Skin cancer
Concurrent chemotherapy	– Head and neck cancer – Ca cervix stage IIb/IIIA onwards – Ca anal canal – Ca nasopharynx
Intracavitary brachytherapy	– Treatement of gynecological malignancies, particularly those of the cervix, vagina, and uterus
Interstitial brachytherapy	– Oral cavity – Oropharynx – Nasopharynx – Neck nodes – Skin cancer – Carcinoma of the prostate – Anal canal – Penis – Carcinoma of the breast as salvage for local recurrence Please note contraindications to interstitial brachytherapy: • Tumor infiltrating or attached to bone. • Presence of active infection within the potential implant volume. • Target volume not definable • Tumor not properly accessible
Brachytherapy for benign disease	– Keloid scars are not only unsightly but often itchy and painful – Pterygium is a condition where a pad of connective tissue with blood vessels grows over the cornea – Peripheral vascular disease – Following balloon angioplasty of stenosed peripheral arteries – Coronary artery disease

Systemic RT
- I-131-Ca thyroid
- Strontium-89 and Samarium-132 = painful bone metastases **(8 Gy in single fraction)**
- Yttrium
- Phosphorus-32 = Polycythemia rubra vera

VARIOUS TUMORS AND VISCERA: DOSE LIMITS

Tumor	Control dose
Leukemic cell	6 Gy
Histiocytosis	12 Gy
Wilms' tumor	20 Gy
Microscopic disease	50 Gy
Seminoma	25 Gy
Lymphoma	36 Gy
Carcinoma	60–70 Gy
Sarcoma	70 Gy
Glioma	55–60 Gy
Pituitary tumor	46 Gy
Ewing's sarcoma	55 Gy
Normal tissue	*Tolerance dose*
Brain	50 Gy
Spinal cord	45 Gy
Eye lens	6 Gy
Eye retina	50 Gy
Lungs	22.5 Gy
Liver	35 Gy
Stomach	45 Gy
Kidney	22.5 Gy
Uterus	250 Gy
Rectum	50 Gy
Bladder	60 Gy

The above levels apply when the radiation is delivered in conventional fractionations, i.e. 1.8 to 2 Gy per day treating 5 days a week (Monday to Friday).

GUIDE TO THE RELATIVE RADIOSENSITIVITY OF NORMAL TISSUE

Radiosensitive
Lymphocytes, bone marrow gonads
Embryonic tissue

Moderately sensitive
Skin, small blood vessels, lens of the eye, growing tissues, lung tissue, salivary glands

Moderately resistant
Skin, thyroid gland, nerve cells

Radioresistant
Muscle bone connective tissue, mature red blood corpuscles.

FOLLOW-UP OF CANCER PATIENTS RECEIVING RADIOTHERAPY

Follow-up in cancer patients is very important part of cancer care. The post treatment visits are based on the tumor biology, aggressiveness, failure pattern and radiation after effects. The cancers involving head and neck areas and other site cancers recur very commonly within first 24 months of treatment. The failures of the treatment are classified as residual disease or recurrent disease. When the disease reappears within 6 months after treatment is called residual disease and when reappears after 6-months of follow-up is called recurrent disease. Metastatic lesions detected on follow-up are called metastatic disease.

Some cancers like breast cancer, prostate cancer and ocular melanomas can fail even after 20 years following treatment. This prolonged relapse of above cancers is explained as due to their biological individuality. Hence, they need follow-up for lifelong. After 2 years the chance of relapse of disease is very minimal. A prototype of follow-up policy in cancer is as follows:

Every 2 months × 2 years
Every 3 months × 3 years
Every six months × 5 years
Every year × 10 years

The follow-up includes clinical examination, tumor marker study and radiological study. In gynecological cancers, follow-up PAP smear is not recommended for first 6 months of follow-up. Because during this time the cellular morphology on cytology is very difficult to differentiate between radiation effect and recurrent malignant tumor. In case of head and neck cancer patients with history of radiotherapy should not undergo dental extraction due to the possibility of osteoradionecrosis.

ns and
Section 4

Newer Advances and Interventional Radiology

Chapter 17

Newer Advances

ADVANCES IN CT SCAN

By permitting radical improvements in z-axis spatial resolution, multislice **CT** enhances CT imaging of submillimeter anatomic and pathologic structures. Subsecond scanning techniques with rapid-volume coverage are enabling new functional imaging methods using CT. Fi- nally, rapid developments of computer technology are enabling radiologists to take advantage of new **3D** and 4D imaging methods, moving CT from a 2D anatomy-only tool to a **3D** tool that can provide functional as well as anatomic information.

Multidetector CT

Refinements in detector technology have allowed production of scanners with additional detectors along the scanning axis (z-axis). These scanners, called *multidetector* CT (MDCT) scanners, can obtain multiple slices in a single rotation that are thinner and can be acquired in a shorter period of time. This results in enhanced resolution and increased image reconstruction ability. As the technology has progressed, higher numbers (2, 4, 6, 8, 10, 16, 32, 40, 64 and currently up to 500) of detectors are used to produce clearer final images. The development of MDCT allows for even shorter breath holds, which are beneficial for all patients but especially children, the elderly, and the critically ill. However, it should be noted that despite the advantages of MDCT, there is an increase in radiation dose compared to single-detector CT to consider. With MDCT, the additional detectors along the z-axis result in improved use of the contrast bolus. In addition, the shorter breath holds secondary to faster scanning times and increased resolution have all led to improved imaging of the pulmonary vasculature and the ability to detect segmental and subsegmental emboli. In contrast to pulmonary angiography, CT pulmonary angiography (CTPA) also allows simultaneous detection of parenchymal abnormalities that may be contributing to a patient's clinical presentation. Secondary to these advantages and increasing availability, CTPA has rapidly become the test of choice for many clinicians in the evaluation of pulmonary embolism; it is considered equal to pulmonary angiography in terms of accuracy, and with less associated risks. With advances in CT scanning, MDCT angiography (MDCTA) is replacing conventional angiography for the diagnosis of pulmonary embolism.

Special applications of MD/multislice CT:
- CT Angiography (a non-invasive study)
- Triple phase CT of liver and pancreas
- Cardiac CT
- Coronary calcium scoring (*"Non-invasive coronary angiography"*); Coronary calcium detected by these imaging techniques is quantified using the **Agatston score** most commonly, which is based on the area and density of calcification.
- CT perfusion
- CT enteroclysis
- Virtual colonography
- CT urography
- CT fluoroscopy

Virtual Bronchoscopy

The three-dimensional (3D) image of the thorax obtained by MDCT can be digitally stored, reanalyzed, and displayed as 3D reconstructions of the airways down to the sixth- to seventh-generation. Using these computed generated reconstructions, a "virtual" bronchoscopy can be performed. Virtual bronchoscopy has been proposed as an adjunct to conventional bronchoscopy in several clinical situations: It can allow accurate assessment of the extent and length of an airway stenosis, including the airway distal to the narrowing; it can provide useful information about the relationship of the airway abnormality to adjacent mediastinal structures; and it allows preprocedure planning for therapeutic bronchoscopy to help ensure the appropriate equipment is available for the procedure. Virtual bronchoscopy can also be used to perform noninvasive follow-up of patients with treated airway lesions. Navigational systems using virtual bronchoscopy have been developed to allow pathfinding to guide the bronchoscopist to a peripheral region within the lung, allowing peripheral lung lesions to be sampled more efficiently. Finally, with the advent of endobronchial lung volume reduction surgery in the management of pulmonary emphysema, virtual bronchoscopy may be able to help target the area of peripheral lung for endobronchial valve procedures. The extent of emphysema in each segmental region together with other anatomic details may help in choosing the most appropriate subsegments. However, software packages for the generation of virtual bronchoscopic images are relatively early in development and their utilization and potential impact on patient care are still unknown. In addition to allowing virtual bronchoscopy, advances in computing capabilities and digital imaging allow the bronchoscopic images obtained through a real bronchoscopic examination to be stored as digital images and reviewed after completion of the procedure.

CARDIAC COMPUTED TOMOGRAPHY

Computed tomography (CT) is fast, simple and noninvasive, and it provides images with excellent spatial resolution and good soft-tissue contrast.

Imaging the heart is a more difficult problem, however, because image acquisition times for conventional CT have until recently been on the order of 1s, far too long to freeze cardiac motion.

Electron-beam CT employs a fixed detector array and radiation source (Generation V CT scan).

The X-rays are generated by an electron beam sweeping continuously across the target anode ring. This is accomplished very rapidly, on the order of 50 to 100 ms (Ultrafast CT scan).

The electron beam can be triggered by the electrocardiogram trace and single static images or cine images are generated with excellent temporal resolution ("Real-time" CT scan).

Clinical Applications

- Pericardial calcification is an important sign of constrictive pericarditis and is easily detected by CT.
- CT is useful in characterizing cardiac masses, particularly those containing fat or calcium.
- The ability to detect small amounts of fat with high spatial resolution makes CT an attractive technique for imaging patients with suspected *arrhythmogenic right ventricular dysplasia.*
- Cine images can be used to evaluate wall motion and determine ejection fraction, end-diastolic and end-systolic volumes and cardiac mass.
- CT angiography (CTA) has demonstrated accuracy similar to MRA in imaging the aorta and great vessels, and CTA is rapidly becoming the examination of choice in the evaluation of patients with suspected pulmonary embolus (Screening tool for aorta but investigation of choice for pulmonary embolism).

- Coronary CTA with multidetector spiral CT is in the developmental stage.
- Both CT and MRI are valuable in delineating the presence and course of anomalous coronary vessels; however, the clinical utility of either technique in detecting and grading coronary artery stenoses has not been widely demonstrated.
- *Coronary calcification:* Calcium in the coronary arteries occurs in atherosclerosis and is absent in the normal coronary artery. CT is very sensitive for the detection of coronary artery calcification and is being promoted as a *noninvasive modality for the screening and diagnosis of CAD*. The amount of coronary calcification (coronary calcium score) is related to the severity of coronary disease.
- However, although CT has a very high sensitivity for the detection of CAD, it has a low specificity. The overall predictive accuracy for angiographic obstructive coronary disease in a typical CAD patient population is similar to other imaging modalities, such as SPECT.
- Due to its low specificity, CT should not be used for the diagnosis of obstructive coronary disease. However, in asymptomatic patients, more severe coronary atherosclerosis (and thus a higher calcium score) is associated with a higher risk of future cardiac events.

Limitations of CT

- Ionizing radiation
- Radiation doses tend to increase as the spatial and temporal resolution improve; however, the dose for cardiac CT is almost always significantly lower than the dose delivered during cardiac catheterization.
- Need for iodinated contrast, which is problematic in patients with renal insufficiency or contrast allergy.

CARDIAC MAGNETIC RESONANCE IMAGING

It is particularly challenging because of the rapid physiologic motion of the heart and coronary arteries. Both static and cine images can be obtained using electrocardiographic triggering, often within a short breath-hold of 10 to 15s **(GATING)**. Cine images can be acquired in any plane with excellent blood-myocardial contrast, and these images can be used to quantify ejection fraction, end-systolic and end-diastolic volumes and cardiac mass with high accuracy and reliability.

Clinical Applications

- The multiplanar capabilities of MRI, coupled with excellent contrast and spatial resolution, are often valuable in defining anatomic relationships in patients with *complex congenital heart disease*.

- *Cardiac masses* can be characterized and their relationship to normal anatomic structures defined. Likewise, MRI is often the examination of choice to determine whether a mediastinal or pulmonary mass has invaded the pericardium or heart.
- The entire pericardium can be visualized in multiple planes and MRI has proved useful in characterization of *pericardial effusions, pericardial thickening and constrictive pericarditis* in patients with indeterminate results on echocardiography.
- MRI is an important technique for evaluation of patients with suspected *arrhythmogenic right ventricular dysplasia*, where fatty infiltration of the right ventricular free wall can be identified, as can right ventricular dilatation and dyskinesis.
- MRA is a standard technique for *imaging the aorta and large vessels of the chest and abdomen*, with results essentially identical to conventional catheter-based angiography.
- MRA of the coronary arteries is a much more difficult challenge, both because of the small size of these vessels and because of their rapid and complex motion during the cardiac cycle. Although promising results have been achieved, coronary MRA is not yet an accurate and reliable clinical technique.
- MRI is a promising technology for the evaluation of myocardial perfusion. *Myocardial perfusion* is evaluated by injecting a bolus of contrast and then continuously scanning the heart as the contrast passes through the cardiac chambers and into the myocardium. Relative perfusion deficits are reflected as regions of low signal intensity within the myocardium.
- *Myocardial viability* may be determined by imaging the heart 10 to 20 min after contrast injection, as infracted tissue retains contrast by virtue of its larger extracellular volume.
- Specialized pulse sequences have been designed to measure the velocity of blood in each pixel of the image, so that flow across valves and within blood vessels may be accurately determined. These techniques may allow *characterization of the severity of valvular disease as well as quantification* of shunt volumes.

Computed Tomography Enteroclysis

Computed tomography enteroclysis consists of bowel intubation with an enteroclysis catheter and instilling a water-soluble contrast agent, a dilute barium suspension, or a methylcellulose suspension followed immediately by CT scanning. Whether a positive contrast agent or a water-density agent together with an intravenous contrast agent to opacify bowel mucosa is superior is not clear. Negative oral contrast agents designed specifically for CT-enteroclysis are also becoming available. Multislice CT performed during a single breath-hold allows three-dimensional (3D) reconstruction.

Computed tomography enteroclysis is a viable alternate in a setting of small bowel obstruction or inflammatory bowel disease and in a search for polyps. It is superior to conventional CT, especially with low-grade bowel obstruction. Whether CT enteroclysis is preferred over conventional enteroclysis is debatable.

Advantages of MDCT (Generation IV CT)

- Shorter scan times
- Reduced patient and organ motion
- The ability to acquire images dynamically during the infusion of intravenous contrast that can be used to construct CT angiograms of vascular structures and CT perfusion images.

Dual-energy CT

- The photoelectric effect and Compton scatter are the primary ways in which X-ray photons interact with matter at the energy levels used in diagnostic imaging. The term photoelectric effect refers to the ejection of an electron from the K shell (the innermost shell) of an atom by an incident photon. An electron from an adjacent shell fills the void, and energy is released in the form of a photoelectron. The photoelectric effect occurs when an incident photon has sufficient energy to overcome the K-shell binding energy of an electron. Organic substances with a low atomic number are affected by Compton scatter, whereas those with a higher atomic number are affected by the photoelectric effect.
- The energy dependence of the photoelectric effect and the variability of K edges form the basis of dual-energy techniques.
- Current dual-energy CT scanners differ in terms of the number of X-ray tubes, the number and arrangement of detector arrays, the energy of fan beams, and the rotation of X-ray tubes and detector arrays, depending on the manufacturer. These machines are rapidly evolving: Some scanners employ two tubes and allow nearly simultaneous data acquisition, some use kilovolt switching techniques, and some use a detector-level scintigraphic approach, in which energy discrimination occurs at the level of the detector. Radiation doses may vary depending on the manufacturer and the dual-energy techniques employed. However, radiation doses similar to those used in single-energy CT have been reported with dual-energy techniques.
- Dual-energy CT provides information about how substances behave at different energies, the ability to generate virtual unenhanced datasets, and improved detection of iodine-containing substances on low-energy images. These capabilities are promising for improved detection and characterization

of lesions in the abdomen and pelvis and for evaluation of vascular structures. Further research is needed to validate the accuracy of some of these techniques before their use becomes widespread. Reductions in radiation dose are possible with dual-energy CT if the need for true unenhanced datasets is eliminated, and if low tube currents are used, radiation doses delivered in dual-energy CT are similar to those used in single-energy CT.
- Current applications of dual-energy CT in the abdomen and pelvis provide information about tissue composition and how tissues behave at different energies, the ability to generate virtual unenhanced datasets, and improved detection of iodine-containing substances on low-energy images.

ECHO-PLANAR MRI: ULTRAFAST MR SEQUENCE

Recent improvements in gradients, software and high-speed computer processors now permit extremely rapid MRI of the brain. With echo-planar MRI (EPI), fast gradients are switched on and off at high speeds to create the information used to form an image. In routine spin echo imaging, images of the brain can be obtained in 5 to 10 min. With EPI, all of the information required for processing an image is accumulated in 50 to 150 ms, and the information for the entire brain is obtained in 1 to 2 min, depending on the degree of resolution required or desired. Fast MRI reduces patient and organ motion, permitting diffusion imaging and tractography, perfusion imaging during contrast infusion, fMRI, and kinematic motion studies.

Newer MRI Applications Principle Utility

Perfusion MRI: Involves the acquisition of EPI images during a rapid intravenous bolus of gadolinium contrast material.
Relative perfusion abnormalities can be identified on images of the relative **cerebral blood volume, mean transit time, and cerebral blood flow**.
- Delay in mean transit time and reduction in cerebral blood volume and cerebral blood flow are typical of infarction.
- In the setting of reduced blood flow, a prolonged mean transit time of contrast but normal or elevated cerebral blood volume may indicate tissue supplied by collateral flow that is at risk of infarction.
- pMRI imaging can also be used in the assessment of brain tumors to differentiate intra-axial primary tumors from extra-axial tumors or metastasis.

Diffusion tract imaging (DTI): Derived from diffusion MRI techniques. Preferential microscopic motion of water along white matter tracts is detected by diffusion MR, which can also indicate the direction of white matter fiber tracts. Great potential in the assessment of brain maturation as well as diseases that undermine the integrity of the white matter.[Q]

DIFFUSION WEIGHTED MRI (DWMRI)

A sequence that detects reduction of microscopic motion of water, is the *most sensitive technique for detecting acute ischemic stroke* and is also useful in the detection of encephalitis, abscesses and prion diseases. CT, however, can be quickly obtained and is widely available, making it a pragmatic choice for the initial evaluation of patients with acute changes in mental status, suspected acute stroke, hemorrhage, and intracranial or spinal trauma.

CT is more sensitive than MRI for visualizing acute bleed, calcific lesions, and fine osseous detail.

FUNCTIONAL MRI

- **fMRI** is Blood oxygen level dependent MRI (BOLD imaging).
- Functional MRI (fMRI) and position emission tomography (PET) have made it possible to investigate cognitive processes such as perception, making judgments, paying attention and thinking.
- **fMRI** uses contrast mechanisms related to physiologic changes in tissue and brain perfusion can be studied by observing the time-course of changes in brain water signal as a bolus of injected paramagnetic gadolinium contrast moves through the brain. More recently, to study intrinsic contrast-related local changes in blood oxygenation with brain activity, **blood-oxygen-level-dependent** contrast has been used to provide a rapid noninvasive approach for functional assessment. These techniques have been reliably utilized in the field of both behavior and cognitive sciences. One example is the use of fMRI to demonstrate physiological study of brain in general. Other examples of the use of fMRI include the study of memory.

MR SPECTROSCOPY (MRS)

Information obtained is in the form of a spectrum which provides the biochemical information contained within a selected voxel of tissue.

Used to detect the absence or presence of a certain compound.
Assists in differential diagnosis when standard clinical radiological tests fail or are too invasive.

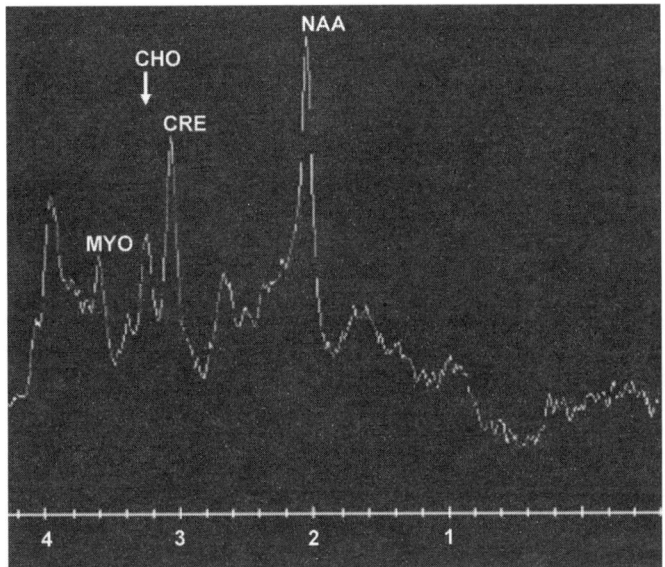

MRS Current Applications

- Multiple sclerosis
- Leigh's
- Huntington's
- Parkinson's
- Alzheimer's
- Epilepsy
- Other dementias
- Metabolic disorders
- Stroke
- Asphyxiation or ischemic injury
- Tumors and intracranial lesions
- Prostate cancer
- Encephalopathies
- Leukodystrophies.

NEAR INFRARED SPECTROSCOPY

Near infrared spectroscopy (NIRS) is a spectroscopic method which uses the near infrared region of the electromagnetic spectrum (from about 800 nm to 2500 nm). It is a noninvasive method for the *in vivo* monitoring of tissue oxygenation. Originally used predominantly to assess cerebral oxygenation, NIRS has gained widespread popularity in many clinical settings in all age groups. Changes in regional tissue oxygenation as detected by NIRS may reflect the delicate balance between oxygen delivery and consumption in more than one organ system.

Chapter 18

Interventional Radiology

DIGITAL SUBTRACTION ARTERIOGRAPHY
- Refinements in radiological imaging have now almost eliminated the need for translumbar aortography.
- Satisfactory imaging of the renal vessels can even be achieved by digital subtraction angiography (DSA) after intravenous injection of contrast medium.
- More precise information can be obtained by intra-arterial injection through a fine catheter inserted into the *femoral artery* using the *Seldinger technique*.
- Arteriography is now rarely used as first investigation of choice.
- It remains "gold standard".

Angiography
- Conventional angiography
- DSA—Best
- CTA
- MRA
  DSA—We can do diagnostic and therapeutic in same setting.

Arteriography
- Catheterization—Femoral artery (large size access to aorta of all its branches)
  FA opposite to side of symptoms

- Bone under local anesthesia
- If FA blocked—axillary or brachial
- Contrast is non-ionic dye (max 4–5 mL/kg)
- Contrast medium—H₂O soluble iodine dye

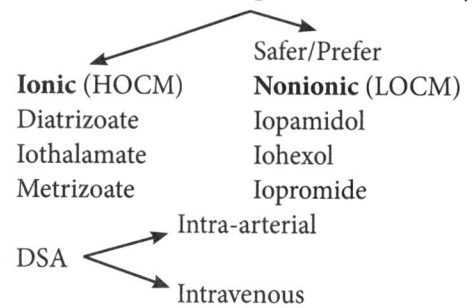

        Safer/Prefer
Ionic (HOCM) **Nonionic** (LOCM)
Diatrizoate   Iopamidol
Iothalamate   Iohexol
Metrizoate   Iopromide

DSA → Intra-arterial / Intravenous

- IADSA—Best type of angiography.

CATHETER ANGIOGRAPHY

Benefits

- Catheter angiography presents a very detailed, clear and accurate picture of the blood vessels. This is especially helpful when a surgical procedure or some percutaneous intervention is being considered.
- By selecting the arteries through which the catheter passes, it is possible to assess vessels in several specific body sites. In fact, a smaller catheter may be passed through the larger one into a branch artery supplying a small area of tissue or a tumor, this is called "superselective angiography".
- Unlike CT or MRI, use of a catheter makes it possible to combine diagnosis and treatment in a single procedure. An example is finding an area of severe arterial narrowing, followed by angioplasty and placement of a stent.
- The degree of detail displayed by catheter angiography may not be available with any other non-invasive procedure.

Risks

- Allergic reaction to the dye and this could lead to skin reaction, a drop in blood pressure, difficulty breathing or even loss of consciousness.

- There is a small risk that blood will form a clot around the tip of the catheter, blocking the artery and making it necessary to operate to reopen the vessel.
- In patients of diabetes or kidney disease, the kidneys may be injured when contrast media is eliminated through the urine.
- Rarely, the catheter punctures the artery, causing internal bleeding. It is also possible that the catheter tip will separate material from the lining of the artery, causing a block "downstream".
- Risk of radiation if patient is pregnant.

| Guidelines for use of intravenous contrast in patients with impaired renal function ||
Serum creatinine, Micromol/L (mg/dl)	Recommendation
<133 (<1.5)	Use either ionic or nonionic at 2 mL/kg to 150 mL total
133–177 (1.5–2.0)	Nonionic; hydrate diabetics 1 mL/kg per hour x 10 h
>177 (>2.0)	Consider noncontrast CT or MRI; nonionic contrast if required
177–221 (2.0–2.5)	Nonionic only if required (as above); contraindicated in diabetics
>265 (>3.0)	Nonionic IV contrast given only to patients undergoing dialysis within 24 h

General interventional radiology	Interventional radiology for cancer	Neurointervention
		Endovascular procedures for:
Imaging-guided biopsies	Preoperative embolization for vascular tumors (e.g. Juvenile angiofibroma, meningioma, hemangiopericytoma, RCC)	Embolization of brain and spinal arteriovenous malformations (AVMs)
Diagnostic angiography		
Angioplasty and/or vascular stenting		
Embolization (BAE, UAE)	Fluid collections drainage	Embolization of dural arteriovenous fistulae (DAVF) and carotid-cavernous fistulae (CCF)
Thrombolysis	Transcatheter chemoembolization (e.g. HCC)	
Transjugular intrahepatic portosystemic shunt		
Uterine fibroid embolization	Tumor ablation	Treatments for vasospasm as a complication of SAH
Vascular access procedures	Pain control procedures	Treatment for arterial atherosclerosis and the treatment for intracranial arteries in acute stroke
Biliary drainage and stenting	Vertebroplasty (PMMA)	
Fallopian tube catheterization	Preoperative embolic occlusion of portal branches (PVE) in patients with hilar cholangiocarcinoma	
Gastrostomy tube insertion		
Urinary tract obstruction		Endovascular repair of aneurysm with platinum microcoils
IVC filters		

Contd...

Contd...

Endovenous ablation of varicosities (LASER/RFA)
Cryoablation
Radiofrequency ablations of tumors

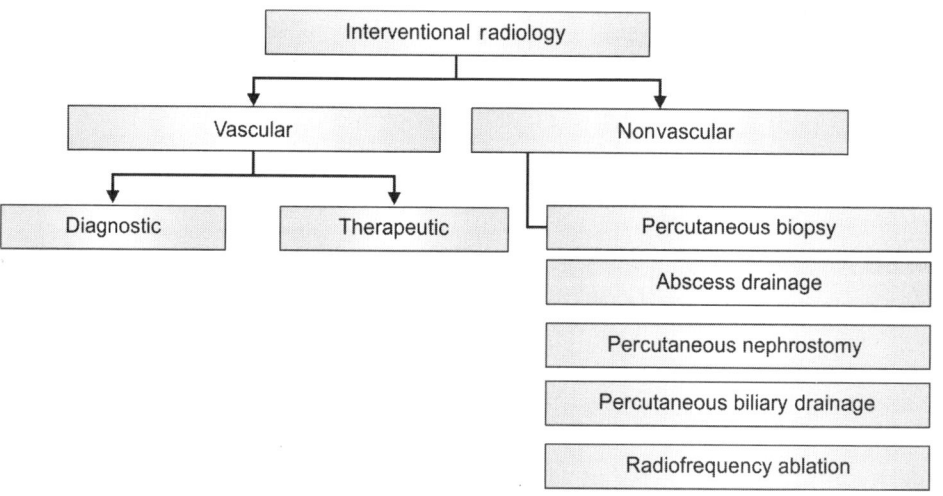

Clinical problems with surgical solutions replaced by minimally invasive solutions		
Clinical problem	*Surgical solution*	*Interventional radiology solution*
Acute abdomen	Exploratory laparotomy	CT- and image-guided drainage
Hydro-and pyonephrosis	Surgical nephrostomy	Percutaneous nephrostomy
Nephrolithiasis	Surgical nephrolithotomy	Lithotripsy, percutaneous nephrostolithotomy
Malignant biliary obstruction	Surgical choledochoenterostomy	Percutaneous biliary drainage, stent placement
Undiagnosed tumor mass	Open surgical biopsy	Image-guided needle biopsy
Symptomatic peripheral arterial disease	Endarterectomy, bypass	PTA and stent placement

Contd...

Contd...

Upper gastrointestinal tract bleeding due to varices	Portocaval shunt creation	Transjugular intrahepatic portosystemic shunt creation
Ostial renal artery stenosis	Bypass, endarterectomy	Renal artery stent placement
Feeding problems	Surgical gastrostomy	Percutaneous (and endoscopic) gastrostomy
Peripheral or pulmonary arteriovenous malformations	Surgical resection	Embolization
Symptomatic uterine fibroleiomyoma	Hysterectomy, myomectomy	Embolization
Lower gastrointestinal tract bleeding (colonic)	Colon resection	Angiography, embolization
Subarachnoid hemorrhage due to aneurysm	Craniotomy, aneurysm clipping	Detachable coil embolization of aneurysm
Severe symptomatic coronary artery disease	Coronary artery bypass graft	Coronary PTA, coronary stent placement

THERAPEUTIC EMBOLIZATION

Arterial embolization may be used in the treatment of
- Acute hemorrhage
- Tumor therapy
- Arteriovenous malformations
- Hypersplenism
- Priapism.

Venous embolization is used for treatment of
- Gastroesophageal varices
- Testicular varicocele
- Deliberate vascular embolization with the aim of occluding a vessel can be achieved using a variety of different materials including:
    - Gelatin
    - Sponge fragments
    - Polyvinyl alcohol foam particles (PVA)
    - Spiral metal coils.

PARTICULATE EMBOLIC AGENTS

Only used for precapillary arterioles or small arteries, these are also very good for AVM deep within the body. The disadvantage is that they are not easily targeted in the vessel. None of these are radiopaque so it makes radiologic imaging difficult to see them unless they were soaked in contrast prior to injection.

Polyvinyl alcohol (PVA): These are permanent agents. They are tiny balls of 50 to 1200 nm in size. The particles are not meant to mechanically occlude a vessel. Instead they cause an inflammatory reaction. Unfortunately they have a tendency to clump together since the balls are not perfectly round. The clump can separate a few days later failing as an embolic agent.

BRONCHIAL ARTERY EMBOLIZATION

- Bronchial artery embolization (BAE) is a well-accepted and effective form of treatment for massive and/or recurrent hemoptysis. Patients most commonly treated by BAE are those with chronic **TB, bronchiectasis and mycetomas** as the long-standing pulmonary inflammation in these patients results in the development of hypertrophied systemic arteries that can be selectively catheterized and occluded. It is, however, rarely employed for management of bleeding from malignant disease.
- In the great majority of patients hemoptysis originates from systemic rather than pulmonary arteries and **the bronchial vessels are almost universally involved and** hence, should be the first to be evaluated and embolized.
- There is considerable variation in the way in which bronchial arteries arise from thoracic aorta but the **commonest is one main right artery from a common intercostobronchial trunk at T5 level, and two left bronchial arteries arising a little lower.**
- While evaluating it is vital to remember that virtually any systemic artery in the chest (from intercostals, inferior phrenic, internal mammary, thyrocervical trunk, costocervical and subscapular vessels and other branches of subclavian and axillary arteries) can contribute to bronchial circulation and be a source of continued hemoptysis after successful embolization of the bronchial arteries and may even be the sole supply to the lesion responsible for hemoptysis.
- The pulmonary arteries are culpable in 5 to 10 percent of patients of chronic disorder like TB with **Rasmussen aneurysm** formation.
- PVA particles are embolizing agents of choice, although at some centers gelfoam is used.

INTERVENTIONAL GI RADIOLOGY

- Angiographic embolization or vasoconstriction decrease bleeding from sites not amenable to endoscopic intervention.
- Dilation or stenting with fluoroscopic guidance relieves luminal strictures.
- Contrast enemas can reduce volvulus and evacuate air in acute colonic pseudoobstruction.
- CT and ultrasound help drain abdominal fluid collections, in many cases obviating the need for surgery.
- Percutaneous transhepatic cholangiography relieves biliary obstruction when ERCP is contraindicated.
- Lithotripsy can fragment gallstones in patients who are not candidates for surgery.
- In some instances, radiologic approaches offer advantages over endoscopy for gastroenterostomy placement.
- Finally, central venous catheters for parenteral nutrition may be placed using radiographic techniques.

INTERVENTIONAL NEURORADIOLOGY

- This rapidly developing field is providing new therapeutic options for patients with challenging neurovascular problems.
- Available procedures include:
  - Detachable coil therapy for aneurysms (edovascular repair of aneurysms with platinum micro coils)
  - Particulate or liquid adhesive embolization of arteriovenous malformations
  - Balloon angioplasty and stenting of arterial stenosis or vasospasm
  - Transarterial or transvenous embolization of dural arteriovenous fistulas
  - Balloon occlusion of carotid-cavernous and vertebral fistulas
  - Endovascular treatment of vein-of-galen malformations
  - Preoperative embolization of tumors (e.g. juvenile angiofibroma in which sphenopalatine or internal maxillary artery is embolized)
  - Thrombolysis of acute arterial or venous thrombosis.
- The highest complication rates are found with the therapies designed to treat the highest-risk diseases. The advent of electrolytically detachable coils has ushered in a new era in the treatment of cerebral aneurysms.
- It remains to be determined what the role of coils will be relative to surgical options, but in many centers, coiling has become standard therapy for many aneurysms.

ABLATION

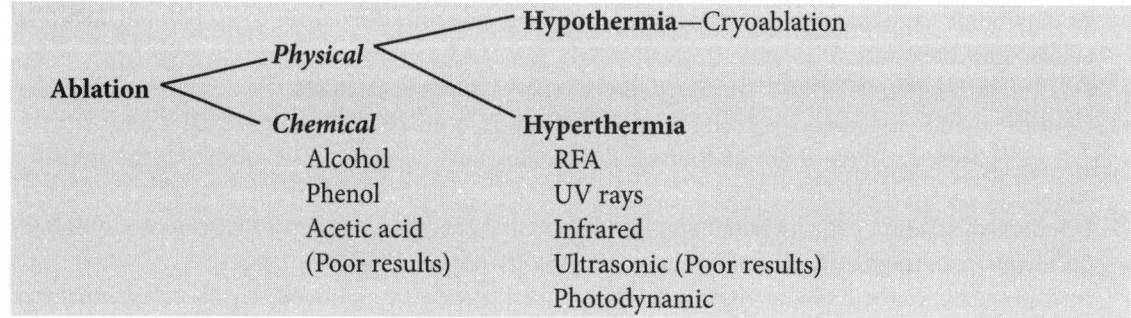

Applications of RFA

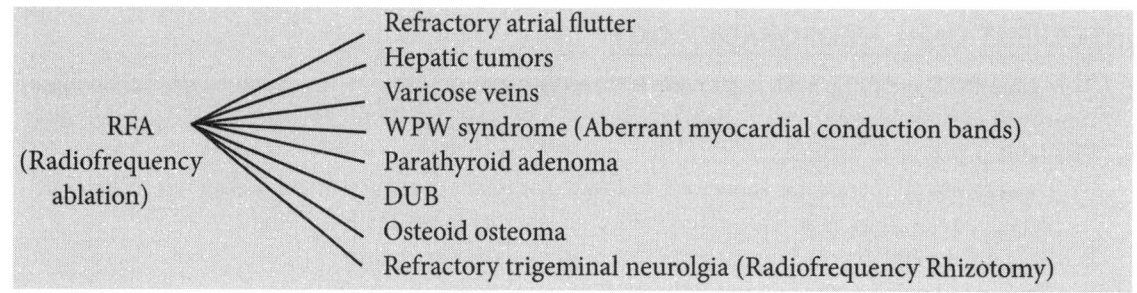

Newer treatment methods for varicose veins are:
- RFA
- SEPS
- Trivex
- Endolaser.

Varicose veins can usually be treated with conservative measures. Symptoms often decrease when the legs are elevated periodically, when prolonged standing is avoided, and when elastic support hose are worn. External compression stockings provide a counterbalance to the hydrostatic pressure in the veins. Ablative procedures, including sclerotherapy, endovenous radiofrequency or laser ablation, and surgery may be considered to treat varicose veins in selected patients who have persistent symptoms, suffer from recurrent superficial vein thrombosis, and/or develop skin ulceration. Ablative therapy may also be indicated for cosmetic reasons. Small, symptomatic varicose veins can be treated with sclerotherapy, in which a sclerosing solution is injected into the involved varicose vein and a compression bandage is applied. Percutaneous, endovenous delivery of radiofrequency or laser energy can be used to treat incompetent greater saphenous veins. Surgical therapy usually involves ligation and stripping of the greater and lesser saphenous veins. Endoscopic perforator surgery (SEPS) is a minimally invasive technique to interrupt incompetent communicating veins.

Algorithm

Therapy for HCC (Flow chart 18.1)
- HCC < 2 cm: RFA ablation, percutaneous ethanol injection, or resection
- HCC > 2 cm, no vascular invasion: Liver resection, RFA, or OLTX (orthotopic liver transplantation)
- Multiple unilobar tumors or tumor with vascular invasion: TACE
- Bilobar tumors, no vascular invasion: TACE with OLTX for patients whose tumors have a response.

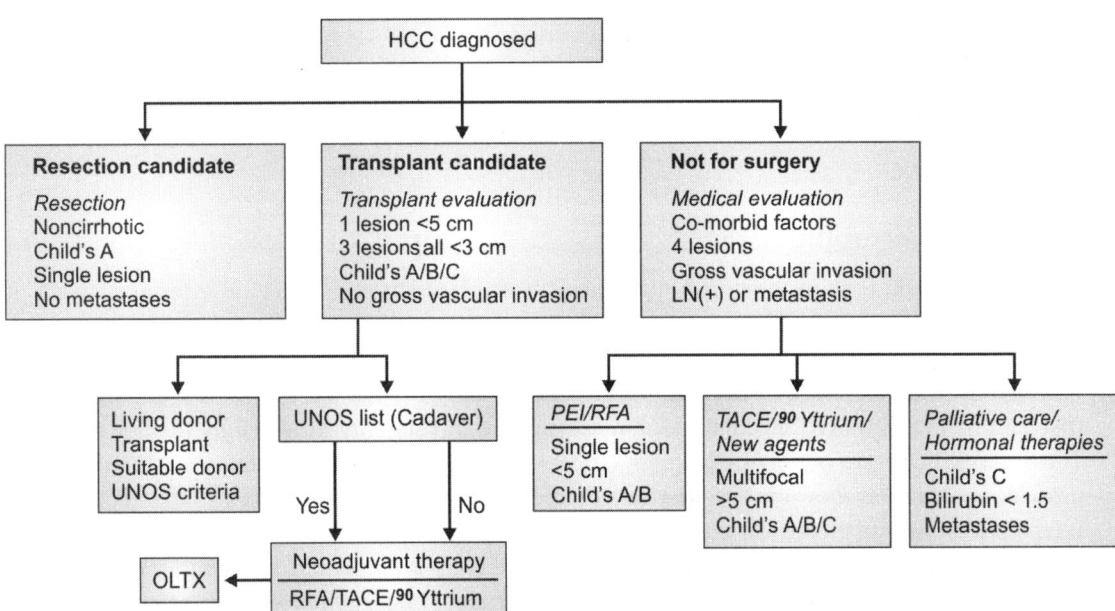

Flow chart 18.1: Hepatocellular carcinoma treatment algorithm

In contrast to the dismal results of systemic chemotherapy, a variety of agents given via the hepatic artery have activity in HCC confined to the liver. Two randomized controlled trials have shown a survival advantage for patients undergoing TACE (DSA-guided selective catheterization of hepatic artery for injecting the chemotherapeutic agent mixed-up with embolizing agent).

Transarterial chemoembolization (TACE) in a selected subset of patients. One used doxorubicin and the other used cisplatin. Despite the fact that increased hepatic extraction of chemotherapy has been shown for very few drugs, some drugs such as cisplatin, doxorubicin, mitomycin C, and possibly neocarzinostatin produce substantial objective responses when administered regionally. Most of the studies on regional hepatic arterial chemotherapy also use an embolizing agent such as ethiodol, gelatin sponge particles (gelfoam), starch (spherex), or microspheres.

CAVITRON ULTRASONIC SURGICAL ASPIRATOR

The cavitron ultrasonic surgical aspirator (CUSA) is an innovative tool for resecting hepatic parenchyma, which reduces intraoperative blood loss and perioperative morbidity.

The CUSA, an instrument designed for neurosurgery (brain surgery), is useful in liver surgery. Its tip selectively fragments liver cells leaving blood vessels and bile ducts exposed. Blood vessels are not fragmented as they are made of firmer fibrous tissue. Once exposed they are then divided, thus, avoiding any significant blood loss which means that it is safe to remove individual segments, one half or even 70 percent of a liver. The remaining liver substance increases rapidly in size as the liver has enormous powers of regeneration.

Percutaneous Vertebroplasty

- It is a newer technique in which acrylic cement is injected through a needle into a collapsed or weakened vertebra to stabilize the fracture. This procedure is effective for treating certain types of painful vertebral compression fractures and some painful or unstable benign and malignant vertebral lesions that fail to respond to the traditional conservative therapies. Most experts believe that pain relief is achieved through mechanical support and stability provided by the bone cement. The semisolid mixture of polymethylmethacrylate (PMMA), an acrylic cement used in orthopedic procedures, has been shown to restore strength and stiffness in vertebral bodies.
- Interventions [percutaneous vertebroplasty (PVP), kyphoplasty] exist for osteoporotic compression fractures associated with debilitating pain. Candidates for PVP should have midline pain, focal tenderness over the spinous process of the affected vertebral body, 80 percent loss of vertebral body

height, and onset of symptoms within the prior 4 months. The technique consists of injection of polymethylmethacrylate, under fluoroscopic guidance, into the affected vertebral body.
- Rare major complications include extravasation of cement into the epidural space (resulting in myelopathy) or fatal pulmonary embolism from migration of cement into paraspinal veins. Approximately three quarters of patients who meet selection criteria have reported enhanced quality of life.

Relief of pain following PVP has also been reported in patients with
- Vertebral metastases
- Myeloma, or
- Hemangiomas.

PERCUTANEOUS TRANSCATHETER VASCULAR OCCLUSION

Over the past 20 years, percutaneous transcatheter vascular occlusion (PTVO) techniques have been applied to an increasing number of medical problems largely driven by innovations and improvements in occlusive agents and catheter delivery systems.

Indications for PTVO techniques can be divided into two main categories: (1) peripheral and (2) head, neck, and spine. These can be further subdivided into neoplastic and non-neoplastic problems.

Peripheral

Neoplastic
Percutaneous transcatheter vascular occlusion techniques have been used to devascularize tumors, for palliative infarction of unresectable tumors and for control of bleeding associated with tumor growth. These techniques are usually reserved for those patients who have failed more conventional forms of therapy including surgery, chemotherapy, radiotherapy, or they are employed in situations where these therapies may be contraindicated. The goal of PTVO under these conditions is to destroy tumor cells through infarction. Polyvinyl alcohol (PVA), surgical gelatin sponge (gelfoam), and microfibrillar collagen are the most commonly used occlusive agents. Dehydrated ethanol, which causes endothelial cell necrosis and sloughing with resultant vessel occlusion, is also commonly used.

Non-Neoplastic
Percutaneous transcatheter vascular occlusion techniques are commonly used to control or alter the vascular supply of non-neoplastic lesions. The techniques and agents utilized are similar to those used for neoplastic lesions.

Hemorrhage

Control of hemorrhage was one of the first applications of transcatheter embolization. Emergent control of hemorrhage from esophageal varices and tumors has been achieved with PTVO techniques.

Vascular Malformations

Vascular malformations represent abnormal connections between the arterial and venous systems, which usually are associated with arteriovenous shunting. These connections can range from a single hole between a major artery and vein to a large tangle of multiple abnormal vessels and shunts.

Liquid agents such as dehydrated ethanol, sodium tetradecyl sulfate, or cyanoacrylate adhesives have been used to treat these lesions. Particulate agents such as PVA, Avitene, Gelfoam, or suture can reach and occlude the nidus of the malformation. Care must be exercised to ensure that embolic materials do not pass into the venous circulation. Cyanoacrylates are not currently approved by the FDA for use in humans in the United States.

Varicoceles

Varicoceles are readily treated with PTVO techniques using coils, detachable balloons, and hot contrast.

Congenital Cardiac Defects

An important area for future development in PTVO therapy involves cardiac applications. Transcatheter technique to deliver PVA material to "plug" a patent ductus arteriosus. Modifications of these procedures may prove useful in closing septal defects.

Organ Function Ablation

Percutaneous transcatheter vascular occlusion techniques have been employed for organ function ablation most commonly involving the parathyroid gland, adrenal gland, kidney, and spleen.

Head, Neck, and Spine

Neoplastic

A number of neoplastic lesions in the head and neck area can benefit from PTVO techniques, most commonly meningiomas and hemangioblastomas intracranially and paragangliomas and juvenile nasopharyngeal angiofibromas extracranially. Hemangiomas and metastatic tumors of the spine also can benefit from PTVO techniques.

Non-Neoplastic

The most common non-neoplastic indications for PTVO treatment in the head, neck, and spine area are for: hemorrhage, most commonly epistaxis, and vascular malformations.

Epistaxis

Arterial bleeding constitutes a medical emergency, and more aggressive therapy may require posterior nasal packing, ligation of the maxillary or ethmoid arteries, or embolization of internal maxillary arterial feeders.

A post-traumatic aneurysm of the petrous or cavernous portion of the internal carotid artery may be permanently occluded by detachable balloons in some cases of massive epistaxis.

Vascular Malformations

Vascular malformations can involve the brain, spinal cord, or extracranial head and neck area. The most common lesions that PTVO techniques are utilized to treat are arteriovenous malformations, dural fistulas, and carotid cavernous fistulas.

MEDICAL TUMOR ABLATION

Hypervascular tumors (renal tumors, juvenile angiofibroma) or large hepatic tumors may require embolotherapy or ablation with ethanol or contrast media prior to surgical resection. This procedure controls hemorrhage as well as decreases the tumor size in nonoperable patients. In addition, splenic artery embolotherapy with antibiotic therapy may be performed prior to splenectomy to control excessive use of blood products and hypersplenism in the pediatric and adult patient. In addition, partial splenic embolotherapy can be performed, and the spleen may remain in place to avoid immunologic compromise in patients that may have hypersplenism.

THERAPEUTIC EFFECTS OF DEEP HEATING

Deep heat causes a temperature rise from the conversion of energy into heat as it penetrates the tissues of the body where the energy is applied.

Energy sources include
- High-frequency currents (shortwave diathermy)
- Electromagnetic radiation (microwaves), and
- Ultrasound (high-frequency sound).

Therapeutic effects of deep heating modalities usually are produced by the conversion of applied energy into heat as it penetrates tissue. Because the temperature distribution varies significantly across different modalities, the clinician should use the appropriate modality for the condition at hand. To provide the greatest therapeutic effect, the temperature rise generated by the modality should be the maximum tolerated by the patient. For a specific localized pathology, the deep heating modality selected must produce a maximum temperature elevation at that specific location.

The following areas are treated selectively by the listed modalities
- Application of shortwave diathermy with capacitor plates or microwave radiation at a frequency of 2456 MHz can provide selective heat for deep subcutaneous tissue and superficial muscle.
- Shortwave diathermy with an induction coil applicator at 27 MHz can heat superficial muscle.
- Microwave diathermy at 915 MHz selectively heats muscle thoroughly.
- Ultrasound at a frequency of 0.8–1 MHz preferentially heats joints, ligaments, tendons, tendon sheaths, fibrous scars, nerve trunks, and myofascial interfaces. Ultrasound is especially useful for heating joints with a thick layer of overlying soft tissues that shortwave diathermy or microwave diathermy cannot penetrate.
- Shortwave diathermy with internal electrodes at 27 MHz can provide selective heat for pelvic organs in cases of chronic pelvic inflammatory disease or management of coccygeal muscle spasms (e.g. of the urogenital diaphragm).

HIGH-INTENSITY FOCUSED ULTRASOUND

Introduction

- High-intensity focused ultrasound (HIFU) is a method of focusing ultrasound waves in the same way as a convex mirror can focus the sun's rays to set light to a piece of paper. Thus, focused ultrasound rays can be directed to highly specific areas of the prostate and be used to kill the tissue on which they are focused by heating them to temperatures of 80 to 100 °C — way higher than normal body temperatures. In short HIFU is the precise reverse of cryotherapy.
- Clinical HIFU procedures are typically performed in conjunction with an imaging procedure to enable treatment planning and targeting before applying a therapeutic or ablative levels of ultrasound energy. When Magnetic resonance imaging (MRI) is used for guidance, the technique is sometimes called Magnetic Resonance-guided Focused Ultrasound, often shortened to MRgHIFU or MRgFUS.

Mechanism

- Mechanical phenomena, in addition to thermal effects, are associated at high intensities but are not present at lower intensities. Mechanical phenomena include cavitation, microstreaming, and radiation forces.

Advantages

- HIFU is often considered a promising technology within the non-invasive or minimally invasive therapy segments of medical technology.
- An important difference between HIFU and many other forms of focused energy, such as radiation therapy or radio surgery, is that the passage of ultrasound energy through intervening tissue has no apparent cumulative effect on that tissue.
- HIFU's capacity to generate in-depth precise tissue necrosis using an external applicator, with no effect on the surrounding structures, is unique.

Disadvantages

- Because HIFU is essentially ultrasound, any artifacts related to ultrasound would apply to HIFU as well, such as acoustic shadowing, reverberation, and refraction.
- With diagnostic sonography, these reflected sound waves are of such low energy that there is no adverse effect from them. However, with HIFU, these reflected waves are very high energy, and they can produce burns in the tissues that lie between the transducer and the target.
- One potential complication of HIFU is the dissemination of malignant cells from the shear forces generated by the procedure.

Current Applications

- To date, studies using animals and human subjects have been published for the treatment of hepatocellular carcinoma (HCC), renal cell carcinoma, pancreatic cancer, sarcomas, urinary bladder tumors, prostate carcinoma and uterine fibroids and breast fibroadenomas.
- HCC is rapidly becoming the most common malignancy worldwide. Surgery, particularly liver transplantation, offers the only real hope for cure; survival rates are only 25–30 percent at 5 years. As a result, noninvasive alternatives to surgery, such as radiofrequency ablation, ethanol injection, and HIFU, have generated increasing interest as alternative or adjunct treatments to surgery.

Index

A

Abdomen radiology 165
Abdominal
  imaging 165
  MRI 59
  plain film 215
  sonogram for trauma 202
  tuberculosis 191
Aberrant left subclavian artery from right aortic arch 178
Aberrant right subclavian artery 178
Abnormal nephrogram 21
Absolute diagnostic ultrasonographic sign 103
Absorbed dose 85
Ace inhibitor scintigraphy 449
Achalasia cardia 176
Achondroplasia 259
Acoustic
  enhancement 30
  neuroma 362
  shadowing 31
Acquiring chest X-ray 87
Acro-osteolysis 255
Acute
  appendicitis 193
  cholecystitis 217
  effects of total body irradiation 506
  hemarthrosis 282
  hemorrhage 31
  pancreatitis 222
  stroke 341
Adamantinoma of long bone 301
Adenoid tissue hypertrophy 374

Adenolymphoma 384
Adjuvant radiotherapy 491
Adjuvere 491
Adnexa 405
Adrenal 312
  adenomas 315
  carcinomas 315
  metastases 315
  scan 449
Adson maneuver 158
Adulthood hypothyroidism 311
Adverse effects of iodinated contrast media 63
AIDS-related cholangiopathy 218
Air 31
  crescent sign 129
  embolism 144
  space edema 135
Airbronchogram 97
Airbronchogram sign 97
AJCC-UICC classification of regional lymph nodes 125
Albers schonberg disease 256
Allergic bronchopulmonary aspergillosis 111
Alpha radiation 4
Alpha-particle emission 431
Ambiguous genitalia 239
Ameloblastoma 301
Amifostine 472
Amipaque 18
Ampullary carcinoma 224
Amyotrophic lateral sclerosis 350
Anatomy of nose 370

Anencephaly 404
Aneurysmal bone cyst 295
Angiography 527
Angiomyolipoma 242
Ankylosing spondylitis 306
Ankylostoma duodenale 187
Annihilation photons 48
Anode 8
Anorectal malformations 195
Anterior
  scalloping of vertebra 391
  wall of rectum 196
Antomic landmarks 175
Aorta 149
Aortic trauma 155
Apart from barium procedures 17
Apical cap sign 154
Apicogram 88
Appendix 193
Apple core appearance 167
Applications of
  hepatobiliary scintigraphy in liver diseases 446
  RFA 534
Arhinencephaly 335
Arnold Chiari I malformation 332
Arrhythmogenic right ventricular dysplasia 521
Arteriography 527
Arteriovenous malformations 100, 345
Asbestosis 115
Ascaris lumbricoides 186
Ascending urethrography 23

Ascites 170
Aseptic bone necrosis 279
Ashman's focus 108
Askin tumor 310
Aspergillus
  antigen 111
  fumigatus mycelia 111
Asymptomatic parotid enlargement 385
Ataxia-telangiectasia 335, 339
Atom 10
Atomic
  number 4, 423, 424
  weight 423, 424
Atrial septal defects 138
Autosomal dominant polycystic kidney disease 231, 232

B

Bare orbit 336
Barium
  enema 190, 195
  studies 17
  sulfate 60
  swallow 161, 165, 174
    study 172
  titanate 29
Barrett esophagus 179
Barriers for radiation 82
Barter's syndrome 235
Basal
  cell nevus syndrome 335
  ganglia calcification 321
Base of skull 372
Basic isotope notation 427
Basics of nuclear medicine 421
Battered baby syndrome 257
Beaded' appearance of fallopes 26
Beaklike abrupt 190
Beak-shaped vertebra 390
Beam-hardening artifact 45

Beams used for external radiotherapy 485
Bechterew disease 306
Beckwith-Wiedemann syndrome 239
Bedford sign 136
Benign
  diseases treated with radiotherapy 507
  esophageal tumors 178
  intracranial hypertension 369
  prostatic hypertrophy 246
  tumor of pancreas 224
Berry aneurysms 344
Beryllium window 27
Beta radiation 5
Beta-particle emission 432
Betatrons 484
Biconcave vertebra 390
Bilateral but asymmetrical 129
Biliary scintigraphic scan 214, 446
Bird of Prey' sign 167
Birefringent monosodium urate crystals 270
Bismuth 204
  germinate crystals 48
Black nephrogram 22
Bladder 243
  cancers 489
  diverticuli 243
Blighted ovum 400
Blood flow velocity 34
Blue-rubber-bleb-nevus syndrome 335
Blunt trauma abdomen 202
Bochdalek's hernia 102
Bohler's angle 276
Bone 31, 507
  densitometry 50
  infarcts 283
  infections 272
  metastases 241, 490

  metastasis with soft tissue mass 288
  metastasis with sunburst periosteal reaction arises 288
  scan 449
  scan features 284
  tumors 286
  within bone 390
Boot-shaped silhouette 140
Bouchard's nodes 303
Bourneville's disease 337
Bow fissure sign 107
Bowtie sign 392
Brachial plexus 157
Brachytherapy 476
  for benign disease 511
Brain
  metastases 490
  scan 438
  stroke 340
  tumors 353, 358, 438
Branchial cyst 381
Breast
  cancers 489
  diseases 415
  imaging 411
  lesion with halo sign 416
  MRI 58, 415
Brodie's abscess 273
Broken collar or neck 278
Bronchial
  artery embolization 126, 532
  coarctation 100
  vessels 532
Bronchiectasis 126
  disease 115
Bronchogenic cysts 100, 105
Broncholobar sign 113
Bronchopneumonia 106
Bronchopulmonary segments 87
Brown tumor 269
Budd-Chiari syndrome 205

Index

Buerger's disease 160
Bulging fissure sign 107, 129
Bull's eye lesions of liver 207
Bulla ethmoidalis 372
Bullet shaped vertebra 389

C

Ca rectum 200
Calcification in
    few breast diseases 417
    spleen 171
Calcification within heart 147
Calcifying bone secondaries arise 288
Calculus disease of kidney 233
Caldwell's view 372
Caliber 186
Calvarial thickening 318
Cancer
    biology 466
    of uterine cervix 489
Candida albicans pneumonia 112
Candidal esophagitis 173
Candle bone disease 257
Candy-cone appearance 188
Caplan's syndrome 118
Carbon 10
Carcinogenesis 72, 77
Carcinoid tumors 193, 224
Carcinoma
    breast in all 413
    colon 200
    esophagus 178
    gallbladder 218
    head of pancreas 222
    prostate 246
Cardiac
    borders on chest X-rays 133
    computed tomography 519
    magnetic resonance imaging 520
    masses 521
    monitoring 131
    MRI 58
Cardiology 49
Cardiothoracic ratio 133
Cardiovascular
    imaging protocols 132
    radiology 131
Caries sicca 274
Carman's meniscus sign 181
Carney's triad 124
Caroli's disease 219
Carotid body tumors 156, 382
Carotid imaging 155
Carpometacarpal joint 303
Cartilaginous
    benign tumors 289
    malignant tumors 289
Castleman's disease 129
Caterpillar sign 180
Catheter angiography 528
Cathode 8
Catterall stages of perthes disease 280
Causes of
    Charcot's joint 308
    congenital hydrocephalus 331
    cortical lesions 254
    cupped and frayed metaphyses 266
    dense metaphyseal bands 254
    honeycombing in lungs 95
    inferior rib notching 150
    left-sided pleural effusion 114
    lesions with blood-fluid levels 254
    lucent metaphyseal lines 253
    multilocular expansile osteolytic lesion of bone 251
    multiple lytic lesions in bone 252
    pneumobilia 216
    pneumoperitoneum 169
    pulmonary edema
        with cardiomegaly 142
        without cardiomegaly 143
    radioactivity 421
    right-sided pleural effusion 114
    secondary achalasia 177
    septal lines 144
    soft-tissue calcifications 310
    superior margin rib notching 151
Cavernous hemangioma 379
    of liver 207
Cavitron ultrasonic surgical aspirator 536
Cecoureterocele 244
CECT
    abdomen 56
    pelvis 56
Cell cycle 466
    and radiation 69
Central nervous system 75
Cerebellar ectopia 332
Cerebelloretinal hemangioblastomatosis 338
Cerebral
    aneurysms 344
    angiography 326
Cerebritis and cerebral abscess 346
Cerebrospinal fluid imaging 440
Cervical
    cancer 486
    spine
        injury 392
        trauma 392
Cervicothoracic sign 130
Changes in leukemia in childhood 284
Charcot's joint 307
Chemical processing of X-ray film 14
Chemodectoma 156, 382
    tumor 382

Chest 260
  MRI 58
Chiari I malformation 332
Chiari II malformation, childhood 332
Chilaiditi's syndrome 168
Childhood hypothyroidism,
    cretinism 311
Cholecystectomy 218
Chondroblastoma 295
Chondrocalcinosis 269
Chondromyxoid fibroma 295
Chondrosarcoma 297
Chordoma 300
Chromosomes and cancer 467
Chronic 341
  adhesive arachnoiditis 18
  hemophilic arthropathy 282
  TB 126
Cingulate gyri 348
Claw sign 167, 190
Clay Shoveler's fracture 392
Cleidocranial dysplasia 258
Cloaca 272
Coarctation of aorta 149
Cobalt-60 486
Cobra head appearance 244
Codman's tumor 295
Coffee bean sign 167
Coiled spring
  appearance 167, 190
  sign 190
Colitis cystica profunda 196
Collateral circulation 149
Collimator 9, 428
Colon and rectum 194
Color Doppler ultrasonography 160
Combo sign 111
Common
  abnormalities noted on CXR 91
  type of bladder rupture 245
Complications of

early pregnancy 400
fibrosing stage 120
HSG 25
Pott's spine 395
radiotherapy 504
Compton scattering 12
Computed tomography
    enteroclysis 521
Concomitant chemoradiation 495
Concurrent
  chemoradiotherapy 492
  chemotherapy 511
Conformation therapy 498
Congenital
  anomalies 138
    of vertebral bodies 388
  cardiac defects 538
  cystic adenomatoid lung
      malformation 103
  diaphragmatic hernia 102
  diseases 230
  dislocation of hip 308
  dysplasia of hip 308
  hypertrophic pyloric stenosis 179
  lesions 100
  lobar emphysema 100, 104
  malformations of brain 331
  skeletal anomalies 255
  syphilis 274
  tracheoesophageal fistula 100
Conical cecum 191
Contents of barium powder 60
Continuous
  diaphragms sign 127
  hyperfractionated accelerated
      radiotherapy 475
Contraindications for HSG 25
Contrast media for nonbarium
    procedures 62
Copper 10
Corkscrew 160
Costoclavicular maneuver 158

Cottage-loaf heart configuration 141
Couinaud 204
Coxa plana 280
Craniopharyngioma 359
Craniospinal irradiation 498
Craniosynostosis 319
Crescent-in-doughnut 190
Criteria of diffuse axonal injury 367
Crohn's disease 197
Cryptococcosis 347
Cryptococcus neoformans 347
Cryptorchidism 239
Crystal-deposition arthropathies 309
CSF seedlings of intracranial 358
Cupola sign 167
Cushing's
  disease 314
  syndrome 313
Cut corner sign 262
CXR
  features atrial septal defect 138
  signs of VSD 139
Cyclotrons 484
Cystic
  adenomatoid malformation 100
  hygroma 381, 402
  lesion in liver 206
  lymphangiectasis 381
Cystosarcoma phyllodes 413
Cytomegalovirus esophagitis 173

D

Dalfopristin 107
Dandy-Walker malformation 333
Declared pregnant workers and
    minors 82
Deep venous thrombosis 161
Deep-dose equivalent 81
Delayed bone age 250
Dense
  nephrogram 22
  persistent nephrogram 22

Dental
  abnormalities 274
  films 13
Dentigerous 301
Dermatological effects 71
Dermoid cyst 409
Descending urethrography 23
Detection of fetal structures by ultrasound 398
Developmental
  dysplasia of hip 308
  hip dysplasia 308
Diagnosis of
  airbronchogram sign 97
  bilateral upper lobe fibrosis 97
  calcific foci in lungs 94
  cavitating pulmonary lesions 94
  chondrocalcinosis 270
  ground-glass haze on X-ray chest in neonate 97
  honeycombing of lungs 95
  linitis plastica 185
  miliary mottling 93
  opaque hemithorax 92
Diagnostic evaluation of gallbladder 209
Diaphyseal aclasis 293
Diethylene triamine penta-acetic acid 448
Difference between radical radiotherapy and palliative radiotherapy 491
Differential diagnosis of hip pain in children 280
Diffuse
  axonal injury 365, 366
  esophageal spasm 176
  idiopathic skeletal hypertrophy 307
  osteosclerosis 250
Diffusion MRI 524
Digital subtraction arteriography 527

Dimercaptosuccinic acid 448
Diminish sensory neuropathies 472
Disadvantages of
  MUGA scan 445
  PACS 16
Discoid atelectasis 113
Diseases of demyelination, acquired 350
Disorders of
  diverticulation and cleavage 334
  hemopoietic system 282
  lymphoreticular system 282
  sulcation and cellular migration 333
Disputed TOS 158
Dissecting aneurysm 153
Dissection of aorta 151
Distal interphalangeal joints 303
Diuretic urography 21
Diverticulosis of colon 199
Dog ears 170
Dollar vertebra 388
Double
  aortic arch 162
  bronchial wall sign 128
  density sign 273, 294
  duct sign 223
  emulsion/coated films 13
Double/triple track sign 180
Double-barrel esophagus 173
Double-wall sign 167
Down's syndrome, skeletal features of 261
Drash syndrome 239
Drop metastases 358
Dual energy X-ray absorptiometry 51
Dual photon absorptiometry 50
Dual-energy CT 522
Duodenal atresia 187
Duodenum 61

Dyschondroplasia 294
Dysostosis 258
Dysphagia lusoria 162, 177

E
Echo-planar MRI 523
Ectopic
  pregnancy 405
  ureterocele 244
Effects in developing
  embryo 77
  fetus 77
Effects of radiation 70
Eggshell calcification 129
EHBA 219
Eisenmenger syndrome 139
  CXR signs of 139
Eister's rule 363
Electromagnetic rays 459
Electron capture 432
Element 423
Ellis-Van creveld syndrome 232
Emphysema 99
  CXR in 99
Empty orbit sign 336
Encephalotrigeminal syndrome 336
Enchondromatosis 294
  with hemangiomas 294
Endocavitary radiotherapy 497
Endocrine imaging 311
Endorectal coil MR 33
Endoscopic grading of esophageal varices 174
Endoscopic retrograde cholangiopancreaticography 52
Endosteal apposition of bone 282
ENT radiology 370
Epilepsy 439
Epiloia 337
Epiphyseal injuries 275
Erectile dysfunction 248

Erythroblastosis fetalis 402
Esophageal
  diseases 173
  duplication cyst 105
  malignancy 178
  motility disorders 175
  varices 174
Esophagus 61, 172
Etanidazole 471
Ewing's sarcoma 300
Exaggerated military position 158
Excretory urography 18
Exostosis 293
Expansile lytic (bubbly) osseous
    metastases 253, 288
External beam therapy machines
    482
Extra-adrenal pheochromocytoma
    316
Extra-axial
  brain tumor 360
  tumor 355
Extracorporeal shock wave
    lithotripsy 51
Extracranial vertebral artery 159
Extralobar sequestration 101
Extraperitoneal bladder rupture 245
Extra-pleural sign 128

F

Face 259
Facial nerve trauma 367
Fan beam DXA scanners 51
Fast neutrons generators 484
Fat 31
  necrosis of breast 413
Fatigue stress fracture 276
Feature of
  breast cancer 413, 414
  cholecystitis on USG 217
  degenerative arthritis 302
  hemophilia 282

hydronephrosis on IVU 235
interstitial pulmonary
    edema 143
mitral stenosis 136
osteoarthritis 302
osteoporosis 267
scurvy 266
sickle cell anemia 282
Feet 259
Feline esophagus 173
Fibroadenoma 413
Fibrolamellar
  carcinoma 208
  hepatic carcinoma 208
Fibrous dysplasia 292
Figure-of-eight appearance 334
First branchial cleft cyst 381
Fish mouth 390
Fistulas 100
Fleischner sign 191
Fleischner's plate atelectasis 113
Flexion rotation injury 392
Floor of maxillary sinuses 28
Flow inversion 135
Flower vase ureters 232
Flushing 65
Focal
  hepatic lesions 206
  nodular hyperplasia 208
Fogarty catheter 164
Follicular cyst 301
Fong's syndrome 260
Football sign 167, 169
Foregut duplication cysts 105
Foreign body aspiration 106
Forestier's disease 307
Four subtypes of
    brachytherapy 476
Four-vessel angiogram 156
Fractionation
  radiotherapy 475
  schedules 474

Fractures of
  first cervical vertebra 393
  second cervical vertebra 394
Friedlander's bacillus 107
Frontal lobe abscess 346
Function preservation techniques
    489

G

Galactoceles 413
Gallbladder and biliary
  apparatus 209
  system pathologies 215
Gallstone ileus 215
Gamma
  gandy bodies 171
  knife 501
  radiation 5
  rays 3
  scintillation camera 428
Gargoylism 262
Gas in biliary tree 216
Gastric
  carcinoma 184
  diverticulum 183
  leiomyomas and leiomyosarcomas
    184
  lymphoma 184
  polyps 183
  volvulus 182
Gastrointestinal
  bleeding 201
    studies 447
  syndrome 75
  tract effects 71
Gendarme's cap sign 278
General aspect and skull radiograph
    317
Genetic dose 81
Genital tuberculosis and HSG 25
Genitourinary radiology 226
Geometric magnification 8

Index

Germinal matrix hemorrhage 342
Gestational trophoblastic neoplasms 406
Ghon's focus 108
Ghost
   cavities 106, 107
   vertebra 390
Giant cell tumor 296
Giardia lamblia 186
Glandular tissues 507
Gleevec 503
Glial tumors 353
Gliotic temporal scarring 439
Glomerulonephritis 239
Glomus
   jugulare 382
   jugulotympanicum tumors 382
   tumor 382
   tympanicum 382
Golden 's' sign 113, 129
Goose neck deformity 191
Gout 270
Greater inherent soft tissue contrast 356
Grid 9
Ground-glass pattern 96
Gut signature sign 182
Gynecology 407
Gyriform enhancement on CT scan brain 326

H

H shaped vertebra 388
Hair on end skull 319
Half axial view 372
Hamartoma 242
Hamburger sign 190
Hands 259
Hand-Schuller-Christian disease, chronic 284
Hands-up signs/inverted 129
HAT sign 167
Hay fork sign 190
HDR brachytherapy 496
Head 538
   imaging 317
   trauma 364
Heart 131
Heberden's nodes 303
Heller's operation 177
Hellmer's sign 170
Hematopoietic syndrome 74
Hemodynamic effects 63
Hemorrhage 538
Hepatic
   adenoma 208
   iminodiacetic acid scan 214
   veno-occlusive disease 205
Hepatobiliary system 204
Hepatocellular carcinoma 208
   treatment algorithm 535
Hepatopetal 205
Hereditary osteo-onychodysplasia 260
Herpes
   esophagitis 173
   simplex encephalitis 348
Heterotopias 334
Hexamethylpropyleneamine oxime 438
Hiatus
   hernia 174, 175
   semilunaris 371
Hibb's angle 276
HIDA scan 214
High dose rate and pulsed dose rate brachytherapy 496
High-intensity focused ultrasound 540
Hila 89
Hilum overlay sign 130
Hirschsprung's disease 194
Hirtz's view 372
Histiocytosis X 284
Holistic approach 495
Holoprosencephaly 335
Honey comb vertebra 388
Horseshoe kidneys 232, 239
Hot
   cross bun skull 274
   filament or coolidge X-ray tube 7
   metal filament 8
Hounsfield units 37
HU value 37
Human placenta 400
Hunter's syndrome 261
Hurler's syndrome 261, 262
Hutch diverticulum 243
Hutchinson's triad 274
Hyaline membrane disease 97, 101
Hydatid disease of lung 110
Hydrocephalus 331, 403
Hydrogen 10
Hyperabduction maneuver 158
Hyperacute stroke 341
Hyperdense brain lesions 325
Hyperflexion injury 392
Hyperfractionation 475
Hyperparathyroidism 269
Hypersensitivity pneumonitis 121
Hypersplenism 172
Hypertension injury 392
Hypertensive
   encephalopathy 345
   hemorrhage 342
Hypertrophic pyloric stenosis 187
Hypodense brain lesions on CT 325
Hypoplasia and aplasia 100
Hypospadias 239
Hyposplenism 171
Hysterosalpingography 24

I

Ideal time to perform HSG 24
ILDs primarily affecting LZs 97
Ileal atresias 187

Iliac horns 260
Imaging in
　dementia 340
　obstructive jaundice 210
　renovascular hypertension 236
Imaging of
　adrenals 312
　carcinoma cervix 408
Imatinib mesylate 503
Immune hydrops fetalis 402
Immunoradiotherapy 502
Incomplete abortion 400
Increased bone density 250
Increment fracture 267
Indications for
　cranial and spinal CT 324
　HSG 24
Industrial disease 115
Inevitable abortion 400
Inflammatory orbital pseudotumor 378
Infrahyoid neck spaces 381
Infusion urography 21
Inherited cystic kidney diseases 230
Insufficiency stress fracture 276
Intense sclerosis 273
Intensifying screens 14
Intensity modulated radiotherapy 500
International
　atomic energy agency 78, 80
　commission on radiological protection 78, 80
Interstitial
　brachytherapy 477, 511
　lung disease 115
　　affecting upper zone 96
　pulmonary edema 135
Interventional
　GI radiology 533
　neuroradiology 533
　radiology 527

Intestinal TB 191
Intra-adrenal pheochromocytoma 316
Intracavitary brachytherapy 477, 511
Intracoronary brachytherapy 497
Intracranial
　calcification, causes 322
　infections 346
　metastases 356
Intralobar sequestration 102
Intraoperative radiotherapy 492, 497
Intraspinal extension 241
Intrauterine
　fetal death 401
　growth retardation 401
Intravascular brachytherapy 477
Intravenous urography 18, 229
Inverted umbrella sign 191
Involucrum 272
Iohexol 18
Ionization 460
Ionizing
　radiation 460
　　cause cancer, how? 464
　　measured, how? 460
　　produce genetic mutations, how? 465
Iopamidol 18
Ioversol 18
Ischemic colitis 196
Isomeric transition 432
Isotopes 425
Ivory vertebra 300

J

Jaffe-Lichtenstein disease 292
Japanese encephalitis 349
Jean-Daniel colladon 28
Jefferson fracture 393
Jejunal or proximal ileum atresia 187

Joint diseases 302
Juvenile
　angiofibroma 533
　bone cyst 293
　chronic polyarthritis 304
　nasopharyngeal angiofibroma 375
　rheumatoid arthritis 304

K

Kerley
　A lines 143
　B lines 143
　lines 143, 144
Kidneys and ureters 230
Kilovoltage range 485
Kirkland sign 180
Kite's angle 276
Klebsiella pneumoniae 107
Klippel-Feil syndrome 261
Klippel-Trenaunay syndrome 335
Kommerell's diverticulum 163, 178

L

Lacunar infarcts 341
Ladd's band 187
Lamina dura 269
Langhans' layer 274
Large bowel 61
Laser scanners 14
Late signs 281
Lateral
　nasal wall 370
　view 114
Law of radiobiology 68
LDR brachytherapy 496
Lead 10
　aprons 83
　zirconate titanate 29, 30
Left
　heart border 133
　subclavian artery 163

Index

Lens dose equivalent 81
Leptomeningitis and meningoencephalitis 346
Letterer-Siwe disease, fulminant 284
Limbs 259
Limbus vertebra 389
Limitations of CT 520
Linear accelerators 483
Linezolid 107
Lipoma of corpus callosum 364
Lissencephaly 334
Liver
  hemangioma 31
  metastasis 208
  scan 445
  tumors in children 209
Loculated pleural effusion 114
Lodwick's classification 289
Looser lines 267
Looser's zones 267
Louis-Bar syndrome 339
Luftsichel sign 113
Lump' sign 154
Lung
  apices 157
  carcinoma 124
  collapse 112
  diseases 40
Lymphadenopathy 119
Lymphangiitis carcinomatosa 117
Lymphangioleiomyomatosis 117
Lymphangioma 381
Lymphoid tissue hypertrophy 374
Lymphoma 414
Lyre's sign 156
Lytic
  bone lesion surrounded by marked sclerosis 251
  expansile eccentric lesions 251, 252
  lesions 253

M

Maffucci's syndrome 294
Magnetism of hydrogen nucleus 42
Major
  advantages of CRS 15
  role of MRI 33
Malabsorption 185
Male pseudohermaphroditism 239
Malignant
  lymphoma and leukemia 129
  ovarian neoplasms 408
  salivary tumors 384
  schwannoma 355
Malrotation of gut 185
Mammography 26
  algorithm 412
Management of benign obstruction 211
Manual afterloading machines 481
Marble bone disease 256
Marfan syndrome 263
Marie-Strumpell disease 306
Maroteaux-Lamy syndrome 262
Marrow hyperplasia 282
Matter 10
Mature cystic teratoma 409
McLeod's syndrome 100, 104
MDCT, advantages of 522
Meckel's diverticulum imaging 447
Meconium ileus atresia 187
Mediastinal
  masses 128
  node in various diseases, characterization of 128
  outline 90
Mediastinum 127
Medical tumor ablation 539
Medullary
  cystic disease of kidneys 231
  sponge kidneys 231, 232
Medulloblastoma 357

Megacalycosis 233
Melorheostosis 257
Meningioma 360
Meningofacial angiomatosis 336
Meniscus sign 190
Mercaptoacetyltriglycine 448
Mesenteroaxial volvulus 183
Mesial temporal lobe epilepsy syndrome 352
Metabolic
  bone disorders 265
  radiotherapy 502
Metaphyseal dysplasias 265
Metastasis
  distal to knee and elbow 287
  occurs late 301
Metastatic tumor in thyroid 312
Metrizamide 18
Metronidazole 471
Micturating
  cystourethrogram 244
  cystourethrography 23
Midgut volvulus 187
Milkman syndrome 267
Miscellaneous musculoskeletal radiology diseases 277
Mismatched perfusion defected 146
Misonidazole 471
Missed abortion 400
Mixed
  bone secondaries 288
  fat and water-density lesion 416
  sclerotic 253
Modalities
  available for abdominal pathologies 165
  for detection of gynecologic lesions 407
Modes of radiotherapy 476
Molar pregnancy 406
Mold brachytherapy 477

Molybdenum target 27
Monads' sign 111
Monophasic 205
Morquio-Brailsford syndrome 262
Mother-in-law sign 361
Moulage sign 167, 186
MR spectroscopy 524
MRI
  breast 415
  in bone tumors 286
Mucopolysaccharidosis 261
  type I 262
  type IV 262
Mucosa 186
MUGA scan, advantages of 445
Multicystic dysplastic kidney 231
Multimodal approach 495
Multiple
  enchondromas 294
  epiphyseal dysplasia 258
  exostoses 293
  gated acquisition scan 445
  myeloma 283
  osteolytic lesions in children 252
  sclerosis 351
Multislice machine and coronal
    sections 374
Musculoskeletal
  disorders, techniques for 249
  MRI 58
  radiology 249
Mushroom sign 180
Mustache sign 129
Mycetoma 126
Mycobacterium
  avium intracellular complex
      infection 109
  tuberculosis infection 108
Mycoplasma pneumoniae 107
Myelography 18
Myocardial
  perfusion studies 444
  scan 443
  viability 521

N

Nail-patella syndrome 260
Naked facet sign 392
Nasopharyngeal carcinomas 376
Nasopharynx 489
Nausea 65
Near infrared spectroscopy 526
Neck 538
  imaging 317, 381
Necrotizing enterocolitis 195
Negative
  contrast 18
  pyelogram 22
Neonatal
  GI obstruction 187
  wet lung disease 100
Neoplasms 122
  of anal canal 201
  of neuroendocrine origin 316
  of spleen 172
Nephroblastomas 239
Nephrocalcinosis 234
Nephrogenic fibrosing
    dermopathy 67
Nephrogram 20
Nephrolithiasis 233
Nephronophthisis 231
Nephrotoxic effects 472
Nephrotoxicity 472
Nervous system 335
Neural tube defects 404
Neuroblast migration 333
Neuroblastoma 241
Neurocutaneous syndromes 335
Neurocysticercosis 349
Neuroenteric cyst 105
Neurofibromatosis 335
Neurology 49
Neurosonography 323

Neurotoxicity 472
Neutron
  number 4
  therapy 511
Newer
  advances 517
  MRI applications principle
      utility 523
Niobium-titanium 44
NMR in bone tumors 286
Nodular pattern 96
Nonbarium studies 17
Non-Hodgkin's lymphoma 503
Noninvasive cardiac output
    monitoring techniques 131
Nonlissencephalic cortical
    dysplasia 334
Nonossifying fibroma 292
Nonradiation workers and public 82
Nonspecific aortoarteritis 161
Normal variants of kidney 230
Nuclear
  medicine 419
  scans 437
  stability and radioactive decay 431
Nutcracker esophagus 176

O

Obstetrics and gynecological
    radiology 396
Old stroke 341
Oligodendroglioma 359
Ollier's disease 294
Omental caking 409
Omnipaque 18
Onodi cells 372
Opacities on plain X-ray 233
Optic
  drum scanners 14
  nerve
    enlargement 377
    gliomas 379

Index

Oral cholecystography 215
Orbital tumor in childhood 354
Organ
   function ablation 538
   preservation 489
Orthoiodohippurate 448
Orthopantomography 27
Orthovoltage range 485
Osler-Weber-Rendu disease 335
Osseous malignant tumor 289
Ossified posterior longitudinal
      ligament 307
Osteitis fibrosa cystica 269
Osteoarthritis in hands 303
Osteoblastic bone lesions 252
Osteoblastoma 293
Osteochondritis 278
   dissecans 279
   of femoral capital epiphysis 280
Osteochondroma 293
Osteogenesis imperfecta 256, 320
   congenita 256
   tarda 256
Osteoid
   osteoma 294
   seams 267
Osteomalacia 267
Osteomyelitis 272
Osteonecrosis 278
Osteopenia 269
Osteopetrosis 256
Osteosarcoma 298
Ototoxicity 472
Ovarian neoplasms 408

P

PACS, advantages of 16
Paget's disease 271, 320, 452
   of bones 271
Palliative radiotherapy 489
Pan lobular emphysema 99
Panacinar emphysema 99

Pancake vertebra 390
Pancoast tumor 126
Pancreas 220
Pancreatic
   cystadenomas 224
   endocrine tumors 224
Panoramic radiography 27
Papile classification 342
Papillary
   cystadenoma 384
   necrosis on IVU 235
Parasitic infestation 186
Parasympathetic paragangliomas 382
Parathyroid
   gland 442
   scan 442
Parenchymal changes 119
Parrot's pseudoparesis 274
Particulate embolic agents 532
Parts of breasts 27
Patchy sclerosis of skeleton 251
Pathological consideration in
      obstetrics USG 400
Pathology of craniovertebral
      junction 320
Patterns of
   bone destruction 289
   interstitial lung diseases 95
Pediatric chest 100
Pelvis 259
Penile
   angiography 248
   Doppler 248
   imaging 248
Penumbra sign 273
Peptic ulcer disease 181
Percutaneous
   transcatheter vascular occlusion 537
   transhepatic cholangiography 212
   vertebroplasty 536

Periampullary carcinoma 223
Pericardial
   effusion 147
   tumors 148
Pericardium 147
Peripheral arterial disease 160
Peristalsis 185
Permeative bone metastasis 288
Perthes disease 280
Phakomatoses 335
Phantom tumor 114
Phase of cell cycle 69
Pheochromocytoma 316
   of adrenal medulla 382
Photodensitometry 50
Photoelectric interaction 10
Photoplethysmography 158
Photosensitive layer 12
Picture frame vertebra 389
Piezoelectric
   effect 29
   materials 30
Pigmented villonodular
      synovitis 277
Pimonidazole 471
Pincer sign 190
PIP joints 303
Pituitary
   bright spot 363
   imaging 363
   tumor 363
Plain
   AXR features of rupture of spleen 171
   KUB film 236
Planning conformal radiotherapy 499
Platybasia 320
Pleomorphic adenoma 384
Pleural
   diseases 113
   effusion 113
   effusion, etiology of 114

Plummer-Vinson syndrome 178
Pneumatoceles 107
Pneumocystis carinii
   infection, CXR of 110
   pneumonia 109
Pneumomediastinum 127
Pneumoperitoneum 168
Pneumosinus dilatans 360
Pneumothorax 114
Polyhydramnios 400
Pores of Kohn and canals of lambert 106
Posterior
   fossa tumor in
      adults 355
      childhood 354
   reversible encephalopathy syndrome 345
   scalloping of vertebra 391
   urethral valves 245, 402,
Postradiation transverse myelitis 72
Potato tumor 156, 382
Pott's spine 394
Predict severe acute pancreatitis 220
Pregnancy related encephalopathy syndrome 345
Prevention of vascular restenosis after angioplasty 507
Primary
   and secondary barriers 82
   bone tumors 289
   diagnostic criteria for allergic bronchopulmonary aspergillosis 111
   gout 270
   radiation 11
   sclerosing cholangitis 217
   TB 108
Principles of radiation therapy 467

Prion disease 351
Prodromal symptoms 506
Properties of X-rays 7
Property of piezoelectricity 29
Prostate
   and testes 246
   cancers 489
Proton
   beam therapy 502
   therapy 511
Pruned tree 217
Pseudofractures 267
Pseudokidney 190
   sign 182
Pseudotumor cerebri 369
Pseudoureterocele 244
Psoriatic arthritis 305
Puhl's lesion 108
Pulmonary
   edema 142
   embolism 145
   hamartomas 99, 123
   infections 106
   lacerations 99
   overcirculation 136
   plethora 136
   radiology 87
   sequestration 101
   tuberculosis 108
   venous hypertension 144
Pulseless disease 161
Purse string stenosis 191
Pyelogram 20
Pyknodysostosis 258
Pyloric teat 180
Pyrex glass 7

Q

Quartz, natural ceramic 29
Quiescent cells 68
Quinupristin 107

R

Radiation 460
   affect humans, how? 462
   hazards and protection 68
   oncology 459
   portals 504
   recall reactions 472
Radioactive
   cobalt machines 483
   decay 433
      chain 422
   half-life 422
   isotopes 436
Radioactivity 421
   measured, how? 421
Radiogrammetry 50
Radiographic
   features of bronchiectasis 115
   sign of acute pancreatitis 220
   signs of increased intracranial tension 318
Radionuclide
   bone scan 299
   considered for bone scanning 450
   imaging 237
Radiopotentiators 472
Radioprotector 471
Radiosensitivity of different tumors 509
Radiosensitizer 471
Radiotherapeutic treatment of painful bone metastasis 478
Radiotherapy in graves disease 508
Ram's horn stomach 167
Rapid sequence IVU 21
Rasmussen aneurysm 127, 532
Rat-tail esophagus 179
Rectal biopsy 195
Regenerative signs 281

Index

Regional ileitis 197
Regulatory limits for occupational exposure 81
Relation between let and RBE of different radiation 471
Remote and manual after loading machines 480
Renal
 cell carcinoma 242
 fascia sign 236
 infections 237
 injuries 243
 scan 448
 TB 237
 tumors 239
Renovascular hypertension 236
Respiratory distress syndrome 101
Retarded skeletal maturity 250
Reticular pattern 95
Reticulonodular pattern 96
Retinoblastoma 379
Retrograde urethrography 23
Rib expansion 91
Rickets 265, 320
Right
 aortic arch 161
 sided aortic arch 163
Rigler's
 double wall sign 169
 sign 167
 triad of gallstone ileus 216
Rim nephrogram 21
Ring
 around artery sign 128
 enhancing lesions in brain on CT scan 326
 of fire appearance 406
Risk factors for carcinoma gallbladder 218
Rituxan 503
Rituximab 503

Robson staging of RCC 242
Role of
 CXR in thoracic trauma 98
 radionuclides in radiotherapy 454
Rotating anode X-ray tube 8
Rounded atelectasis 113
Rugger-Jersey spine 268

S

Saber
 sheath trachea 91
 tibia 274
Salivary gland
 scan 440
 tumors 382
Salmonella osteomyelitis 283
Sandwich sign 190
Sanfilippo syndrome 262
Sarcoidosis 119, 129
Saw-toothed appearance 167
Scalenus anticus muscle 158
Scattered radiation 11
Schedule of radiotherapy 474
Scheie's syndrome 262
Schizencephaly 334
Schuller's view 373
Scintigraphic scan for neuroendocrine tumors 453
Scleroderma 173
Scottish terrier sign 278
Scotty dog 278
Screw hair cut skull 319
Seborrheic keratosis 413
Secondaries in bone 287
Secondary
 chondrosarcoma arises 297
 diagnostic criteria 111
 gout 270
 radiation 11
Segmental liver anatomy 204
Seldinger technique 527
Seminal vesicle 248

Senile ankylosing spondylitis 307
Septal pattern 96
Sequestra 272
Sequestration of lung 100
Serum cold agglutinins 107
Shallow-dose equivalent 81
Shoulder joint 274
Sialography 18
Sialosis 385
Siderotic nodules 171
Sigmoid volvulus 199
Sign of
 enlarged right ventricle on CXR 134
 frostburg 167
 gallstone ileus 216
 left atrial enlargement on CXR 134
 pneumomediastinum on CXR 127
 pneumoperitoneum 169
Silhouette sign 98
Silicosis 115
Simon's focus 108
Simple
 bone cyst 293
 hepatic cysts 206
 ureterocele 244
Single
 emulsion/coated films 13
 photon emission computed tomography 438
Sjögren's syndrome 118
Skeletal
 dysplasias 255
 metastasis 287
 in children 288
 trauma 275
 tuberculosis 273
Skin 335
 cancers 489
Skull 259
 fractures 365

Small
  bowel 61
    obstruction 187
    cell tumors of lung 125
    intestinal 185
      neoplasms 192
Snake head appearance 188
Soap bubble
  appearance 187
  nephrogram 22
Soft
  tissue 310
    tumors 310
Solitary
  bone cyst 293
  pulmonary nodule 122
  rectal ulcer syndrome 196
Special signs of collapse 113
Specific
  cardiac configurations and
    signs 137
  nonstochastic effects 74
Spina
  ventosa 274
Spinal
  meningioma 361
  myeloma 283
Spine 538
  imaging 317
  MRI 57
  radiology 385
Spinnaker sail 128
Spleen 171
Splenic
  trauma 171
  vein thrombosis 171
Spondylolisthesis 277
Spontaneous
  aseptic bone necrosis 279
  CSF leak 369
  pneumothorax 114
Sporadic aniridia 239

Spring onion 244
Square-shaped vertebra 389
Stag antlers sign 129
Staphylococcal pneumonia 97, 106
Stationary anode tube 8
Steeple sign 129
Steinberg sign 263
Stenoses 100
Stenver's view 372
Step-ladder appearance 188
Stereotactic radiotherapy 501
Stierlin's sign 191
Still's disease 304
Stockholm 'C' view 372
Stomach 61, 179
Stones 31
Strangulating obstruction 189
Strategies for preventing contrast
    induced nephropathy 64
Stray radiation 11
Streaky lucencies 128
Street of stone 168
Striated nephrogram 22
Stricture in bile duct 218
String
  of beads
    appearance 236
    sign 167, 188, 189
  sign 180, 192
  of kantor 167
Stroke and vascular disorders 340
Strongyloides stercoralis 186
Sturge-Weber syndrome 335, 336
Subacute stroke 341
Subarachnoid hemorrhage 343
Subchondral resorption 269
Subclavian steal syndrome 159
Subdural and epidural
    empyemas 347
Subfrontal region 348
Submentovertical view 372
Subperiosteal bone resorption 269

Subphrenic abscess 113
Subtypes of thoracic outlet
    syndrome 158
Sugar-icing 357
Sunburst nephrogram 22
Sunburst/spoke-wheel pattern 361
Superadded bone infection 283
Supervoltage range 485
Suprahyoid neck spaces 381
Swiss cheese nephrogram 22
Swyer-James syndrome
Symptom of double micturition 243
Syndromic association of few cardiac
    lesions 138
Synthetic ceramic 29

T

Takayasu's aortoarteritis 161
Target sign 190
Target/Bull's eye sign 190
Targeted radiotherapy 502
Tear
  drop bladder 243
  sign 180
Technetium 444
Technetium-99m 435
Teicoplanin 107
Teletherapy 482
  machines 482
Temporal
  bone imaging 40
  lobe abscess 346
  lobes 348
Temporomandibular joints 28
Tension pneumothorax 115
Tertiary esophageal
    contractions 173
Testicular
  scan 449
  tumor 247
Tetralogy of Fallot 140
Thallium 444

Index

Theoretic safety risks from ultrasound 32
Therapeutic
  effects of deep heating 539
  embolization 531
  uses 454
Thermoluminescence dosimeter 84
Thermoradiotherapy 501
Thoracic
  aorta 162
  outlet syndrome 157
    etiology of 157
Thornwaldt cyst 374
Thromboangiitis obliterans 160
Thumb sign 129
Thumb-print sign 167
Thymic sail 128
Thymus 100
Thyroid 311
  scan 441
TNM staging for lung cancer 126
Tolerance doses 77
Torus aorticus 149
Total anomalous pulmonary venous
    connection 97
  drainage 141
Total
  effective dose equivalent 81
  natural radiation 70
Towne's view 372
Toxic synovitis of hip 281
Toxoplasmosis 348
Trachea 90
Tracheoesophageal fistula 174
Transarterial chemoembolization 536
Transesophageal echocardiography 34
Transient
  synovitis of hip 281
  tachypnea of newborn 100
Transitional zone 188

Transrectal ultrasonography 32
Transtentorial herniation 366
Transvaginal sonographic landmarks 397
Trapezioscaphoid joint 303
Traumatic facial nerve palsy 367
Treatment verification 489
Trichuriasis 187
Tricuspid atresia 140
True magnification 8
Tubercular
  meningitis 348
  spondylitis 394
Tuberculosis or fungal infection 129
Tuberculous
  dactylitis 274
  lymphadenopathy 192
  salpingitis 25
  subgluteal bursitis 395
Tuberous sclerosis 337
Tubular artery sign 128
Tulip bulb aorta 138
Tumor
  and treatments of choice 508
  like conditions 286
  localization of GI NETs 224
  of thyroid 312
  on bone scans 451
  volume delineation 488
Turner's syndrome 232, 260
Types of
  anomalous pulmonary venous connection 141
  cancers treated with conformal radiotherapy 499
  emphysema 99
  grids 9
  histiocytosis x 285
  ionizing radiation 461
  OGI 256

ovarian malignancies 408
PACS 15
radiations 4
radiotherapy treatment 489

U

Ulcerative colitis 197
Ultrafast MR sequence 523
Ultrasonography in pregnancy 396
Ultrasound markers of trisomy 403
Umbau zones 267
Umbilical cord 399
Umbrella sign 180
Unicameral bone cyst 293
Unilateral
  hyperlucent lung syndrome 104
  hypertranslucent of lung 92
  megalencephaly 334
Upper and lower jaws 28
Ureterocele 244
Urethra 243
Urethral strictures 244
Urethrography 23
Urinary bladder 244
Useful terminologies 425
Uses of
  iodinated water soluble contrast media 63
  nuclear scan in GI diseases 202
Uterus 405

V

V sign of naclerio 128
Vanishing tumor 114
Variations of normal sella 317
Varicoceles 538
Various
  atresias 100
  breast diseases 412
  tumors and viscera 512

Vascular
  coarctation 100
  intraorbital tumors 378
  malformations 538
  rings 161
  TOS 158
Vein of galen malformation 331
Ventilation-perfusion scan 146
Vertebra plana 388
Vertebral lesions 387
Vesicoureteral reflux 232
Vestibular schwannoma 362
Villous adenomas 201
Virtual bronchoscopy 518
Vital topics 68
Vocal cord cancer of larynx 489
Voiding cystourethrography 23
von Hippel-Lindau disease 230, 338

W

Wafer thin vertebra 388
Waldenstrom
  legg calve perthes disease 280
  sign 280
Warthin's tumor 384
Water soluble
  contrast medium 195
  iodinated contrast media 18
  radiological media 62
Water's view 372
Weaver's bottom 395
Wedge-shaped vertebra 390
Wegener's granulomatosis 118
WES triad 31
Whirlpool sign 185
Wilm's tumor 232, 239
  versus neuroblastoma 241

Wilson's disease 351
Wimberger sign 274
Winking-owl eye sign 391
Wormian bones 319

X

Xanthogranulomatous
  pyelonephritis 238
Xeroradiography 26
X-knife 501
X-ray
  beam restrictor 9
  tube 7

Z

Zone of cartilage hypertrophy 275
Zuckerguss 357